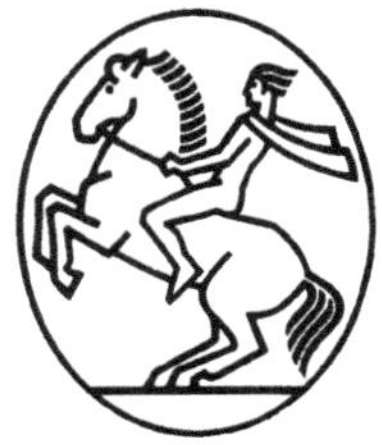

H. F. M. Peters, W. Hulstijn (eds.)

Speech Motor Dynamics in Stuttering

Springer-Verlag Wien New York

Herman F. M. Peters, Ph. D.
Department of Speech Pathology
University Hospital
University of Nijmegen
Nijmegen, The Netherlands

Wouter Hulstijn, Ph. D.
Department of Experimental Psychology
Psychological Laboratory
University of Nijmegen
Nijmegen, The Netherlands

Printed in Austria

With 107 Figures

ISBN 3-211-81971-1 Springer-Verlag Wien-New York
ISBN 0-387-81971-1 Springer-Verlag New York-Wien

Preface

The present book arose from a conference on Speech Motor Dynamics in Stuttering held at the University of Nijmegen in Nijmegen, the Netherlands from June 13-15, 1985. The conference was organized on the occasion of the 25th anniversary of the Department of Speech Pathology of the University Hospital.

The topic selected for the conference and now developed within this book, Speech Motor Dynamics in Stuttering, was judged to be particularly timely and especially relevant to an emerging body of work on stuttering. For over ten years there had been no conferences that brought together researchers who have worked on stuttering from perspectives stressing the dynamics of motor processes. Yet during that time major changes have occurred in research on stuttering which signify a growing level of scientific maturity within the problem area. This book attempts to characterize a number of major trends in research on speech motor processes in stuttering.

There has been a lessening in the postulation of causes of stuttering in the form of global hypothesis which have tenuous ties to empirical data. New ideas about speech motor processes in stuttering have been stimulated by researchers who have done productive work on more general issues of motor control.

This book therefore directs our attention to a number of models of speech production which are relevant to stuttering. Numerous researchers have recognized that the resolution of observations ascertained by unaided senses are not sufficient for effective progress toward either the objective description of the phenomena in stuttering or the understanding of the problem.

Significant developments in methods of physiological and psychological measurement have revealed important new regularities in stuttered speech. In particular, multiple, parallel physiological and behavioral measurements enable us to describe relationships between oral articulation, laryngeal activity and respiration in both stutterers and normally fluent speakers. New computer software and sophisticated forms of signal analysis now extend the techniques by which stuttering can be examined. The book makes a particular effort to report on these progressions.

The developments just mentioned, when taken together, present critical mass of concepts, research methods and data, signifying a new era in stuttering research which forms the subject of this book. The book is organized around five topic areas: 1) a historical review of work on speech motor activity in stuttering; 2) the presentation of a number of models of speech production which appear to be of relevance in our understanding of speech motor processes in stuttering; 3) an examination of methodological considerations in the study of complex speech processes; 4) research reports dealing with the coordination and timing of speech motor events and 5) research reports concerned with acoustic analysis of speech signals and other reviews dealing with the relationship between acoustic analyses and the perception of speech signals. Each topic area with the exception of Starkweather's Historical Review, begins with an introduction to the ideas, methods and findings relevant to the area and also includes a brief summary of the contents of the section.

As described by Starkweather in the first part, recent ideas on speech motor activities during stuttering can be attributed to three general historical sources. First, there was Wingate's vocalisation hypothesis which resulted from his examination of conditions under which stuttering was ameliorated. Second, there were experiments which examined reaction times in stutterers and nonstutterers and other experiments in which electromyographic and photoglottographic measurements were made of laryngeal activity. Finally, the direction of research has been influenced by the development of new perspectives in the control of speech production. One of these developments is the emergence of action theory, in which the coordination and timing of the many movement components of speech is stressed. Another important development has been initiated by Zimmerman in conceiving stuttering as a disorder of movement. In Starkweather's chapter, recent studies in speech motor control, acoustic analysis and linguistic relations are discussed and a number of directions is suggested for future research.

A substantial part of the conference was devoted to the basic know-how on theories on speech motor behavior and methodological aspects of research in speech motor production. Part two of this monograph adresses the current models on speech motor behavior in relation to stuttering. In research on speech motor processes in stuttering the lack of guidance by theory may be considered as a great omission. During the last years, results from fundamental research and developments in the theory on gross motor behavior have become incorporated in speech motor theories and at this moment they are finding increasing application in speech pathology and stuttering. There is also growth in the basic know-how concerning the validity of measurement methods. In Part three, therefore, much attention is paid to the methodological aspects of simultaneous measurement and the relationship between physiological parameters and acoustic analysis.

Part four and five of the monograph present a large range of current experimental work on speech motor behavior in stuttering. In Part four recent research on the coordination and timing of speech motor processes is presented. In these studies speech physiological processes are studied in the aerodynamic, laryngeal and supralaryngeal domain and in the coordination between these domains. The final section of the book deals with a range of studies in which a large number of new developments in acoustic methods are presented. It appears that a number of methods in the acoustic analysis of the speech signal can add specific information to our understanding of the speech motor processes in stuttering.

ACKNOWLEDGEMENTS

The conference was organized by the Department of Speech Pathology in close cooperation with the Department of Experimental Psychology, the Institute of Phonetics and the Interfacultary Research Unit for Language and Speech from the University of Nijmegen.

The organization of the conference would not have been possible without the help of many people. We would particularly like to mention Ineke van Dielen, Yolande Hennink, Piet Kooyman and Gerrie Westerlaken from the executive committee.

Special thanks are also due to Ben Salemans and Willy Peters who provided the camera-ready lay-out of the manuscript, Cor de Bruin who adapted the figures and Elly Cloudt for her general assistance. Louis Boves and Ron Webster assisted in the editorial work. Judith Abma-Hill helped with parts of the English text.

Without the financial support of the Department of Otorhinolaryngology at Nijmegen University and Hollins Communication Research Institute it would not have been possible to prepare the manuscript for this book.

Nijmegen, The Netherlands
June 1987

Herman F.M. Peters
Wouter Hulstijn

Contents

PART FIVE

Acoustic Analysis of Speech Production

List of contributors

James H. Abbs, *Speech Motor Control Laboratories, University of Wisconsin, Madison, Wisconsin 53706-2208, U.S.A.*

Joseph G. Agnello, *University of Cincinnati, 331 Braunstein, M.L. 379, Cincinnati, Ohio 45246, U.S.A.*

Peter J. Alfonso, *Haskins Laboratories, 270 Crown Street, New Haven, Connecticut 06510, U.S.A.*

Ann-Marie Almé, *Institute of Linguistics, University of Stockholm, S-106 91 Stockholm, Sweden*

Barbara J. Amster, *Department of Pediatrics, Medical College of Pennsylvania, 26 Eldon Road, Lansdowne, Pennsylvania 19050, U.S.A.*

Joy Armson, *Department of Speech, Temple University, Philadelphia, Pennsylvania 19122, U.S.A.*

Thomas Baer, *Haskins Laboratories, 270 Crown Street, New Haven, Connecticut 06510, U.S.A.*

Klaas Bakker, *Department of Special Education, Murray State University, Murray, Kentucky 42071, U.S.A.*

Günther Bergmann, *Department of Psychology, Justus-Liebig-Universität Giessen, Otto Behagel Strasse 10, D-6300 Giessen, West-Germany*

Gloria I. Borden, *Department of Speech, Temple University, Philadelphia, Pennsylvania 19122, U.S.A.*

Louis Boves, *Institute of Phonetics, University of Nijmegen, Erasmusplein 1, 6500 HD Nijmegen, The Netherlands*

Gene J. Brutten, *Department of Communication Disorders and Sciences, Southern Illinois University, Carbondale, Illinois 62901, U.S.A.*

Maurice W. Cannon, *Hollins Communication Research Institute, Hollins College, Roanoke, Virginia 24020, U.S.A.*

Anthony J. Caruso, *Speech Motor Control Laboratories, University of Wisconsin, Madison, Wisconsin 53705-2280, U.S.A.*

Edward G. Conture, *Department of Communicative Disorders, Syracuse University, 805 S. Crouse Ave., Syracuse, New York 13210, U.S.A.*

Michael Dames, *Max-Planck-Institut für Psychiatrie, Kraepelinstrasse 10, 8000 München 40, West-Germany*

Nirit El-Janiv, *Department of Psychology, University College London, Gower Street, Londen WC I E 6BT, England*

Terese Finitzo, *Callier Center for Communication Disorders, University of Texas, 1966 Inwood Road, Dallas, Texas 75235, U.S.A.*

Marie Christine Franken, *University Hospital Nijmegen, Department of Speech Pathology, University of Nijmegen, 6500 HB Nijmegen, The Netherlands*

Francis J. Freeman, *Callier Center for Communication Disorders, University of Texas, 1966 Inwood Road, Dallas, Texas 75235, U.S.A.*

Vincent L. Gracco, *University of Wisconsin, Speech Motor Control Laboratories, Madison, Wisconsin 53706-2208, U.S.A.*

Jonathan Harrington, *University of Edinburgh, Department of Linguistics, Centre for Speech Technology Research, Edinburgh EH8 9LL, England*

Katherine S. Harris, *Haskins Laboratories, New Haven, Connecticut 06510, U.S.A.*

Kathy E. Herbrich, *Stuttering Center, Department Neurology, Beylor College of Medicine, Houston Texas 77030, U.S.A.*

Peter Howell, *Department of Psychology, University College London, Gower street, London WC I E 6BT, England*

D.B. Hoyt, *Stuttering Center, Department Neurology, Baylor College of Medicine, Houston Texas 77030, U.S.A.*

Wouter Hulstijn, *Department of Experimental Psychology, University of Nijmegen, 6500 HE Nijmegen, The Netherlands*

Peggy Janssen, *Phoniatric Department, University Hospital, University of Utrecht, 3511 GV Utrecht, The Netherlands*

Robert McAllister, *Institute of Linguistics, University of Stockholm, S-106 91 Stockholm, Sweden*

Briant T. Morgan, *Hollins Communication Research Institute, Hollins College, Roanoke, Virginia 24020, U.S.A.*

Harvey B. Nudelman, *Stuttering Center, Department Neurology, Baylor College of Medicine, Houston Texas 77030, U.S.A.*

Herman F.M. Peters, *University Hospital Nijmegen, Department of Speech Pathology, University of Nijmegen, 6500 HB Nijmegen, The Netherlands*

Kenneth D. Pool, *University of Texas at Dallas, Callier Center for Communication Disorders, 1966 Inwood Road, Texas 75235, U.S.A.*

David J. Powell, *Department of Psychology, University College London, Gower street, London WC I E 6BT, England*

David B. Rosenfield, *Stuttering Center, Department Neurology, Baylor College of Medicine, Houston Texas 77030, U.S.A.*

Paul Schäfersküpper, *Max-Planck-Institut für Psychiatrie, Kraepelinstrasse 10, 800 München 40, West-Germany*

Howard D. Schwartz, *Department of Communicative Disorders, Northern Illinois University, Decalb, Illinois, 60115-2899, U.S.A.*

C. Woodruff Starkweather, *Department of Speech, Temple University, Philadelphia, Pennsylvania 19122, U.S.A.*

Courtney Stromsta, *Department of Speech Pathology and Audiology, Western Michigan University, Kalamazoo, Michigan 49008, U.S.A.*

Louise Vause, *Department of Psychology, University College London, Gower street, London WC I E 6BT, England*

Ben C. Watson, *Callier Center for Communication Disorders, University of Texas, 1966 Inwood Road, Dallas, Texas 75235, U.S.A.*

Ronald L. Webster, *Hollins Communication Research Institute, Hollins College, Roanoke, Virginia 24020, U.S.A.*

George Wieneke, *Phoniatric Department, University Hospital, University of Utrecht, Catharijnesingel 101, 3511 GV Utrecht, The Netherlands*

Mark Williams, *Department of Psychology, University College London, Gower street, London WC I E 6BT, England*

Part One

Historical Review

Chapter 1

Laryngeal and Articulatory Behavior in Stuttering: Past and Future

C. Woodruff Starkweather

HISTORICAL BEGINNINGS

The purposes of this chapter are to describe the history from which the current ideas relating stuttering to concepts of speech motor control have been derived, to review some current studies, and to look ahead to the future of research in this area. It all began with Wingate's (1976) review of the conditions under which stuttering is wholly or partially relieved, an area we have come to call "fluency enhancement". Wingate concluded that what the fluency enhancing conditions had in common was a tendency to produce speech that prolonged and emphasized vocalization. For a while, there was a spate of research on laryngeal behavior in stuttering. As it turned out, Wingate's review failed to make clear that in addition to altered laryngeal behavior, most of the fluency enhancing conditions also altered the rate of speaking. Later, in a comprehensive experimental study of the speech changes produced by fluency enhancing conditions, Andrews (1982) would show that altered rate of speaking was also common to fluency enhancement conditions and that changes in vocalization were likely to be a by-product of changes in rate. However, it was also evident that two conditions - metronomically paced speech and chorally supported speech - enhanced fluency not because they slowed the rate of speech but because they provided external rhythmic support. One area of future investigation that constitutes a challenge to the current ideas relating stuttering to motor control is the further analysis of fluency-enhancing conditions to find out why the support of another speaker or a regular external rhythm enhances fluency.

Several attempts to verify Wingate's hypothesis were made. Adams and Reis (1971) constructed a passage containing all voiced sounds and asked stutterers to read it aloud. They observed less stuttering on the experimental passage than on a normal passage. The study was later replicated but was nonetheless criticized on a number of methodological grounds (Young, 1975; Starkweather, 1982). Other researchers performed phonemic analyses of stutterers' spontaneous speech and found evidence that stuttering was likely to be located where voicing adjustments were made (Wall, Starkweather, and Harris, 1981), although it was not entirely clear, in my opinion, that these locations were ultimately based on linguistic factors. Indeed, a clear separation of linguistic and motoric factors related to stuttering remains one of our chief difficulties.

Wingate's review led a number of us to examine the vocal reaction times of stutterers and to compare these reaction times to those of nonstutterers (Adams and Hayden, 1976; Starkweather, Hirschman, and Tannenbaum, 1976; Prosek et al., 1979). In our zeal to confirm Wingate's "vocalization hypothesis", we failed at first to control for the possibility that stutterers might have had slower reaction times in nonlaryngeal behavior as well. Luper and Cross (1978) however, demonstrated that the manual reaction times were correlated with the vocal reaction times. These findings were later challenged on methodological grounds by Reich, Till and Goldsmith (1981), who failed to replicate the earlier finding. Ultimately, the differences between stutterers and nonstutterers in manual reaction time was independently confirmed (Starkweather, Franklin, and Smigo, 1984), although the correlation between manual and vocal reaction times was not. From the results of this last study, it was evident that there was a greater difference between manual and vocal reaction times in the stutterers than in the nonstutterers. We interpreted this to mean that stutterers had a general motoric deficit which slowed their reaction time, but that in addition they had learned habits of tension and struggle that were specific to the speech mechanism. The presence of this additional muscular tension acted as a drag on the coordinative structures of speech and slowed the vocal reaction time even further. Later, we'll see that another explanation of this finding may also be tenable. It should be noted that the reaction time literature shows a clear and replicable difference between stutterers and nonstutterers in vocal and nonvocal reaction times, but it does very little to explain what might cause such a difference. In any event, the reaction time research led several researchers to begin to consider the possibility that stutterers may not have the same level of speech motor control that nonstutterers have.

Other findings led to the same conclusion. Freeman and Ushijima (1975), Shapiro (1980), and Conture, McCall, and Brewer (1977) began to look at laryngeal behavior more objectively than the early reaction time studies, trying simply to document laryngeal physiology during stuttering. These studies made it evident that laryngeal behavior during stuttering is at least as disrupted as oral behavior is, but a number of other ideas emerged from this line of investigation that in the long run may prove of more theoretical importance. First was the finding by Freeman and Ushijima, later confirmed by Shapiro, that during stuttering, muscle activity was abnormally high, poorly timed, and that muscle systems which usually functioned reciprocally were, during stuttering, simultaneously active. This nonreciprocity formed an interesting explanation of the reaction time results described earlier. If stutterers, in performing a reaction time task, were attempting a gesture, laryngeal or manual, for which antagonistic muscles were simultaneously active, it stands to reason that they would perform the gesture more slowly, since the antagonistic muscles would stiffen the entire coordinative structure and act as a drag on its movement. Second, these first EMG studies showed a large number of tokens that were judged to be fluent acoustically but showed high levels of muscle activity and nonreciprocity similar to that found in the stuttered tokens. This observation called into serious question a well established body of literature on the perceptually fluent speech of stutterers. Perhaps these earlier studies had not succeeded in excising stuttered speech from the samples they examined but had instead retained tokens that were physiologically nonfluent even though they were perceptually (acoustically) not stuttered. At first we called these tokens examples of "subclinical stuttering". Now, experimenters seem to be calling them "physiological stuttering". They could also be called a most unpleasant thorn in the flesh of a large body of literature, a thorn which a number of current experiments have not controlled for.

It seems to me that these subclinical stutterings also raise an interesting question about what stuttering is. How shall we define it? Are these physiological abnormalities stuttering or something else? Whatever answer emerges to this essentially philosophical question, it is clear that when stutterers talk, physiological events are occurring that appear discoordinated and ill timed but which do not result in overt stuttering.

The early interest in reaction time and the emergent interest in motor control led naturally to a consideration of the rate of speech. If stutterers could not react quickly to external stimuli, it followed that they might also be unable to react quickly to internal stimuli such as might be needed to sequence a series of speech gestures. This interest in speech rate was also supported by a review of the nature and development of fluency in normal speakers (Starkweather, 1981), from which it became evident that the rate at which speakers can produce meaningful speech is an important sign of the effort that speech production requires. When coupled with the evidence that stutterers may be attempting to talk with a mechanism slowed and stiffened by overly active muscle systems, the implication was obvious that the supposedly "fluent" speech production of stutterers might be slower than that of nonstutterers. Several studies of this question had already been done (Zimmermann, 1980; Starkweather and Myers, 1979), and the results seemed to make clear that stutterers, even in their perceptually fluent speech, were slower than nonstutterers. Of course, there was now a question about whether perceptually fluent speech was genuinely fluent speech. It was clear, however, that the speech of stutterers was being slowed by a stiffened system, perhaps the result of subclinical stuttering. Other implications of raised muscle tonus were less immediately apparent - for example raised tonus should also make the speech mechanisms of stutterers move less smoothly, an implication that is yet to be confirmed.

A similar question, however, was the variability, particularly the temporal variability of stutterers' speech. Kent (1983) reported that he and a number of his colleagues had examined the variability of speech segment durations in stutterers and nonstutterers and found that the stutterers produced segments that were more variable in their duration. These results were later presented in a conference at Temple University by Kent (1984) and were interpreted with appropriate caution by the presenter. However, the presence of a generally raised level of muscle activity could also be used to explain such a result since the temporal location of a gesture would be less sure if movements initiating and terminating the segment were made less smoothly.

Meanwhile, Conture continued his investigation of the laryngeal behavior of young stutterers, using the electroglottograph. This method yielded more precise and empirically verifiable results than the earlier fiberoptic studies. The EGG technique provided a visual record that was a close analogue of glottal opening and with filtering could be used to assess both the rapid movements of vocal fold vibration and the slower movements of glottal abduction and adduction. Conture (1983) presented a number of different results, but striking among them was one that related directly to the level of muscle activity in the larynx. This result was the observation that the turnaround time taken by the vocal folds in the transition from the opening to the closing phases of vocal fold vibration was more rapid in the stutterers than in their nonstuttering peers. As the stutterers' vocal folds reached the point of their widest excursion away from the midline, they tended to "snap back", decelerating their abductory motion and accelerating their adductory motion more quickly than in the nonstutterers. This observation was clearly in keeping with the possibility that the vocal folds at least were intrinsically more tense and springy in the children who stuttered.

It should be noted that all of this evidence regarding higher levels of muscle tension during stuttering has no necessary relationship to etiology. It is entirely possible that the higher tension levels are a result, not a cause, of the disorder.

TWO BROADER IDEAS

Superimposed on these observations and interpretations were two broadly theoretical notions which influenced the direction of research. The first of these ideas was that enunciated most elegantly by Kelso (1981): that established principles of kinematics could be profitably applied to speech production. The chief benefit of such an application was an understanding of the speech mechanism as a mass-spring system, in which the passive forces of mass and tension play an important role in constraining the movements used to produce speech sounds. Although there is no question that these passive forces need to be taken into account in any explanation of speech movement, it is sometimes difficult to derive predictions from them because the more active forces of muscle contraction naturally also play a role in determining muscle movement, particularly with regard to temporal measures. A case in point is the matter of development. As children grow, their speech structures become larger and more massive. In addition, the spaces are enlarged and the distances that moving parts need to travel to achieve targets are increased. Muscle lengths are also increased, and in the case of the vocalis muscle this change is dramatic, particularly so in men. Yet all these changes are ones that decrease the springiness of the coordinative structures of speech and lower the resonant frequencies of the oscillators of the speech mechanism. Taken by themselves, they would predict that as children grow, the rate of speaking slows, that vocal reaction time slows, and that segmental durations become longer. Of course, the opposite is the case, and we are forced to conclude that the passive elements of the speech production mechanism are less important in determining temporal phenomena than the more active ones.

The second broad theoretical notion was presented by Zimmermann (1980). The idea was that stuttering should be regarded as a disorder of movement and that the principles of motoric behavior established in a rich history of inquiry be brought to bear on the problem. Essentially, Zimmermann was saying about stuttering what Kelso was saying about normal speech production. Zimmermann, however, went on to make a number of observations, one of which was particularly important. This was the idea that at the level of the motor neuron a number of inputs from diverse sources are integrated, and that the sum of these inputs determines the background tonus and triggering thresholds for coordinated structures. This suggestion provided, for the first time in my opinion, a physiological principle that could be used to explain a number of diverse stuttering phenomena that had hitherto been explained only psychologically. Specifically, Zimmermann's idea explained the phenomena of situational variability in stuttering and the common report that fluency is improved during periods of self-confidence. These phenomena had previously been related to "anxiety" or some other ill-defined and hard-to-observe construct, and it was not known how the motoric behavior of stuttering could be related to these more general and less observable events. Attempts had been made of course (Brutten and Shoemaker, 1967; Wischner, 1950), but none seemed to be reconcilable with other kinds of variability that seemed more obviously related to motoric factors, variability such as that seen with differences in speech rate, or with adaptation, or with choral speech.

Zimmermann's idea explained how all the different sources of variability could not only coexist under the same theoretical roof but further how their influence on stuttering could be a result of their pooled effects. That seemed to me to be a major contribution. Zimmermann's idea that background tonus and triggering thresholds were distinct aspects of motor control also helped in explaining the two sources of fluency change in fluency enhancement conditions that Andrews et al. (1982) had identified - slowed rate and external rhythmic support. The first of these seemed most closely related to background tonus and the second more closely related to triggering. It remains to be shown, however, how slower speech rate reduces muscle tonus (although it seems likely that it should), and it also remains to be shown how external rhythmic support can influence the triggering thresholds of movement.

A PROBLEM FOR MOTORIC EXPLANATIONS

The idea that stuttering behaviors may arise and perhaps develop in their characteristic way through interaction with the environment as a result of increased muscle background tonus raises a problem that is an ancient one for explanations of stuttering based on physiological (non-emotional) constructs - why does the disorder affect only the speech physiology? If general muscle tonus is raised, there should be some observable effect on other aspects of stutterers' motor performance. I think there is one answer to this problem that deserves investigation: It may be that the effect of increased tonus is limited to small muscles. This limitation could occur if the background tonus is generally elevated but not in a way that is proportional to muscle size. Essentially, this means, as Zimmermann would have suggested, that the problem is not located in the muscle fibers themselves, in which case large muscles would be affected more, but proportionately equally, because of their greater numbers of muscle fibers, but rather that the problem is located less peripherally in the inputs to the motorneuron, so that background tonus is raised nonproportionally to muscle size. As a result the effect on large muscles would be negligible. Of course, such an explanation predicts that the small muscles of the body that are unrelated to speech production - the oculomotor musculature, the eyelid musculature, the muscles of the middle ear, and to a lesser extent the muscles of the hands and fingers - should also show differences in function or reactivity in stutterers. There may be other small muscle systems in the body that should also be explored, but the list just given is presented because in each of these cases there is evidence to suggest that motoric functioning in these muscle systems is abnormal in stutterers. To quickly review this literature, Barret and Stoeckel (1979) presented a paper that I have always thought was particularly interesting. They asked stutterers and nonstutterers to wink one eye while they videotaped the movement of both eyes. They performed what amounted to a time-motion study of the eye contralateral to the winking eye and showed clearly that stutterers were more likely to show movement in the contralateral eye. That is, they were less able to keep the contralateral eye relaxed and still while lowering the winking one. I remember thinking at the time that the results were similar to the observations of Freeman and Ushijima (1975) and Shapiro (1980) in that they both showed an inability on the part of the stutterers to inhibit the muscle activity of functionally related muscles.

With regard to oculomotor behavior, recall the study by Brutten and several Dutch scientists (Brutten et al., 1984) in which the eye movements of young stutterers and nonstutterers were recorded while they read silently. The stutterers showed more extraneous movement - more eye fixations and regressions - than the nonstutterers. The authors interpreted this observation as related to the expectation of stuttering that the children had when they encountered words that they had fears about. In addition, the stuttering children showed fewer correlations among the various measures of eye movement than the nonstutterers did. The authors interpreted this finding very cautiously as evidence simply for a different pattern of eye movement in stuttering children. It seems reasonable, however, to interpret both of these findings as evidence of raised muscle tonus and perhaps also altered levels of triggering thresholds in the oculomotor musculature. This interpretation seems to fit well with the correlational differences as well as with the differences in the frequency of fixations and regressions. The inability to inhibit the movements of functionally related eyelid movements would tend to introduce a randomness to the patterns of movement that might be reflected in fewer intrinsic correlations.

A similar interpretation can be offered for two studies of the middle ear muscles in stutterers. Delaney (1979) found greater amounts of middle ear muscle activity during contractions and more frequent contractions among stutterers than among nonstutterers. The result was interpreted as suggestive of a feedback disturbance, but could as easily have been a by-product of generally raised muscle tonus evident in the small muscles of the middle ear. Similarly, Horowitz et al. (1978) reported that induced anxiety lowered the threshold of the acoustic reflex in stutterers but not in normal speakers. This finding could be taken as an example of the summation of inputs to the motor neuron pool of the kind that Zimmermann suggested may be operating in stutterers.

In several studies previously mentioned (Luper and Cross, 1978 Starkweather, Franklin, and Smigo, 1984) slower manual as well as slower vocal reaction times were found in stutterers than in nonstutterers. It seems correct to say that the manual reaction time difference is harder to document and smaller in extent than the vocal reaction time. In the interpretation of our results, Sharon Franklin, Therese Smigo, and I felt that the larger group difference for vocal than for manual reaction times reflected the combined effects of a general deficit of motor control onto which an additional deficit was superimposed as a result of the stutterers' experiences with the disorder. However, the difference between the two systems could also be a function of the average size of vocal tract muscles as compared with the average size of hand and finger muscles.

RECENT WORK IN MOTOR CONTROL

I am going now to look at just a few of the more current studies in this area, restricting myself to studies that illustrate certain points which I consider important.

Klich and May (1982) asked seven male stutterers to produce a randomized sequence of /hVd/ with three different vowels and then to read a passage in the presence of an experimental assistant who was apparently familiar with the experimental purpose. There were five different conditions of fluency enhancement - normal, whispered, DAF, rhythmic pacing, and noise. Stuttered tokens, as judged acoustically, were excised. A number of measures were made, including vowel duration, duration of formant transitions, relative duration of formant transition (duration of transition/ duration of vowel), F1 and F2 frequencies at steady state, and the mean rate of formant transition (extent of frequency shift/transition duration). Fluency enhancement was not as extensive as previously reported for the noise condition. They found a complex pattern of results, in which significant differences were observed for vowel duration between the normal and the rhythmic pacing conditions. Other conditions lengthened the durations of some vowels but not all. The results for formant transition duration and rate were also somewhat mixed as were those for steady-state formant frequencies, but the authors summarized the results as indicating that stutterers showed more centralized vowels than those reported for nonstutterers, particularly when the context was reading as compared with nonsense syllables, and that the vowel articulation of stutterers is more restricted temporally and spatially than that of nonstutterers. However, the results of this study cannot easily be used either to support or refute theoretical positions for several reasons. The authors acknowledge that the sample of stutterers was too small, the reading task too unlike spontaneous speech, and the severity range too narrow for much generalization. They also acknowledge that comparisons with nonstutterers are not valid until a matched sample of nonstutterers is observed under the same experimental conditions. But the results need also to be questioned because the demand characteristics of the experiment were compromised by the presence of an assistant, visible to the subjects, who was familiar with the purpose of the experiment. The assistant could easily have sent nonverbal cues to the subjects contingent on their speech characteristics. The assistant was, in any case, taking note of their disfluencies in their presence, which would surely have influenced their speech. The authors also fail to acknowledge the possibility that stuttering-like behavior may have been present at a physiological level but undetected by the method they used to identify and excise stuttered tokens from the subjects' speech. As a consequence, many of the tokens may actually have been "stuttered" in a subclinical way, and the presence of these tokens makes it particularly difficult to accept their conclusion that the findings "support Zimmermann's suggestion that stutterers use restricted articulatory adjustments to control their speech". Stutterers may well have restricted articulation - indeed I suspect that they do - but we cannot accept the results of this study as evidence for that assertion, particularly when the assertion is made about the "fluent" speech of stutterers.

The work of Andrews and his colleagues (1982) on fluency enhancement has already been briefly described. Another study on fluency enhancement has provided some fascinating results and a considerable challenge to motoric explanations of stuttering. Martin et al. (1984) compared the frequency of disfluency, vocal intensity, and rate of 24 stutterers and matched nonstutterers under conditions of noise, amplified sidetone, and quiet. The two groups showed similar reactions to the experimental conditions insofar as vocal intensity was concerned, and rate of speaking was slower for the stutterers than for the nonstutterers in all conditions. What was unexpectedly observed, however, is that the fluency of stutterers is enhanced by the presence of amplified sidetone if and only if that condition is preceded by exposure to noise, a finding which has recently been confirmed in a study that will be forthcoming. For motor control theories of stuttering, this observation presents a considerable challenge since it is necessary to show how exposure to noise can produce a change in the manner of speech production that disappears after the noise is removed yet is brought back by the presence of amplified sidetone. The finding cannot be explained by temporary threshold shift, since the noise exposure was too brief and too moderate to cause this phenomenon. Further study of the effects of noise on speech production are clearly in order.

ACOUSTIC ANALYSIS

Healey and Gutkin (1984) were interested in observing the laryngeal behavior of stutterers under a variety of controlled conditions. Specifically, they were interested in observing voice onset time differences between stutterers and nonstutterers. They asked 10 stutterers and an equal number of matched control subjects to read lists of utterances containing a variety of monosyllabic words and nonsense syllables. Sentences that included stuttering, as judged by acoustic observation, were excised from the samples. It was important, the authors felt, to the measurement of VOT that the samples be equivalent in the rate at which they were produced, since VOT varies with rate of articulation. To assess rate, the authors measured the duration of each of the utterance. They then performed an analysis of variance on the utterance duration and found no significant difference between the two groups. They concluded that the "potential group differences in VOT scores could not be attributed to differences in rates of articulation". This is, in my experience, the most common error made by experimenters in our field, that of concluding, on the basis of no significant difference, that two measures are equivalent. Equivalence and nonsignificant difference are of course not the same thing. As Carl Sagan puts it, "the absence of evidence is not evidence for absence". In addition, these authors did not succeed in assuring readers that the tokens they analyzed were completely fluent, since acoustic observation was the basis on which the excisions were made. They found that for the voiceless stops the stutterers did not have significantly longer VOT than nonstutterers although they showed a wider range of fundamental frequencies than the nonstutterers.

For the voiced stops, however, the difference in VOT was significant but not the Fo difference. These observations, however, do not seem to meet scientific standards as evidence for the idea that stutterers have slower VOT than nonstutterers, since the differences could have been produced by differences in rate between the two groups and because they could have been produced by the presence of subclinical stuttering in the samples.

In their discussion, the authors noted that their results were different from those of Healey (1984), who found no significant differences between stutterers and nonstutterers in Fo in an experiment that was identical in method except that the target words were placed in the middle rather than at the beginning of the phrase as in the present study. Although it is probably true that laryngeal behavior in stutterers is more likely to be different from that of nonstutterers at locations earlier in the sentence, particularly when there is the possibility of physiological stuttering in the sample, it is not appropriate to draw this conclusion by comparing two different studies, however similar their method might have been. The difference could also be attributable to the subject samples that were used. One other problem should be noted. In this study, as in the one by Klich and May described earlier, an attempt is made to infer motoric behavior from acoustic analysis. It is well known that such inferences are dangerous because of the wide variations in motoric behavior that may be responsible for similar acoustic results.

LINGUISTIC RELATIONS

One of the tasks that must be accomplished before motor control explanations of stuttering can be accepted is an understanding of how the relations between stuttering and various linguistic variables (Starkweather and Gordon, 1983) can be accounted for in physiological terms. Jayaram (1984) examined language variables in stuttering in what was in many ways quite an elegant experiment. He asked ten monolingual and ten bilingual stutterers to read lists of sentences. The bilingual stutterers read two lists, one in each of two languages. The sentences differed in the following way. One set of sentences was short, a second set of sentences was long but contained the short sentences as the first clause, and a third set of sentences was long but contained the short sentences as the second clause. Thus a direct comparison between the length of the sentence and the position of the clause in the sentence was possible. The results showed that there was significantly more stuttering on the sentence when it served as the first clause of a long sentence than there was when it stood alone, and there was significantly more stuttering on the sentence when it stood alone than there was when it was the final element in the long sentence. There were no differences between the two language nor between the monolingual and bilingual stutterers. The author concluded that "in addition to sentence length, the factor of clause position also influences stuttering". Although this study is elegant in its designed simplicity, it fails to control for one important variable that would make it possible to distinguish, perhaps, the linguistic from the motoric influences on stuttering. The uncontrolled variable is speech rate. Since the rate of speech is faster at the beginnings than at the ends of sentences (Umeda, 1975; 1977) and faster on longer than on shorter utterances (Malecot, Johnston, and Kizziar, 1972), it is possible that the higher frequencies of stuttering observed in this study are attributable to variations in the rate of speech production. I think it is often difficult for researchers to see stuttering and for that matter normal fluency from both a linguistic and a motoric point of view, yet that is exactly what must be done if fluency and its disorders are to be completely understood, since fluency seems to combine both motoric and linguistic elements, and since stuttering seems to be influenced both by linguistic and motoric variables. Certainly, a major challenge for those who would explain stuttering as a motoric disorder is to explain the linguistic variations of stuttering in motoric terms.

SIMULTANEOUS MEASUREMENT

A current trend in the literature seems to be the simultaneous measurement of related physiological events. There are two types of simultaneous measurement. One type is the simultaneous measurement of events at different anatomical locations, an approach to stuttering introduced by Ford and Luper (1975) and currently used by Borden, Baer, and Kenney (1985). The other type of simultaneous measurement is measurement of the same speech events at different levels of measurement, e.g., acoustic, kinematic, and neuromotor. These two types of simultaneous measurement have different purposes. The first type - simultaneous measurement of different systems - gets at the question of coordination, specifically the idea suggested by Perkins et al. (1979) that stuttering was a discoordination of the different systems of speech. Borden, Baer, and Kenney (1985) tested this idea by measuring oral movement with an Optical Tracking System and laryngeal movement with the Fourcin laryngograph simultaneously during the execution of speech sequences. In the stuttered tokens of their sample, they observed a well coordinated pattern of stuttering, that is, oral movements were in phase with laryngeal movements, even during the rapid oscillations of glottal ab- and adductions associated with laryngeal repetitions. They concluded that the vocal tract functioned as a coordinated whole, even during stuttering and rejected the hypothesis that stuttering resulted from a discoordination of different systems.

The study by Ford and Luper (1975), however, painted a somewhat different picture. They simultaneously assessed the intraoral air pressure, subglottal air pressure, lip EMG, and acoustic signals of four different stutterers. They found that each of the different subjects had a different pattern, which they suggested was characterized by a focus of tension at one location or another. The difficulty the stutterers had in making the systems work together seemed to result not from an intrinsic discoordination but from their attempt to adjust other systems in response to the system that had the focus of tension.

Peters and Boves (1984) measured subglottal pressure and vocal fold movements as they had stutterers produce isolated words as quickly as possible in response to a visual presentation. In one condition the words were produced normally. In another, they were produced with an easy voice onset, and in a third they were produced with a gentle articulatory contact. Stuttered tokens, as judged visually and acoustically, were excised from the sample, introducing a difficulty in the interpretation of the results, which had been noted previously. No significant differences were found between the stutterers and the nonstutterers for glottal activity before the start of phonation. In the build-up of subglottal pressure, five different patterns were identified and their frequency of occurrence was counted. Two of the types, identified as being abnormal in their temporal relation to the onset of phonation, were more frequently present in the fluent speech of the stutterers. They did find that the gentle voice onset condition was more conductive to fluency than the gentle articulatory contact condition. They also found that the pressure build-up pattern associated with a gradual build-up of subglottal pressure was clearly associated with the easy onset condition.

As with other studies mentioned previously, this one suffers from having used tokens judged acoustically to be free of stuttering. This is particularly bothersome in this case, because stuttered tokens could have been judged physiologically. Also, of course, the single word condition is not easily generalized to spontaneous speaking. Furthermore, it would have been interesting to have some reporting of the different speech rates which the various conditions produced.

Baer and Alfonso (1982), noting the problem referred to earlier of deriving information about movement from acoustic observation, also note the similar difficulty of deriving information about muscle activity from observations of movement. As a solution they suggest simultaneously measuring speech events at different levels. When a few studies of this kind have been done, it may be that we will be able to derive some rules of inference, known limits of variance, etc., so that in the future such inferences can be made with at least a known margin of error. As an illustration of the usefulness of this procedure they describe an experiment of their own. The experiment is not much related to the role of motor control in stuttering, so I will not review it here, but it should be noted that their point is made. Simultaneous measurement of neuromuscular, movement, and acoustic events has the potential for resolving a number of important questions in the area of stuttering.

THOUGHTS FOR THE FUTURE

This brief look at past and current research in this area suggests a number of directions that future researchers might wish to investigate. First, an explanation of the reaction time differences would be useful. One avenue of research that might lead to such an explanation is the simultaneous measurement of different physiological levels during the reaction time paradigm. This is a direction already begun by Peters and Boves (1984).

Certainly one of the important areas for motor control theories is a resolution of the language connection in motoric terms. One suggestion, which I have made on more than one occasion, is that there are changes in the rate of speaking at the linguistic locations where stuttering is more likely to occur. This goes beyond the tendency for stuttering to occur at the beginnings but not at the ends of sentences, where the duration of segments suggests that articulatory rate speeds up and slows down respectively. It also may be used as an explanation for the word frequency and word length effects, as well as the sentence length effects. The only "linguistic" location of stuttering that does not seem to be explicable in terms of rate change is the strong tendency for stuttering to occur on stressed syllables, which are if anything more "slowly" produced than unstressed syllables. However, I think it may turn out, and I would appreciate some evidence in support of the idea, that rapid rates of speech are physiologically similar to syllable stress, specifically with regard to rapid changes in subglottal air pressure, which are associated with stress but not, insofar as I am aware, with changes in rate. What needs to be done to make the case that linguistic effects depend on rate is to achieve a better understanding of the speech physiology associated with alterations of rate in normal speakers. This is part of our general lack of interest in speech rate, which I think has been unfortunate for the understanding of stuttering. I would like to suggest, however, that the experimental investigation of speech rate not be undertaken by assessing the speech physiology during speeded and nonspeeded speech. Speeded speech seems to differ from nonspeeded speech in more ways than its rate. There is overarticulation in order to achieve intelligibility too. What would be more helpful is to create or observe conditions under which rate is likely to speed up or slow down naturally, and then assess simultaneously the various levels of measurement suggested by Baer and Alfonso (1982). With a more thorough understanding of the physiology of speech rate variation, I suspect we will be in a better position to explain the linguistic locations of stuttering.

A similar problem faces explanations of fluency enhancement based on motor control. In the past the tendency for certain conditions to reduce or eliminate stuttering has been explained by distraction, reductions in anxiety, changes in vocalization, and changes in audition. The challenge for motor control theories is to explain these phenomena in motoric terms. I don't think it will be difficult. First, it is already evident from the Andrews et al. (1982) evaluation that rate is a potent factor, explaining all but two of the fluency enhancing conditions. Those two - choral speaking and metronomic pacing - seem to have their fluency-enhancing effects even when speech occurs at normal or faster than normal rates. Since these two conditions share the characteristic of having an external source of rhythmic support, it suggests that in order to achieve a unified explanation of fluency enhancement, it is necessary first to document the physiological changes associated with speech under conditions of external rhythmic support (and for this purpose singing might also be considered). This physiological assessment should be made, as with speech rate, with simultaneous measures at different locations. Then, when we understand how speech is changed physiologically under conditions of external rhythmic support with that for rate alterations. If there are common characteristics between these two fluency enhancing variables, a unified explanation of fluency enhancement compatible with motor control theories of stuttering will be at hand.

I would like to suggest an approach to the investigation of speech physiology during external rhythmic support. Choral speaking is a powerful fluency enhancer and has the advantage of being controllable by varying both the intensity and the rate of the model's speech. As this is done, the stutterer will usually continue to talk fluently at a normal or rapid rate for a brief period of time until the stuttering returns. With a little practice the period of unsupported fluency can be extended. What would be interesting would be not only to assess the physiology of fluency under this condition but also to assess the physiological changes that occur as stuttering slowly returns. We would get a unique opportunity to see just which systems at simultaneously different levels of measurement begin to show different patterns. Essentially the same thing could be done with metronomically paced speech, gradually fading the support at a slower than normal rate, as well as at a normal rate, and at a faster than normal rate.

REFERENCES

Adams, M.R. & Hayden, P. (1976). The ability of stutterers and nonstutterers to initiate and terminate phonation during production of an isolated vowel. *Journal of Speech and Hearing Research, 19,* 290-96.

Adams, M.R. & Reis, R. (1971). The influence of the onset of phonation on the frequency of stuttering. *Journal of Speech and Hearing Research, 23,* 639-44.

Andrews, G., Howie, P., Dozsa, M. & Guitar, B. (1982). Stuttering: speech pattern characteristics under fluency inducing conditions. *Journal of Speech and Hearing Research, 25,* 208-16.

Baer, T. & Alfonso, P. (1982). *On simultaneous neuromuscular, movement, and acoustic measures of speech articulation.* Status Report on speech research. New Haven, CT: Haskings Laboratories.

Barret, R.S. & Stoeckel, C.M. (1979). Unilateral eyelid movement control in stutterers and nonstutterers. *Asha, 21,* 769. (Abstract)

Borden, G., Baer, T. & Kenney, M. (1985). Motor control and stuttering. *Journal of Speech and Hearing Research, in press.*

Brutten, G., Bakker, K., Janssen, P. & Van der Meulen, S. (1984). Eye movements of stuttering and nonstuttering children during silent reading. *Journal of Speech and Hearing Research, 27,* 562-66.

Brutten, G. & Shoemaker, D. (1967). *The modification of stuttering.* Englewood Cliffs, NJ: Prentice Hall, Inc.

Conture, E.G.(1984). *Diamond Conference,* Temple University, Philadelphia, Pa.

Cross, D.E. (1978). Finger reaction times of stuttering and nonstuttering children and adults. Poster session, ASHA.

Cross, D.E. & Cooke, P.A. (1979). Vocal and manual reaction times of adult stutterers and nonstutterers. Convention address, ASHA (1979). Abstract in *ASHA, 21,* 693.

Delaney, C.M. (1979). The function of the middle ear muscles in stuttering. *South African Journal of Communication Disorders, 26,* 20-34.

Ford, S. & Luper, H. (1975). Aerodynamic, phonatory, and labial EMG patterns during fluent and stuttered speech. Convention address, ASHA.

Freeman, F. & Ushijima, T. (1975). Laryngeal activity accompanying the moment of stuttering: a preliminary report of EMG investigation. *J. Fluency Dis., 1,* 36-45.

Healey, E.C. & Gutkin, B. (1984). Analysis of stutterers' voice onset times and fundamental frequency contours during fluency. *Journal of Speech and Hearing Research, 27,* 219-25.

Horowitz, L. Johnson, S., Pearlman, R., Schaffer, E. & Hedin, A. (1978). Stapedial reflex and anxiety in fluent and disfluent speakers. *Journal of Speech and Hearing Research, 21,* 762-67.

Jayaram, M. (1984). Distribution of stuttering in sentences: relationship to sentence length and clause position. *Journal of Speech and Hearing Research, 27,* 338-41.

Kelso, J. (1981). Contrasting perspectives on order and regulation of movement. In J. Long & A. Baddeley (Eds.), *Attention and Performance.* IX. Hillsdale, NJ: Erlbaum.

Kent, R.D. (1983). The segmental organization of speech. In P.F. MacNeilage, *The Production of Speech.* New York: Springer-Verlag.

Klich, R. & May, G. (1982). Spectrographic study of vowels in stutterers' fluent speech. *Journal of Speech and Hearing Research, 25,* 364-70.

Luper, H.L. & Cross, D.E. (1978). Relation between finger reaction time and voice reaction time in stuttering and nonstuttering children and adults. Convention address, ASHA.

Malecot, A., Johnston, R. & Kizziar, P.A., (1972). Syllabic rate and utterance length in French. *Phonetica, 26,* 235-51.

Perkins, W.H., Rudas, J., Johnson, L. & Bell, J. (1976). Stuttering: discoordination phonation with articulation and respiration. *Journal of Speech and Hearing Research, 19,* 509-22.

Perkins, W.H., Bell, J., Johnson, L. & Stocks, J. (1979). Phone rate and the effective planning time hypothesis of stuttering. *Journal of Speech and Hearing Research, 22,* 747-55.

Peters, H.F.M. & Boves, L. (1984). Timing of aerodynamics and laryngeal functions in stuttering. Convention address, ASHA.

Reich, A., Till, J., Goldsmith, H. & Prins, D. (1981). Laryngeal and manual reaction times of stuttering and nonstuttering adults. *Journal of Speech and Hearing Research, 24,* 192-96.

Shapiro, A. (1980). An electromyographic analysis of the fluent and dysfluent utterance of several types of stutterers. *JFD, 5,* 203-31.

Starkweather, C.W. (1981). Speech fluency and its development in normal children. In N. Lass (Ed.), *Speech and language: advances in basic research and practice, Vol. 4.*

Starkweather, C.W. (1982). Stuttering and laryngeal behavior: a review. *ASHA monograph,* # 21.

Starkweather, C.W., Franklin, S. & Smigo, T. (1984). Voice and finger reaction times: differences and correlations. *Journal of Speech and Hearing Research, 27,* 193-96.

Starkweather, C.W. & Gordon, P. (1983). Stuttering: The Language Connection. Short course, ASHA, 1983.

Starkweather, C.W., Hirschman, P. & Tannenbaum, R.S. (1976). Latency of vocalization: stutterers v. nonstutterers. *Journal of Speech and Hearing Research, 19,* 481-92.

Starkweather, C.W. & Myers, M. (1978). The intervocalic interval in stutterers and nonstutterers, a close analysis. Convention address, ASHA.

Umeda, N. (1975). Vowel duration in American English. *Journal of the Acoustical Society of America, 58,* 434-45.

Umeda, N. (1977). Consonant duration in American English. *Journal of the Acoustical Society of America, 61,* 846-58.

Wall, M., Starkweather, C. & Harris, K.S. (1981). The influence of voicing adjustments on the location of stuttering in the spontaneous speech of young child stutterers. *JFD, 6,* 299-310.

Wingate, M. (1976). *Stuttering: theory and treatment.* New York: Irvington Pub.

Wischner, G. (1950). Stuttering behavior and learning: a preliminary theoretical formulation. *Journal of Speech and Hearing Disorders, 15,* 324-35.

Young, M.A. (1975). Letter to the editor. *Journal of Speech and Hearing Research, 18,* 600-602.

Zimmermann, G. (1980b). Articulatory behaviors associated with stuttering: a cinematic analysis. *Journal of Speech and Hearing Research, 23,* 108-21.

Zimmermann, G. (1980c). Stuttering: A disorder of movement. *Journal of Speech and Hearing Research, 23,* 122-36.

Part Two

Models in Speech Motor Production

Overview

One of the aims of this book is to describe and encourage research on stuttering that is based on, or inspired by, current theories of motor control. This part of the book presents three different theoretical perspectives for stuttering research. Two of them represent the two main streams in the motor control literature, i.e. action theory and motor programming. The third view is a very elaborate theory about speech production, that stresses the importance of sensory information in motor control. Each of these chapters ends with a few specific questions about the nature of stuttering originating from these theories. These questions and suggestions for research have already given shape to a few experiments. This and other research, stemming from the ideas given in this section, will be described in Part four of this book.

In Part one, Starkweather's review of the recent history of stuttering research sketches developments, starting with investigations directed towards the conditions that lessen stuttering and moving on to demonstrations of abnormal speech, f.i. longer reaction times, in nonstuttered, perceptually fluent speech. As Starkweather pointed out, these longer reaction times as such do not explain very much. What should be done instead, is to base these differences in 'fluent' speech, between stutterers and nonstutterers, on theories of motor control. A second trend noted in the preceding chapter, is the increase in simultaneous measurements of related physiological events. These events appear to be discoordinated in stutterers, even in what is heard as fluent speech. As is also the case with reaction times, these problems in coordination should not simply be measured from an empirical perspective, but moreover investigated in association with theories on motor coordination.

The last ten or fifteen years have shown a remarkable increase in theories and research on motor control. Naturally, this has led to many different views. However, two main approaches can be distinguished: theories proposing a motor program - in which the commands to the individual muscles are organized centrally by some sort of plan or program - and action theories, that reject such a computer analogy and instead describe motor control in terms of 'coordinated structures'. Historically, this latter approach was the first to develop its implications for a theory on speech production. Therefore, this part of the book opens with a chapter which is intended to give an impression of the latter concept. It is followed by an account of the different perspectives on motor programming. The relevance of these views to the understanding of speech and stuttering, mainly arising from the study of nonspeech movements, are sketched. The section is ended by a chapter in which more or less similar programming notions are used in a very detailed and hierarchical model for speech production.

In Chapter 2, Harris opens by contrasting action theory with the older program notions. She then briefly describes the origins of action theory. The next part is devoted to a description of the evolution in theorizing on the alternative for motor programs, i.e. 'coordinated structures'. Their flexible assembly is stressed and their temporal characteristics are given in detail. It is clear that the timing relationships of some elements in the pronunciation of a word are linear. This is partly the result of a statistical flaw and the author describes an alternative analysis - in a phase plane representation - to overcome these objections. These theoretical developments lead, in a following part of this review, to the detailed formulation of a task-dynamic model of speech movement. This model is designed such a way that, although movements generally involve a large number of muscles (the model has six variables), their trajectory is usually rather simple, with a single velocity peak. In simulations, the model behaves in the same way as normal motor actions, i.e. if a perturbation of the movement is introduced no recomputation of the trajectory is necessary. However, this model has been criticized and three classes of objections are discussed. The chapter ends with potential clinical observations. These center around those characteristics of speech that are most salient according to action theory, i.e. the temporal organization of speech movements and their resistance to perturbation.

One of the criticisms of action theory is that it argues against views on programming that are out of date. Therefore, in the next chapter (Chapter 3) Hulstijn discusses different views on the nature of programming and the optimal experimental paradigm to study it. A short review is given of the experimental literature in which the old question is brought up: whether more complex actions require more elaborate programming, thus causing a longer delay in starting the action. The author presents data from both his own laboratory and other investigators that suggest an interesting difference between speech and typewriting and speech and handwriting. It is suggested that in handwriting and a few other tasks, the number of elements per unit time is much lower than in speech, which possibly induces another strategy in programming. Speech differs in yet another aspect from a great majority of laboratory motor tasks: its elements are highly overlearned. Research on handwriting in which overlearned and relatively unknown movement patterns were compared indicates that the programming is different for each. These observations suggest a concept on the planning of rapid speech utterances in which two levels can be distinguished: low level programming of the muscle commands and high level planning of the order of the units, against which during execution, the progress of the utterance is being checked or monitored. Speech reaction time data and EMG data are presented, suggesting that this planning may partially overlap response execution. Finally some implications of these views for the explanation of stuttering phenomena are given.

The following chapter (Chapter 4, by Gracco) builds on the same ideas, although terms like 'plan' and 'program' have a slightly different meaning. The review gradually works toward a very detailed hierarchical model of speech production, of which the schematic representation is given in the last, summarizing section. Gracco not only specifies each of the levels of this model, but he also explicitly considers the importance of sensory information in the planning, programming and execution of speech movements. First, a great many studies - speech motor as well as anatomical and psychophysical studies - are reviewed which point to the importance of sensors. Data are presented showing that the combined action of the upper lip, lower lip and jaw in oral closure is much less variable than the individual movements of these articulators. This suggests that articulatory movements are not planned individually but that at the planning stage an overall goal-like oral closure is determined. The author proposes that this goal is specified in terms of the sensory information that is specific to that goal. With regard to the next level in the hierarchy, he makes a similar distinction as can be found in the previous chapter, i.e. between a program and programming. This distinction is made in order to explain the results of perturbation studies, suggesting that a dynamic process (programming) must be postulated in which sensory signals are used to (re)parameterize the actions of the individual articulators. Data are presented that support the speculation that this sensory information can be picked up in time to effect the programming of the subsequent movement, since predictive information from the earlier part of the previous movement might be used. Finally the sensory-motor mechanisms are described that may be of significance during the speech motor execution stage.

Chapter 2

Action Theory as a Description of the Speech Process

Katherine S. Harris

A LITTLE HISTORY

Lashley and his Descendants

"Action Theory" evolved as a response to some problems in the description of motor control and coordination. While the theory has been used as a way of specifying appropriate approaches to behavioral description (see, e.g. Turvey, 1977), the goal of this chapter is to sketch the historical evolution of the theory and to indicate a relevant approach to normal and disordered speech production.

In many ways, modern theories of speech production begin with Lashley's (1951) paper "The problem of serial order in behavior". His view was that the behavioral elements of language, such as sounds, or words, must exist as stored elements in the nervous system, as a spatial array, in which temporal order is replaced by a spatial order. When speech is actually produced, these serially ordered elements emerge, having been given some kind of temporal realization by an internal timing program. Thus, the element of acts and their timing are different parts of a system, which are somehow brought together for behavior in the real world.

Lashley explicitly had speech in mind when he constructed this model of behavior. Perhaps for this reason, it is easy to make an analogy between the serially ordered, timeless elements of Lashley's action plans and the phonological units of linguistic analysis, which are, as well, timeless, and ordered from left to right on a page.

The important point to note here, however, is that Lashley's model has at least two stages; that is, the elements of speech exist both before and after assembly with the timing program.

Many modern theories of speech production can be considered logical descendants of Lashley's serial ordering views - two theories that may be mentioned are the theory of tongue slips of Shattuck-Hufnagel (1983), and Hencke's theory of anticipatory coarticulation (1966). In the former theory, the units of an upcoming message are laid out in some form of mental buffer; a "slip of the tongue" occurs because the elements in the buffer become misordered. The fact that the slip is presumed to be adapted to its new environment in such characteristics as duration is attributed, in this model, to the fact that the elements slip before the temporal plan is instantiated.

A somewhat similar model, used to account for the facts of anticipatory coarticulation, is that of Hencke (1967). In this model, the phonological unit is decomposed into its component features. These bundles of features are more or less identified with the features of Chomsky and Halle (1968). Each phone is specified as positive, negative or unspecified with respect to each feature. When phonological units are assembled into strings in a buffer, the units are scanned ahead, and a feature may slip its position into association with an earlier segment.

Some Origins of Action Theory

An opposing point of view is represented by a paper of Fowler, Rubin, Remez and Turvey (1980). Their work stemmed from two threads in the (then) existing literature. The first of these was the work of Bernstein and his colleagues (1967). Bernstein was concerned with the "degrees of freedom" problem as represented in the control of action. Briefly, the point of view is that such a system, with a large number of degrees of freedom, cannot be successfully organized by a central executor, who plans each aspect of the execution at the lower levels of the system. Each muscle that acts, for example, at a joint affects the consequences of contraction of every other muscle. The effects of a given muscle's activation will be altered by the environmental field in which the action occurs. For this reason, it is essential that some aspects of the behavior of the system be delegated, so that the many degrees of freedom are regulated by a very few. Muscle systems are marshalled in the service of various aims in functional groupings, called "coordinative structures". The relationships among the muscles covary in terms of a relatively fixed relationship, the "equation of constraint".

A second source for the ideas of "action theory" is what has been called "neo-Gibsonianism," after the work of Gibson (1950). His views were developed as an account of visual perception. Very briefly, he argued that visual objects are perceived directly, rather than computed - in somewhat different terms, vision is set up in such a way that events are perceived as such, rather than inferred from a reconstruction. By analogy, Fowler et al. suggest that speech is perceived as a series of gestures of the vocal tract. From a production point of view, then, speech is produced as overlapping consonant and vowel gestures, generated by overlapping consonant and vowel coordinative structures; from a perception point of view, these gestures are extracted directly from the time-varying acoustic stream.

THE EVOLUTION OF THE COORDINATIVE STRUCTURE

The Flexibly Assembled Coordinative Structure

The concept of the coordinative structure has evolved in various ways since it was initially proposed. Thus, in Easton's (1972) view, coordinative structures were essentially reflex based. The present formulation at Haskins Laboratories assumes that they are flexibly assembled, even though many of the building blocks for structures in the adult organism may have their origins in the reflexes of the neonate (Fukuda, 1961). The current view is illustrated by a recent experiment (Kelso, Tuller, Bateson & Fowler, 1984), showing the variable effects of an unexpected perturbation of the jaw during articulation. When the jaw was perturbed during its upward movement towards the final /b/ closure in "bab", both upper and lower lips increased their excursions to compensate for the reduced contribution of the jaw to the attainment of closure, as had been previously found by Folkins and Abbs (1975; 1976). The movement increases in the lower lip probably arose, at least in part, from passive shearing of the lower lip from the jaw, as a consequence of momentum created by clamping the jaw. However, compensation in the upper lip arose from active muscle contraction. The two movements together resulted in the attainment of lip closure for the /b/. When the perturbation was applied to the jaw during closure for /z/ in the syllable "baz", there was no active upper lip compensation, but activity in the genioglossus muscle of the tongue increased, evidently to increase tongue raising for appropriate shaping of the groove for /s/ frication, given the lowered position of the jaw. Further studies of the effects of perturbing the jaw at various times during "bab" production showed that compensatory closing occurred only when it was appropriate. The conclusion is, then, that the linkages among muscles are functional, rather then hard-wired. It might be remarked here, that this finding might have been anticipated because since the time of Sherrington, (1906), it has been recognized that there are functional influences on the unfolding of even the most classic simple reflexes.

A number of studies show that the structural field of a group of muscles cooperating in an action is quite broad - if we define that field in terms of the ensemble of muscles whose activity is modified by a disturbance to one member of the ensemble. Thus, Marsden, Merton and Morton (1983) showed that if a perturbation was applied to the thumb of a subject performing a thumb-tracking task, very rapid responses will be observed in the arm muscles of the non-perturbed side. These responses will differ, depending on the posture of that side. Thus, in speech and non-speech acts, local and remote responses are task-specific.

The Temporal Characteristics of Coordinative Structures

The fact that tasks are spatially distributed over a large number of cooperating muscles has been noted above. However, temporal organization can be identified, as well. For example, Kots' work (1977) on the Hoffman reflex shows that, prior to any movement, conditions arise in the potential agonist and antagonist muscles that tend to bias the muscular system to produce an appropriately specified class of movements. Thus, coordinated activities can be considered to have temporal, as well as spatial properties. Indeed, it may be proposed that coordinative structures should have invariant properties over various kinds of metrical change.

The idea of constancy of timing relationships over metrical change is not new; it has been shown for such skilled motor activities as walking (Grillner, 1975) and handwriting (Viviani & Terzuolo, 1980). We have conducted analogous investigations for speech. The experimental paradigm is quite simple. Subjects were asked to produce simple disyllables with the stress on the first or second syllable, and with varying speaking rates. The temporal relationships among consonant and vowel over changes in stress and speaking rate were then examined. Although subjects adopt differing strategies for varying stress and for varying speaking rate (Harris, 1978; Tuller, Harris & Kelso, 1982; Kuehn & Moll, 1976), nonetheless, it was shown that the time of onset of gestures specific to consonant articulation was tightly linked to the timing of gestures specific to the flanking vowels. These results were obtained at two levels; for the onsets of electromyographic activity of consonant and vowel related muscles, (Tuller, Kelso & Harris, 1982), and at the level of the onsets of consonant and vowel-related articulator movements (Tuller & Kelso, 1984), similar results were noted by Gentil (1986).

The original analysis can be illustrated with an example. We examined the relationship between the time from the onset of vowel-related activity, such as the jaw lowering for the first vowel, in "papap" to the onset of lip raising for the consonant (the latency) and the time from jaw lowering for the first vowel to jaw lowering for the second vowel, the "period". A linear relationship between period and latency over stress and speaking rate conditions was found. Note that the relationship is linear, but not ratiomorphic; the latency-period ratio was not a constant.

The motivation for making the period latency analysis in its original form was because of the analogy of the analysis to those used in studies of other forms of movement, such as gait. The analysis is limited by the fact that it has a statistical flaw, as discussed by Barry (1983), by Munhall (1985) and by Benoit and Abry (1986) and perhaps more importantly, the analysis is incomplete, in that only movement onsets are represented.

The statistical flaw arises from the fact that latency and period are not independent. The latency is included in the period; that is, if the latency is represented by an interval a, the period can be represented by $a + b$. Thus, a correlation between a and $a + b$ can be predicted, based on the relative sizes of a and b, and the correlation between period and latency is significant only to the extent to which it exceeds that predicted value.

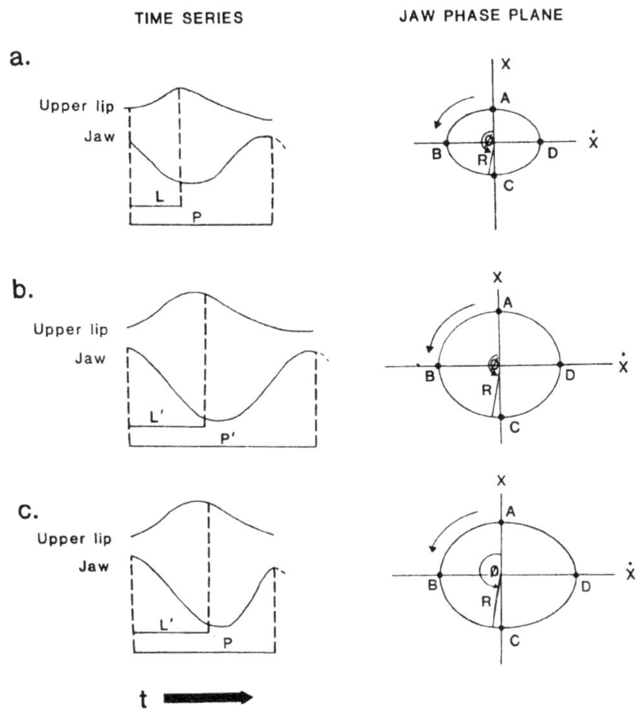

Figure 1. Series representations of idealized utterances. On the left are shown periods and latencies for three utterances that are not linearly related. However, as can be seen in the phase plane representations (right column) they show identical phase plane onset relations. (From Kelso & Tuller, in press).

Most recently, these experiments have been reanalyzed in a way that represents the data more completely and avoids this problem (Kelso, Tuller & Harris, 1985, Kelso, Saltzman & Tuller, 1986). In this analysis, the movements of (as in the example above) the jaw and lip are represented in the phase plane. In a phase plane analysis, a movement trajectory is shown as a function of its normalized instantaneous articulatory position and velocity. Figure 1 shows time series and phase plane representations of two hypothetical utterances. In making the phase plane representation, the absolute amplitude of jaw and lip amplitudes are normalized to a unit value, so that, for example, the absolute amplitude differences in jaw movement between stressed and unstressed syllables is eliminated. It is then possible to compute the phase angle between lip and jaw movement. Preliminary data showed that mean phase angle of upper lip lowering relative to the jaw cycle was constant over changes in stress and speaking rate, although this result appears too simple, in the light of subsequent, ongoing studies. Clearly this analysis is related to, but not identical with the relative timing description. As in Figure 1, it is possible for two utterances to have identical period/latency relationships, but different phase relations.

TASK DYNAMICS

The Model

A result of the experiments and conceptualizations discussed above has been the formulation of a task dynamic model of speech movement (Saltzman, in press; Kelso, Saltzman & Tuller, 1986 and in press). Originally, this model was developed with reference to limb movements (Saltzman, 1979; Saltzman & Kelso, in press) later, it was extended to speech, especially to vocal tract construction formation. In both cases, it was designed to account for two phenomena, trajectory shaping and immediate compensation. The "trajectory shaping" characteristic refers to the fact that, while movements generally involve large numbers of muscles, an end effector such as the hand moves in a simple trajectory like that of a damped mass-spring, with a single velocity peak. The "immediate compensation" property refers to the fact that if a structure is perturbed on its path towards target attainment, its members will coordinate to attain that target, without a recomputation of the trajectory path. Thus, in a reaching task, if the shoulder is clamped, the elbow will increase its amplitude of movement so that the end effector, the hand, attains its original target.

In the model, there are three steps in simulating coordinated movements, as shown in Figure 2. The first step is to specify the functional aspects of the gesture in a *task space*. In the case of speech, this first step involves specifying a constriction in an idealized vocal tract, in two dimensions; constriction location and constriction degree. A discrete speech gesture will have damped second order system dynamics along each axis in the task space. The constriction formation is independent of any particular set of articulators.

The second step is to transform the task space into a two-dimensional *body space;* for example, in the case of lip closure, body space variables might be lip aperture and lip protrusion, defined in the midsagittal plane of the vocal tract, centered on the axis of rotation of the jaw.

The third step is to transform the two dimensional tract variables into the coordinates of a four-dimensional *model articulator space*. The model articulators have lengths, but are massless. In creating the task dynamic model for speech, it has been assumed that the movements of the articulators will be defined with respect to the dimensions of the vocal tract as they are represented in the Haskins Laboratories' articulatory synthesizer (Rubin, Baer & Mermelstein, 1981). There are six variables in the synthesizer model; the position of the velum, jaw, hyoid bone, tongue body center, tongue tip, and lips (see Figure 3). The positions of the second set of variables are dependent on the movement of the jaw, while movements of the tongue tip depend on tongue body. In the case of lip constriction, the articulator movements involved are jaw rotation, vertical displacements of upper and lower lip relative to upper and lower teeth, and horizontal displacements relative to the teeth.

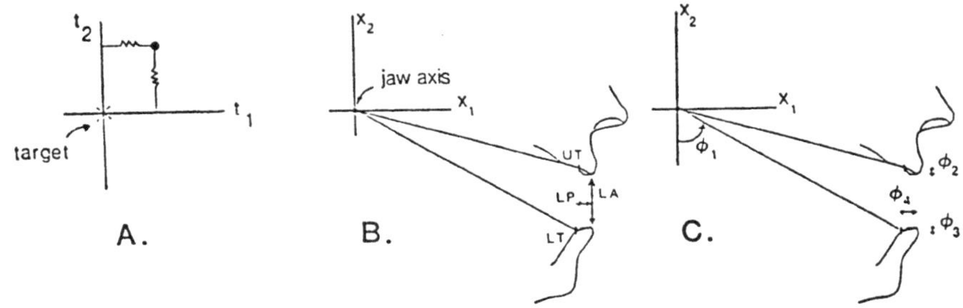

Figure 2. Bilabial tasks:
A. *Task space*. Closed circle denotes current system configuration. The dynamics for each axis are represented in lumped form.
B. *Body space*. The local tract variables of lip aperture and lip protrusion are expressed relative to the coordinates of the jaw. UT and LT denote positions of upper and lower front teeth, respectively. Note that upper and lower lip protrusions are equal in the present model, for simplicity.
C. *Model articulator space*. For lip aperture, jaw rotation (0}2{ and lower lip (0}3{ must be specified. For lip protrusion horizontal displacements of the lips (0)}4{ must be specified (from E. Saltzman, in press).

The transform from body space to model articulation space is made using two matrix components; a matrix that relates motions of the articulators at their current configuration to corresponding tract-variable motions, and an articulator weighting matrix. The elements of the first matrix vary with articulator position; the elements in the second matrix are constant for a given gesture, and specify weights for the contribution of a given articulator to aperture shaping. Thus, for a given closure, by a given speaker, weighting could be greater for the jaw than the lips, either because of the context of the lip closure, or because that particular speaker tends to make greater use of jaw raising than lip raising.

This model, in its preliminary form, produces perceptually satisfactory synthesized speech when model parameters, estimated from running speech are used to drive the articulatory synthesizer (Browman, Goldstein, Kelso, Rubin & Saltzman, 1984). Furthermore, it can be shown that, in simulations, the model displays motor equivalence, that is, trajectory shaping is specified in such a way that no recomputation of trajectory is necessary if a perturbation is introduced in the course of target attainment. The model reaches the same target position in simulated perturbed and unperturbed trials, although with different final positions of the articulators. The way the model functions in compensation does not require reparameterization; it is inherent in the way forces at the tract-variable level are distributed at the model articulator level (see Kelso, Saltzman & Tuller, 1986; Saltzman, in press).

Criticisms of Task Dynamics

Three general classes of objections have been posited to task dynamics, as it now exists.

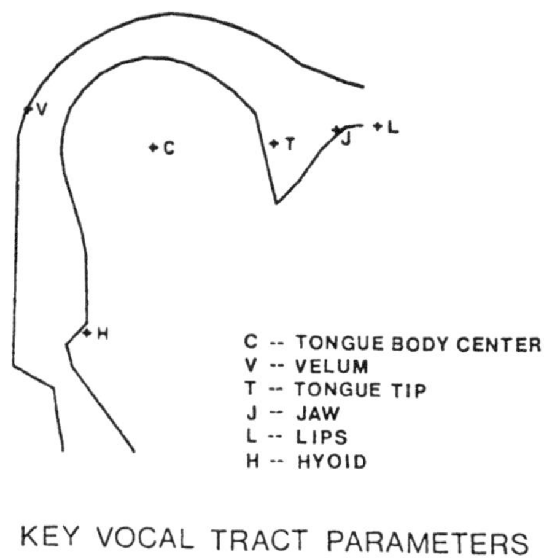

Figure 3. The idealized vocal tract in midsagittal section, as represented in the Haskins Articulatory Synthesizer. From Rubin, Baer and Mermelstein (1981).

First, while it is clear that action theory rejects the notion of a motor plan, and a central agent, it is not specific about what units will be organized. Thus, Kelso and Tuller (in press) state: "Rather, we wish to understand the generation of pattern and form without assuming a priori that there is a *generator* that possesses some kind of representation, neural or mental, of the pattern before it appears". In some sense, this quotation harks back to early criticisms of Lashley's serial ordering description of behavior (Fowler et al., 1977). However, the objective has since become a quite general effort to bring the notions of self organizing systems into experimental psychology (Turvey, 1977).

It can be pointed out that a great deal of current theorizing the motor system and speech can be considered a restatement of obtained results either in the form of a computer metaphor, or a posited neurological mechanism. Thus, Shattuck-Hufnagel proposes the existence of a model for slips of the tongue with, among other components, a serial order processor, and a scan-processor. While the model has obvious computer-based antecedents, it functions in her work simply to organize the facts abouts slips of the tongue, and generate predictions. Presumably, the precise nature of the proposed mental mechanism is not crucial in determining the usefulness of the metaphor. Alternately, computer-program writing can be a way of "testing theories of mental processes by stringently mimicking them" (Steedman & Johnson-Laird, 1980). However, all too many computer models for human processes do not amount to more than a paraphrase of observed facts.

The same kind of criticism can be made of some examples of neurophysiological theories. Thus, it is possible to posit neural generators for rhythmic activities, such as gait, where the sole property of the proposed circuit is the generation of the behavior which led to the proposal of the neural circuit.

A strong reason for a rejection of posited central components, whether computers or unspecified neural circuitry, as an "explanation" for observed behavioral regularities is that the explanation is empty unless it generates further predictions, or leads to direct investigation in the field in which the analogy was made. Curiously enough, given the protagonists involved the rejection of mentalism embodied in the above quotation carries a faint echo of Skinner's objections to mentalism from a behaviorist perspective (Skinner, 1938).

However, although some critics (e.g. Lindblom & MacNeilage, in press) agree that task dynamics may be a healthy reaction to too much mentalism, the positing of task dynamics does not, admittedly, solve the problems of defining intentions, or their origins (Kelso, Saltzman & Tuller, in press). Thus, we can make systematic observations of the production of the word "bob", by asking a subject to say it; and presumably, thus infer important properties of articulation. In principle, the laws governing the formation of the produced entities could be gainfully studied, as well. However, as task dynamics was formulated at the level of observation of skilled movement, it has very little to say directly about the emergence of new entities.

It should be noted that just as a user of the term "coordinative structure" does not necessarily wish to carry all the conceptual baggage with which it has been laden, so a user of the term "plan" may be using it in a sense that refers to a time distributed series of events, rather than an elaborate cognitive computation. Indeed, "plan" and "cognitive structure" terminology could both be used in description of acts unfolding in place and time. Since there is now a substantial body of established fact on movement control, different theories are bound to intersect (Schmidt, 1985).

A second objection to task dynamics in the formal modeling sense is that the present equation structure has a great many free variables (Gottlieb, personal communication). Hence, the model is presently under-constrained and it may become difficult to distinguish between real progress and a successful curve-fitting exercise. It also is incomplete as a model for running speech, as control regimes for successive speech entities overlap (Saltzman, in press). However, it seems reasonable to let modeling constraints develop as the work proceeds, rather than to anticipate them by over-confining the model.

A related point is that the model makes use of second-order systems, curve fitting by means of manipulating mass, damping and stiffness parameters. A question whether this choice is a pragmatically useful decision, or whether the choice has deeper origins in motor organization. This kind of objection, however, can be raised against any model. Our own view is that by careful, systematic exploration of goodness of fit of model to data, we will be able to constrain the model further (Browman & Goldstein, 1985).

A third criticism of the general working assumption of our modeling efforts, is that speech has no special properties at an organizational level. It is the contention of MacNeilage, Studdert-Kennedy and Lindblom (1985) that speech shares with bimanual coordination and no other system a special organizational mode, such that its unit gestures, vowel and consonants are fitted into a larger structure (the syllable) in a special way. The evidence for this special motor organizational mode is that unit reversals, the slips of the tongue, occur in such a way that when reversals occur, the reversals preserve the larger structure. Unit reversals in other forms of action slip are believed to have a different structure. It seems to us that, while slips of the tongue have been extensively examined at a perceptual level, there is, as yet, no analysis of slips of the tongue with an appropriate analysis of the corresponding articulation. Consequently, a detailed answer to the question of whether, or not, the slip of the tongue is evidence for a special style of organizations is presently moot.

POTENTIAL CLINICAL OBSERVATIONS

While the account of action theory presented above is quite fragmentary, it identifies two salient properties of normal speech organization, which must be altered in some way in stuttering, and other forms of pathological speech.

Temporal Cohesion

We have discussed above the short-term temporal cohesiveness of speech. It has long term cohesive properties, as well. Speakers typically inhale to about 60 or 70% vital capacity (Hixon, Goldman and Mead, 1973). This enables them to emit short sentences, or syntactic clauses, using the elastic recoil forces of the lungs efficiently. Of course, air can be inhaled to a greater percent of vital capacity, or exhaled to greater levels than it usually is, but either maneuver involves using greater muscle forces, and is thus, less efficient. If this maneuver is executed successfully, speech will be output with a characteristic overall intonation contour shape, the declination curve, on which local intonation perturbations may be superimposed (see, e.g. Fujisaki & Hirose, 1982).

Research is now in progress to attempt to improve our understanding of just how intonation is controlled physiologically. There are two well-known mechanisms; controversy surrounds their relative importance. The first mechanism is the activity of the laryngeal muscles, especially the cricothyroid; the second is subglottal pressure. Present evidence suggests that the cricothyroid is active for the local perturbations of subglottal pressure which accompany stresses, and raising the overall level of fundamental frequency. However, the overall shape of declination is controlled by the level of subglottal pressure, which is under general respiratory control (Collier, 1975; Gelfer, Harris, Collier & Baer, 1983). Thus, at the beginning of a breath group, appropriate conditions for articulation are "set up" by the activity of the respiratory apparatus. The respiratory apparatus apparently controls pressure, rather than flow, according to recent research (Gelfer, et al., 1983).

What happens to stutterers during respiratory posturing? It is well known that young stutterers are most likely to stutter at the beginnings of utterances (Bloodstein, 1974; Wall, Starkweather & Harris, 1982). This phenomenon can be explained in either of two ways. First, it may be that it is the syntax of the utterance, per se, which is associated the locus of the disfluency - that is, the utterance is organized into syntactic units, and stuttering is more likely to occur at the points in the utterance where syntactic components are relatively weakly linked. Another possibility is that the moment of stuttering is more closely tied to respiratory events, than to syntax per se. Typically, pauses occur at syntactic boundaries, whether in spontaneous or read speech. The pauses, in turn, are often linked to inspiration. The question then becomes "What does the association between utterance onset and stuttering have to do with syntactic or cognitive organizational features, or does it depend more directly on the associated respiratory events?" Watson (1983) has provided us with evidence that stutterers do not coordinate respiratory events as normals do. Obviously, temporal coordination over short time intervals should be investigated, as well.

Resistance to Perturbation

A second property of speech is that it is, in normals, resistant to perturbation; that is, if the articulators are (within limits) subjected to either a static deformation, or a dynamic perturbation during articulation, the speaker can compensate.

One might reason that, if fluent speech is characterized by resistance to perturbation, then disfluent speech should be characterized by a reduced resistance to perturbation. I do not know any relevant studies on stutterers. It should be pointed out, however, that there is evidence that other types of disfluency may be accompanied by failures to compensate for at least static perturbation. For example, Tobey (1981) has shown that very mild aphasics may fail to learn to compensate for jaw, as normals do; Tye, Zimmerman and Kelso (1983) have shown that deaf speakers do not compensate completely for the presence of a bite block, in producing static vowels.

Thus, while experimental evidence is extremely spotty, one might posit that as long- and short-term temporal organization, and compensation for perturbation is the hallmark of normal, fluent production, so are their breakdowns the hallmarks of disfluent production. However, it seems fairly obvious that this characterization alone is inadequate, since at least three types of disfluency, aphasia, deafness and stuttering are very different, both in the perceptual characteristics of the output speech and in the underlying causes even though they are often described as organizational breakdowns. We need to investigate such speech disorders in parallel paradigms, to better specify what we mean by speech organization.

Let me summarize, then, by suggesting that we must concentrate, in analyzing disfluency, on those properties of speech that are robust characteristics of normal production.

REFERENCES

Barry, W. (1983). Some problems of interarticulator phasing as an index of temporal regularity in speech. *Journal of Experimental Psychology: Human Perception and Performance, 9,* 826-828.

Benoit, C. & Abry, C. (in press). *Vowel-consonant timing across speakers.* 72nd International Congress of Acoustics, Toronto, 1986.

Bernstein, N.A. (1967). *The Coordination and Regulation of Movements.* London: Pergamon Press.

Bloodstein, O. (1974). The rules of early stuttering. *Journal of Speech and Hearing Disorders, 39,* 379-394.

Browman, C. & Goldstein, L. (1985). Dynamic modeling of phonetic structure. In V. Fromkin (Ed.), *Phonetic Linguistics.* New York: Academic Press.

Browman, C.P., Goldstein, L., Kelso, J.A., Rubin, P. & Saltzman, E. (1984). Articulatory synthesis from underlying dynamics. *Journal of the Acoustical Society of America, 75,* S22-S23 (A).

Chomsky, N. & Halle, M. (1968). *The sound pattern of English.* New York: Harper & Row.

Collier, R. (1975). Physiological correlates of intonation patterns. *Journal of the Acoustical Society of America, 58,* 249-255.

Easton, T.A. (1972). On the normal use of reflexes. *American Scientist, 60,* 591-599.

Folkins, J.W. & Abbs, J.H. (1975). Lip and jaw motor control during speech: Responses to resistive loading of the jaw. *Journal of Speech and Hearing Research, 18,* 207-220.

Folkins, J.W. & Abbs, J.H. (1976). Additional observations on responses to resistive loading of the jaw. *Journal of Speech and Hearing Research, 19,* 820-821.

Fowler, C.A., Rubin, P., Remez, R.E. & Turvey, M.T. (1980). Implications for speech production of a general theory of action. In B. Butterworth (Ed.), *Language Production.* New York: Academic Press.

Fujisaki, H. & Hirose, K. (1982). Modeling the dynamic characteristics of voice fundamental frequency with applications to analysis and synthesis of intonation. *Preprints of papers, Working Group on Intonation.* The XIIIth International Congress of Linguistics, Tokyo. 57-70.

Fukuda, T. (1961). Studies on human dynamic postures from the viewpoint of postural reflexes. *Acta Oto-Laryngologica, 08,* Suppl. 161.

Gelfer, C.E., Harris, K.S., Collier, R. & Baer, T. (1983). Speculations on the control of fundamental frequency declination. *Haskins Laboratories Status Report on Speech Research, SR-76,* 51-63.

Gentil, M. (1986). *Organisation temporelle de systeme articulatoire: Contributions musculaires des gestes labiaux, linguaux et mandibulaires.* Unpublished doctoral dissertation, Strasbourg.

Gibson, J.J. (1950). *The perception of the visual world.* Boston: Houghton-Mifflin.

Grillner, S. (1975). Locomotion in vertebrates. *Physiological Reviews, 55,* 247-304.

Harris, K.S. (1978). Vowel duration change and its underlying physiological mechanisms. *Language and Speech, 21,* 354-361.

Hencke, W. (1967). Preliminaries to speech synthesis based on an articulatory model. *Conference Preprints: 1967.* Conference on Speech Communication and Processing (Air Force Cambridge Research Laboratories, Bedford, Massachusetts.) 170-177.

Hixon, T., Goldman, M. & Mead, J. (1973). Kinematics of the chest wall during speech production: Volume displacements of the rib cage, abdomen and lung. *Journal of Speech and Hearing Research, 16,* 78-115.

Kelso, J.A.S., Saltzman, E. & Tuller, B. (1986). The dynamical perspective on speech production: data and theory. *Journal of Phonetics, 14,* 29-59.

Kelso, J.A.S., Saltzman, E. & Tuller, B. (in press). Intentional contents, communicative context and task dynamics: A reply to the commentators. *Journal of Phonetics, 14,* 171-196.

Kelso, J.A.S. & Tuller, B. (1983). "Compensatory articulation" under conditions of reduced afferent information: A dynamic formulation. *Journal of Speech and Hearing Research, 26,* 217-224.

Kelso, J.A.S. & Tuller, B. (in press). In E. Keller (Ed.), *Sensory processes and language.* Hillsdale: Erlbaum.

Kelso, J.A.S., Tuller, B. & Harris, K. (1984). A theoretical note on speech timing. *Haskins Laboratories Status Report on Speech Research, SR-79/80,* 161-166. (Also in J.S. Perkell & D.H. Klatt (Eds.),(1985). *Invariance and variability of the speech processes.* Hillsdale: Erlbaum.

Kelso, J.A.S., Tuller, B., Bateson, E. & Fowler, C.A. (1984). Functionally specific articulatory cooperation following jaw perturbations during speech: Evidence for coordinative structures. *Journal of Experimental Psychology: Human Perception and Performance, 10,* 812-832.

Kots, Ya.M. (1977). *The organization of voluntary movement.* New York: Plenum.

Kuehn, D. & Moll, K. (1976). A cineradiographic study of VC and CV articulatory velocities. *Journal of Phonetics, 4,* 303-320.

Lashley, K.S. (1951). The problem of serial order in behavior. In L.A. Jeffress (Ed.), *Cerebral mechanisms in behavior.* New York: John Wiley.

Lindblom, B.E.F. & MacNeilage, P. (1986). Action theory: problems and alternative approaches. *Journal of Phonetics, 14,* 117-132.

MacNeilage, P., Studdert-Kennedy, M. & Lindblom, B. (1985). Planning and production of speech: An overview. In J. Lauter (Ed.), Proceedings of the conference on planning and production of speech by normally hearing and deaf people. *ASHA Reports, 11.*

Marsden, C.D., Merton, P.A. & Morton, H.B. (1983). Rapid postural reactions to mechanical displacement of the hand in man. In J.E. Desmedt (Ed.), *Motor control mechanisms in health and disease.* New York: Raven Press.

Munhall, K.G. (1985). An examination of intra-articulator relative timing. *Journal of the Acoustical Society of America, 78,* 1548-1553.

Rubin, P., Baer, T. & Mermelstein, P. (1981). An articulatory synthesizer for perceptual research. *Journal of the Acoustical Society of America, 70,* 321-328.
Saltzman, E.L. (1979). Levels of sensorimotor representation. *Journal of Mathematical Psychology, 20,* 91-163.
Saltzman, E. (in press). Task dynamic coordination of the speech articulators. *Experimental Brain Research Supplements.*
Saltzman, E. & Kelso, J.A.S. (in press). Skilled actions: A task dynamic approach. *Psychological Review.*
Schmidt, R.A. (1985). "Motor" and "action" perspectives on motor behavior: some important differences, mainly common ground. Paper for the conference *Perspectives on motor behavior and control,* Bielefeld, West Germany, November, 1985.
Shattuck-Hufnagel, S. (1983). Sublexical units and supra-segmental structure. In P. MacNeilage (Ed.), *The production of speech.* New York: Springer-Verlag.
Sherrington, C.S. (1906). *The integrative action of the nervous system.* London: Constable.
Skinner, B.F. (1938). *The behavior of organisms.* New York: Appleton, Century, Crofts.
Steedman, M.J. & Johnson-Laird, P.N. (1980). The production of sentences, utterances and speech-acts: Have computers anything to say? In B. Butterworth (Ed.), *Language Production. V1: Speech and Talk.* New York: Academic press.
Tobey, E. (1981). *Motor speech adaptation: An acoustic study of temporal and spectral reponse patterns in subjects with focal cortical lesions.* Unpublished doctoral dissertation, City University of New York.
Tuller, B., Harris, K.S. & Kelso, J.A.S. (1982). Stress and rate: different transformations of articulation. *Journal of the Acoustical Society of America, 71,* 1534-1543.
Tuller, B. & Kelso, J.A.S. (1984). The timing of articulatory gestures: evidence for relational invariants. *Journal of the Acoustical Society of America, 76,* 1030-1036.
Tuller, B., Kelso, J.A.S. & Harris, K.S. (1982). Interarticulator phasing as an index of temporal regularity in speech. *Journal of Experimental Psychology: Human Perception and Performance, (8), 460-472.*
Turvey, M.T. (1977). Preliminaries to a theory of action with reference to vision. In R. Shaw & J. Bransford (Eds.), Perceiving, acting and knowing: Toward an ecological psychology. Hillsdale: Erlbaum.
Tye, N., Zimmermann, G. & Kelso, J.A.S. (1983). "Compensatory articulation" in hearing-impaired speakers: A cinefluorographic study. *Journal of Phonetics, 11,* 101-115.
Viviani, P. & Terzuolo, V. (1980). Space-time invariance in learned motor skills. In G.E. Stelmach & J. Requin (Eds.), *Tutorials in motor behavior.* Amsterdam: North-Holland.
Wall, M., Starkweather, C. & Harris, K.S. (1981). The influence of voicing adjustments on the locus of stuttering in the spontaneous speech of young child stutterers. *Journal of Fluency Disorders, 6,* 299-310.
Watson, B. (1983). *Simultaneous fiberoptic, transillumination, respitrace, and acoustic analysis of laryngeal reaction time in*

stutterers and nonstutterers. Unpublished doctoral dissertation, University of Connecticut.

Chapter **3**

Programming of Speech and Nonspeech Motor Activity

Wouter Hulstijn

INTRODUCTION

The idea that at least part of our movements (and in particular the fast ones) are planned or programmed before their initiation is an old, and in the research area of motor control, well accepted idea. Particularly the successive rapid movements that are so characteristic of fluent speech are considered by many to be prepared in one form or another before they are uttered. In this chapter an impression will be given of the evolution of theorizing on motor programming.

This will be done for the motoractivity involved in speech and also for other nonspeech behavior, in particular that of handwriting. Handwriting and speech share the same characteristics of complexity, variability, context dependency and continuity. However, handwriting is much slower and easier to record. This quality may be the reason why the most convincing and most cited arguments for programming come from handwriting studies. Therefore, more data will be presented on the movements of a pen than on the motor activity of the mouth and larynx.

The vast amount of literature on motor programming leads to an interesting suggestion about the nature of stuttering. Speech utterances are supposed to be programmed before their initiaton, this means that longer words or longer utterances require more programming. Stuttering mostly occurs at the beginning of a word or an utterance and the frequency of stuttering at the initiation of longer utterances is much higher. This suggests that a programming process may be involved in or is responsible for the origination of stuttering.

The latter idea will be taken up at the end of this chapter (and in the chapter by Peters and Hulstijn). In the next section a few different views on the nature of this programming process will be discussed.

MOTOR PROGRAMS AND FEEDBACK

The concept of a motor program has a long history. As with so many things in psychology, it started with James (1890). Papers by Lashley (1917, 1951) during the first half of this century were very influential, but the most frequently cited definition was the one give by Keele. According to him a motor program is "a set of muscle commands that are structured before a movement sequence begins, and that allows the entire sequence to be carried out uninfluenced by peripheral feedback" (Keele, 1968, p. 387).

Note that the program concept in this definition contrasts with the main rival idea at that time, which viewed all movements as being controlled by feedback. The first line of evidence in favour of a program concept is simply that for very fast movements the processing of feedback is too slow. If, for example, during or even just before a rapid arm swing to hit a tennis-ball a signal arrives saying that this movement does not have to be made, then the movement can only be stopped after a normal reaction time interval of about 150 msec. So, in spite of the 'stop' signal the movement continues without interruption. (Henry & Harrison, 1961). In rapid execution skills like typing or speech, the successive movements follow each other within 100 msec, so there is simply not enough time to use the feedback in the selection of the next movement element.

The second line of evidence comes from studies in which the feedback is eliminated or much reduced by deafferentation. In animals this is done by surgically cutting the dorsal roots on the posterior side of the spinal cord. Lashley (1917) studied a patient with a typical gunshot wound which had caused just about the same effect. Other research has been done on humans, the most notable being that of Laszlo (1967), in which deafferentation of the hand was brought about by a pressure cuff or local anaesthetic. All these research findings lead to the same conclusion: although the movements were impaired, often lacking precision, they could nevertheless be carried out fairly well.

A final, more positive argument for the existence of movement control without feedback comes from a whole series of experiments started by Henry & Rogers in 1960 and, in another paradigm, initiated by Klapp in the seventies, showing that movements could be planned in advance. More complex responses, apparently requiring more elaborate planning or preprogramming were found to have longer initiation times. We will return to these experiments later in this chapter.

These three forms of evidence were the topic of hot debates some 10 years ago. At present the controversy has been much reduced between the peripheralists, who advocate a feedback type of motor control and the centralists who argue that movements are centrally controlled by a motor program. Now theories on motor programming, i.e. those of Schmidt (1975, 1982a), Keele (1982), Rosenbaum, Inhoff and Gordon (1984) and Sternberg, Monsell, Knoll and Wright (1978) all stress the importance of feedback in their program concepts. Although a program can run on without the use of feedback this is not what normally happens. Schmidt (1982b) distinguished two kinds of errors when trying to integrate feedback and motor program concepts: response selection errors and response execution errors. If the wrong response is selected (for example a forehand swing in tennis while a backhand return would have been more appropriate) the person must issue a new motor program which consumes a normal initiation time. But, if an error in execution occurs (for example the correct tennis stroke is programmed but the ball bounces more slowly than expected on the wet gravel) than the correction can be far more rapid. This correction is a reflex-based process, involving the muscle spindles. Their primary goal is, to quote Schmidt, "to keep the movement 'on track'" (Schmidt, 1982b, p. 295). In addition, feedback will be used before the movement occurs - to determine the initial position of the limb - and after the movement has taken place - to evaluate the correctness of the response. This last function of feedback is the more commonly known, but, as stated before, also during its execution feedback may influence the movement in adjusting the force or speed and in monitoring for errors.

FROM PROGRAM TO PROGRAMMING

In addition to the integration of feedback, the motor program concept has evolved on yet another dimension: it has become 'abstract', which means that the program itself does not specify which muscles should be used. Both Keele (1982) and Schmidt (1982b) used the same illustration material, taken from Raibert (1977), to demonstrate this principle. In this experiment the same sentence was written several times using a different set of muscles: firstly, the finger muscles of the right hand, secondly, these (finger) muscles were held stiff and the shoulder - and elbow - muscles were mainly involved, thirdly, the left hand was used, in the fourth stage the pen was held between the teeth and lastly it was taped to the foot. Although there were marked differences in the size and "fluency", remarkable similarities were observed especially with regard to the shapes of the letters. These were such that it was possible to recognize an individual writer by the particular shape of his characters, irrespective of the sets of muscles he used to write these characters. To explain these similarities between the different sets of muscles Schmidt (1975, 1976) introduced the concept of a 'generalized' motor program. This program is considered to be an abstract entity, which needs values for certain parameters in order to specify: which muscles have to be used, the size of the letters, where they must be positioned on the paper and so on. This view led to the introduction of a new term: 'programming'. This programming involves a process in which a generalized or abstract program is retrieved from motor memory. Or, if the movements are new, this program is assembled from existing smaller programs. In the next stage this generalized program must be supplied with its parameters and, much like a computer program or subroutine, must be translated into instructions, i.e. muscle commands.

Now, if the program is abstract, what exactly does it specify? What are its elements and what is the best description of its parameters? The answer very much depends on the model of lower level control that one adopts. Schmidt (in: Schmidt, Zelaznik & Frank, 1978, and Schmidt, Zelaznik, Hawkins and Quinn, 1979) presents his 'impulse-timing' model, in which muscles are thought to be activated by force impulses with a specified onset time, duration and force. According to this model the generalized program specifies three aspects: first, the order of the elements, next the temporal structure, or the phasing of the elements and lastly the relative force of the elementary impulses. But Schmidt (1982a) and Keele (1982) both leave room for the alternative for the impulse timing model: the mass-spring analogy. In this view, which is described in detail by Kelso, Holt, Kugler and Turvey (1980) and in a more introductory manner by Tuller, Turvey and Fitch (1982), the dynamic physical properties of the limbs and the environment are 'better' used. If these mass-spring models are correct then the program will specify spring-like properties such as stiffness and oscillatory features.

Both major proponents of the programming concept stress the hierarchical nature of the program (Greene, 1972). On a high level, a program can be seen as a structure or organization just like a 'coordinative structure' which, according to Kelso, Tuller and Harris (1983, p. 139), is a grouping of muscles "that are constrained to act as a single unit". But exactly how this high level structure proceeds to lower and lower levels is still the subject of debate.

One problem in this debate is that the impulse timing view and the theory on coordinative structures both point to the same empirical evidence: 'relative timing'. According to the impulse timing view the overall duration of a movement sequence may change (overall duration is a parameter that has to be supplied to the program) but the relative duration of its elements remain equal. The time intervals between definite moments in the movements can be measured and a number of studies report equal relative times in spite of large changes in the total duration. Viviani's and Terzuolo's (1980) study of the writing of the letter 'a' at different speeds and sizes is a often cited study in this context. The separate strokes which make up that letter take about the same relative time to draw, irrespective of the total duration of the writing. However, one of the main properties of a coordinative structure is that the temporal patterning of muscle activities or movements are preserved during changes in the overall duration and magnitude of writing (Kelso, Tuller & Harris, 1982, Harris, Chapter 2 in this volume). Therefore, since both opposing views predict the same time relationships it is hard to choose between them on the basis of this type of data.

PROGRAMMING IN SIMPLE REACTION TASKS

It has already been mentioned that one class of data supporting the programming view are reaction-time data. Particularly the increased reaction or initiation time when longer or more complex movements are initiated have been taken as evidence that movements are prepared or programmed in advance. Although there is very substantial evidence in favour of the relationship between the movement complexity and reaction time, there are large controversies about the optimal paradigm to study programming. Firstly, data gathered in a so called simple reaction time task will be presented. In a later section choice-reaction data will be reviewed.

EXPERIMENTS IN SPEECH

In a simple reaction-time type of task the subject knows well in advance what he has to do, for example to pronounce a specific word, but he or she has to wait for a 'go'-signal to start the movement sequence. The most cited results with this type of task are those obtained by Sternberg, Monsell, Knoll and Wright (1978) and Sternberg, Wright, Knoll and Monsell (1980). In their experiments, either natural numbers, or the days of the week, or lists of one- or two-syllable words had to be recited as soon as possible after the go-signal. In different conditions the number of words that had to be recited was varied, i.e. from one to five, and the order of the sequence was changed. In each of these experiments the same results were found, i.e. a linear increase in reaction time with sequence length. In the experiment with one- and two-syllable words it was not the number of syllables that seemed to determine this increase in reaction time but the number of words or 'stress groups'. The concept of programming put forward by Sternberg et al. (1978) is that the whole motor sequence is prepared in advance, before the go-signal and stored (broken up into basic units) in a motor buffer. After the go-signal has been detected, this motor buffer is searched for the correct unit. If there are more units in the motor buffer this search is assumed to take more time, which explains the greater reaction time found in longer sequences. After this retrieval stage, the unit (the 'stress group') has to be 'translated' into movement commands - Sternberg uses the term 'unpacking'. This second unpacking stage takes a little bit longer if there are more syllables or constituents in a unit. This explains the slightly greater reaction time that was found for each sequence length in the two-syllable condition. In the final stage, the command stage, the unit is initiated.

These types of results were also found in typewriting with the number of key strokes (or letters) as the independent variable. In our laboratory we tried to duplicate this finding with handwriting.

EXPERIMENTS WITH HANDWRITING

First, a selection of the data gathered by Teulings, Mullins and Stelmach (1986) will be given. In this particular experiment the number of strokes was varied as indicated in Figure 1 above the X-axis. Figure 1 clearly demonstrates that the expected increase in reaction time using longer sequences did not occur.

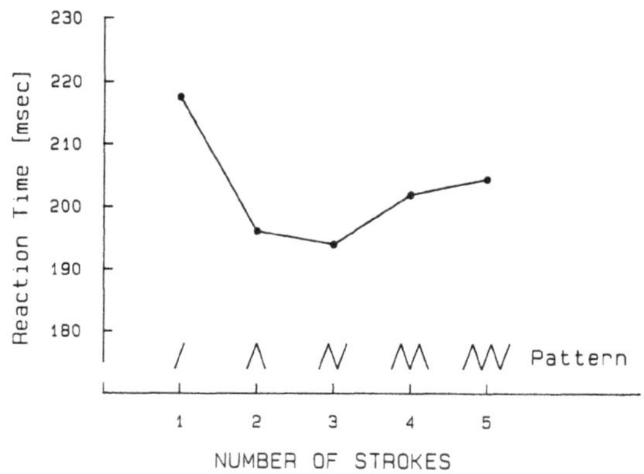

Figure 1. Reaction time as a function of the number of strokes. The patterns that had to be 'written' are shown just above the X-axis.

The second opposing piece of evidence comes from a series of experiments conducted by Hulstijn and Van Galen (1983) in which letters or digits were used as elements. We did find a small increase in reaction time when longer character sequences had to be written (see Figure 2) but these increases were much smaller than those obtained by Sternberg et al. (1978) (for words and key strokes). Moreover, in successive sessions the positive slope dropped from an initial 12 msec per letter to a final 1.5 msec letter in the last series of the third experiment.
The data presented in Figure 2 were obtained in a second experiment, which consisted of two conditions. In both conditions a sequence of one to four digits had to be written as fast as possible. In the so-called overlearned condition these digits were written in a normal way, but in the 'unfamiliar' condition the digit had to be initiated at an unusual starting point (see Figure 2b).

It is quite clear from the figure that the reaction times in the unfamiliar condition were no different from the overlearned condition. Although there is a slightly steeper increase in the unfamiliar condition this effect was not significant. Therefore, the initiation of the first unfamiliar movement pattern was not slower. However, the start of the second unfamiliar movement (in a sequence of two or more) was delayed by more than 100 msec. This can be most easily seen in Figure 3, in which the time to write the digits (the movement time) and the duration of the intervals in which the pen

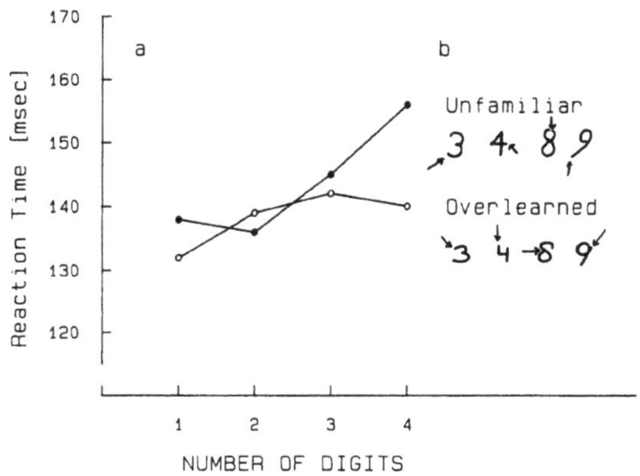

Figure 2. Reaction time for writing the digits, '3', '4', '8' and '9' in a normal, 'overlearned' way and in an newly learned, 'unfamiliar' way. In Figure 2b the starting points in these conditions are marked with an arrow.

was lifted between the digits (inter digit interval) is displayed. Particularly, the interdigit intervals - the lower part of Figure 3 - are considerably higher in the unfamiliar condition.

DISCUSSION

What can be concluded? The first unfamiliar movement pattern had the same reaction and movement time as the overlearned movements. So the first digit was probably completely programmed in advance. But the high interdigit intervals in the unfamiliar condition suggest that this advance programming is restricted to only the first digit. This and similar data support a view in which two levels of programming can be distinguished. One has to do with the movement trajectory itself, i.e. with the order of the separate movements or strokes that make up a familiar or an unfamiliar character. The second and higher level is concerned with the order of the digits.

If it is assumed that a low level motor program for the familiar digit already exists in memory, then the higher level plan only has to contain the memory addresses of these programs. Just before the start of the movement sequence the higher level plan is loaded, which might take slightly more time if the plan is longer. The repeated finding in speech and typewriting that the reaction time for longer sequences is larger (10 msec per unit, instead of our final 1.5 msec for handwriting) may be explained by allowing some overlap between the higher level programming process and the execution process. A few years ago Monsell and Sternberg (1981) described a few versions of their theory, differing in the amount of overlap between programming and execution. In speech and type-

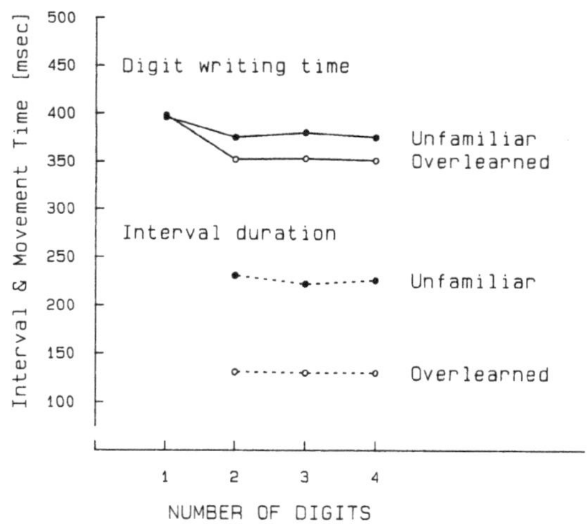

Figure 3. Movement time of writing the first digit and duration of the interval between the first and second digit as a function of sequence length.

writing, where the succession of the various elements is much faster than in writing, there cannot be very much overlap, but in handwriting in which even the fast production of letters takes at least 300 to 400 msec, the writer can easily do two things at once.

Let us add another speculation. Why is this high level program (that specifies the order of the units) only loaded after the go-signal and not well before, as is the case in low-level programming for the unfamiliar trajectory? If it is assumed that this high level program not only serves to initiate the movement, but also to check or monitor the progression of the movement, then it makes sense that this "feedforward"-plan should precede the execution of the movement as closely as possible. If, (as is common in motor behavior) we do two things at once: for example writing and thinking about what to write, then we must have to keep track of what has been written and think ahead about what to write next. This suggests that the motor programming studied by Sternberg et al. (1978) is primarily concerned with the pre-movement set up of a program of order, where the movement sequence can be monitored during its execution.

However, before these ideas can be worked out, data on movement programming in a slightly different experimental paradigm have to be considered.

PROGRAMMING IN CHOICE-REACTION TASKS

Klapp is the most outspoken advocate of the choice-reaction paradigm to study motor programming. He and his coworkers showed that movement complexity influences the choice-reaction time in a long series of experiments starting in 1973 (Klapp, 1977, 1981;

Klapp, Abbott, Coffman, Greim, Snider & Young 1979; Klapp, Anderson & Berrian, 1973; Klapp & Wyatt, 1976; Klapp, Wyatt & Lingo, 1974). In their best known experiment (Klapp & Wyatt, 1976) the subjects had to press a Morse-code key either for a short press - Klapp called this a 'dit' response - or for a longer key press - the 'dah' response. Since the dah-response required an extra 'hold' element, this response was assumed to be more complex. Thus, as expected, the time to start a 'dah' was about 25 msec longer. This difference disappeared (in Klapp's experiments) when the task was changed to a simple reaction-time task, in which the subject knew, before the go-signal whether a 'dit' or a 'dah' press was required, and was encouraged to plan the movements in advance. These and similar findings have been taken by Klapp (1980, 1981) to mean that motor programming cannot be found and studied in the single reaction time paradigm used by Sternberg et al. (1978), described previously.

EXPERIMENTS WITH HANDWRITING

Before commenting on this aspect, some unpublished choice-reaction time data using handwriting and drawing as the motor tasks will be presented. In the first experiment the drawing of a novel grapheme (which was practiced by the subjects a hundred times) was compared to the drawing of only the first stroke. The four novel graphemes used in the experiment are presented in Figure 4. As expected, the time to program the more complex patterns was much longer (592 msec compared to 457 msec) than

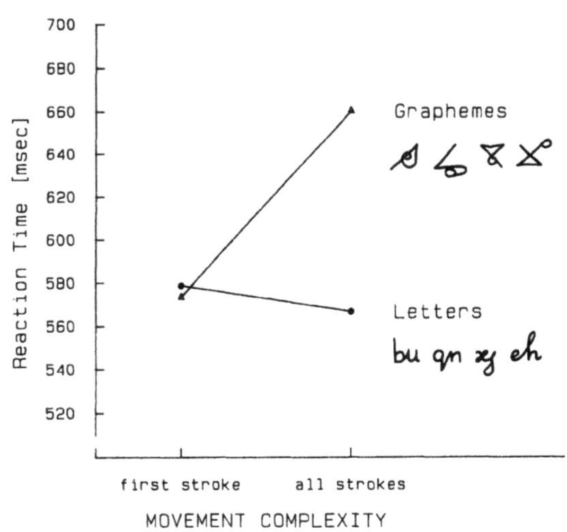

Figure 4. Reaction time for writing either the first stroke or the complete pattern of a novel grapheme or a lettercombination. The four graphemes and the four lettercombinations that were used in the experiment, as well as their first strokes are displayed.

that for a simple stroke. In the second experiment these novel 'graphemes' were compared to letter combinations that also differed in the direction of the first stroke. These letter combinations and the novel graphemes were of at least equal complexity (as measured by the number of strokes). In order to check on possible differences in the time necessary to detect and recognize the stimuli they were also presented in a condition in which only the first stroke of the grapheme or letter had to be made.

Figure 4 gives the most important data of the second experiment. This figure shows quite clearly that there is not only a difference in reaction time between the novel grapheme and the production of one single stroke, but also between these novel patterns and the equally complex letter combinations. It is remarkable that the production of only the first stroke of the letter pairs required a slightly longer time, as though the subjects initiated the program for the first letter but then had to program an extra cancellation for the rest of the program after the first stroke. So we might conclude that although the novel graphemes were practised quite a number of times, there were no stored motor programs and they therefore, had to be 'programmed' at each trial, whereas for the simple lines, programs were used which already existed and could be simply triggered irrespective of their length. Our most recent results illustrate the same point even more clearly.

In this experiment there were not two or four, but fifteen alternative stimuli that either came from a set of letters (see the second line under the X-axis in Figure 5) or from a set of well known symbols (depicted on the line just below the X-axis in Figure 5). These symbols were easy to recognize but no motor programs were stored on how to draw these figures. If we look at the reac-

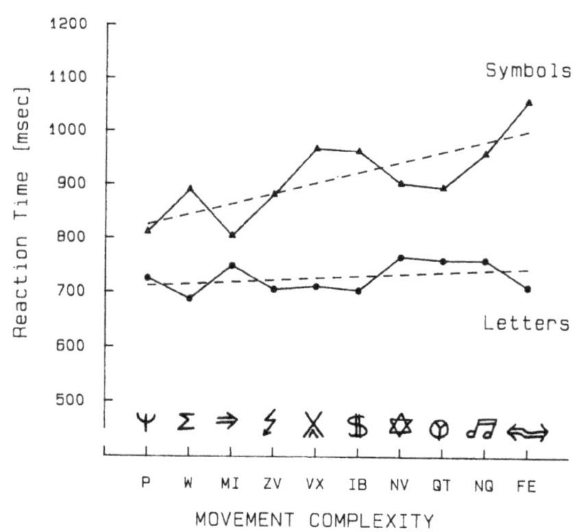

Figure 5. Individual reaction times for letters and symbols, as well as the best fitting straight lines through the ten data points of each condition.

tion times, the important point is not so much that these reaction times are longer for the symbols, but that in going from left to right, the increasing complexity (or the increasing number of strokes) hardly has any effect on the letter reaction times, but strongly influences the reaction times for the symbols. This suggests that the programming of letters is not dependent on their length or complexity: the stored motor program is simply activated as a whole.

DISCUSSION

With respect to the Klapp - Sternberg controversy (the question of whether simple reaction times or choice-reaction times are the best indicators of programming) these data suggest that both paradigms reveal different types of programming. Recently-learned reactions like 'dit'-'dah' key presses can better be studied in a choice-reaction paradigm, since their simple reaction time does not reveal their low level programming. Remember that recently learned or unfamiliar ways to write a digit had no longer reaction times in the simple-reaction paradigm. However, the process called high level programming can probably better be studied using a simple reaction paradigm with long sequences of well learned elements.

CONCLUDING REMARKS

The foregoing introduction on motor programming can best be summarized by presenting a last set of data, coming from an experiment by Peters and Hulstijn (which will be dealt with more fully in one of the following chapters of this book). Only a few data from the nonstutterers control group are relevant in this context.

The subjects saw one-syllable words, three-syllable words or sentences on a screen. They had to read these words or sentences aloud either immediately, which can be compared to a choice reaction time situation, or they had to delay their utterance untill the go-signal was presented - the simple-reaction paradigm. The upper lines in Figure 6 show the voice reaction times. In the choice-reaction task the increase in reaction time for more complex movement sequences was much greater than in the simple paradigm. However, it is quite obvious that part, if not all, of these increased reaction times may be due to the extra time required for reading the longer words or sentences. Interestingly, and in line with Sternberg's results in the simple reaction-time condition, a small but significant increase in reaction time with movement complexity was found.

If Figure 6 is read from top to bottom, which means that the time is running from the top most curve down to the X-axis, the different events within a reaction period are aligned according to voice onset. Three intervals can be distinguished in Figure 6. The first is the interval between the presentation of the stimulus and

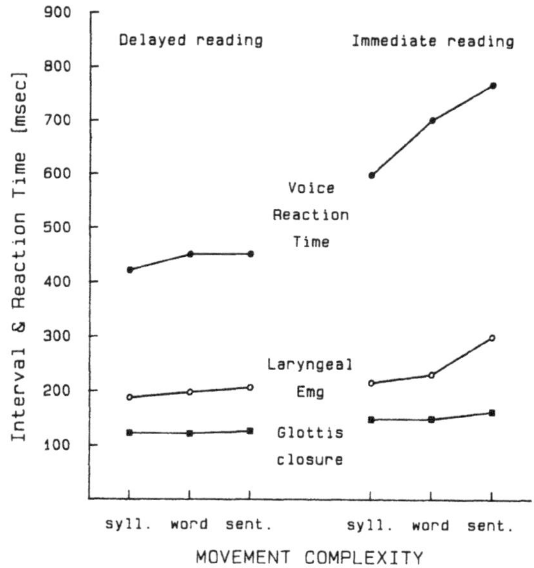

Figure 6. Voice reaction time, as well as intervals within the voice reaction time as a function of utterance length, given separately for two reaction tasks. The intervals are measured backwords from speech onset to Focal-fold closure (lowest curves) and to the start of laryngeal EMG-activity (middle curves).

the start of laryngeal activity. The second interval runs from the start of laryngeal activity to the closure of the glottis and the third interval incorporates the period from the moment that the glottis is closed until the onset of speech. This last interval remains almost constant: it is not influenced by the type of task and sequence length. The first interval shows the effects of both programming variables to the greatest extent. But note that the second interval shows some effects of sequence length (which were highly significant). This means that not all the programming has been completed before the first elements of the movement (in this case the laryngeal emg activity) were initiated. Thus, these data are a demonstration of what has been suggested earlier, i.e. that programming and execution can be done in parallel.

SUMMARY

In the first part of this chapter different views on the nature of programs and programming were introduced which incorporate the processing of feedback in their latest versions. Programs concerned with highly-learned activities are rather abstract. This means that different levels of programming can be distinguished: the low level programming of relatively novel movements and the higher-level programming in which particularly the order of the units are planned. The units in such a plan can only be well learned movement sequences like letters or words. It is suggested that a distinction between these levels of programming can bring together the different views on the optimal paradigm to study programming. In the final section some evidence was presented to show that programming and response execution may occur simultaneously.

At the outset of this chapter the suggestion was made that stuttering may be caused by ineffective motor programming. The often reported findings that disfluencies occur for more than 90 per cent at the start of a word and that the frequency of stuttering dramatically increases with word length, form one type of evidence. Another type of evidence is given via the reaction-time results of fluent utterances by stutterers and nonstutters (more fully presented in chapter 12 by Peters and Hulstijn). It is shown that the fluent words and sentences spoken by stutterers, although they are fluent, still have a longer reaction time than those from nonstutterers. Moreover, the effect of complexity on reaction time is much larger for the stutterers. Both these group differences are mainly confined to the first interval as described in Figure 6, which is the "silent" period between the presentation of the stimulus and the first recordings of speech-related activity. This is the period in which the utterance is programmed.

Do stutterers have more difficulties with the low level programming of motor commands or is the higher level planning of the order of the elements more problematic in stuttering? The difference in reaction time data between simple and choice paradigms should provide the answer. The data given by Peters and Hulstijn, in particular the finding that the differences between stutterers and nonstutterers were equal in both types of task, make it quite clear that it is the low level, motor command programming that is non-optimal in stutterers.

REFERENCES

Greene, P.H. (1972). Problems of organization of motor systems. In R. Rosen & F.M. Snell (Eds.), *Progress in theoretical biology: Vol. 2* (pp. 304-338). New York: Academic Press.

Henry, F.M. & Rogers, D.E. (1960). Increased response latency for complicated movements and a "memory drum" theory of neuromotor reaction. *Research Quarterly, 31*, 448-458.

Hulstijn, W. & Van Galen, G.P. (1983). Programming in handwriting: Reaction time and movement time as a function of sequence length. *Acta Psychologica, 54*, 23-49.

James, W. (1890). *The principles of psychology: Vol. 1.* London: MacMillan.

Keele, S.W. (1982). Learning and control of coordinated motor patterns: The programming perspective. In J.A.S. Kelso (Ed.), *Human motor behavior: An introduction* (pp. 161-186). Hillsdale, NJ: Lawrence Erlbaum Associates.

Kelso, J.A.S., Holt, K.G., Kugler, P.N. & Turvey, M.T. (1980). On the concept of coordinative structures as dissipative structures: II. Empirical lines of convergency. In G.E. Stelmach & J. Requin (Eds.), *Tutorials in motor behavior* (pp. 49-70). Amsterdam: North-Holland.

Kelso, J.A.S., Tuller, B. & Harris, K.S. (1983). A "dynamic pattern" perspective on the control and coordination of movement. In P.F. MacNeilage (Ed.), *The production of speech* (pp. 137-173). New York: Springer Verlag.

Klapp, S.T., Abbott, J., Coffman, K., Greim, D., Snider, R. & Young, F. (1979). Simple and choice reaction time methods in the study of motor programming. *Journal of Motor Behavior, 11,* 91-101.

Klapp, S.T. (1977). Reaction time analysis of programmed control. *Exercise and Sports Sciences Reviews, 5,* 231-253.

Klapp, S.T. (1981). Motor programming is not the only process which can influence rt: Some thoughts on the Marteniuk and MacKenzie analysis. *Journal of Motor Behavior, 13,* 320-328.

Klapp, S.T. & Wyatt, E.P. (1976). Motor programming within a sequence of responses. *Journal of Motor Behavior, 8,* 19-26.

Klapp, S.T., Anderson, W.C. & Berrian, R.W. (1973). Implicit speech in reading, reconsidered. *Journal of Experimental Psychology, 100,* 368-374.

Klapp, S.T., Wyatt, E.P. & Lingo, W.M. (1974). Response programming in simple and choice reactions. *Journal of Motor Behavior, 6,* 263-271.

Lashley, K.S. (1917). The accuracy of movement in the absence of excitation from the moving organ. *American Journal of Physiology, 43,* 169-194.

Lashley, K.S. (1951). The problem of serial order in behavior. In L.A. Jeffress (Ed.), *Cerebral mechanisms in behavior: The Hixon symposium* (pp. 112-146). New York: Wiley.

Laszlo, J.I. (1967). Training of fast tapping with reduction of kinaesthetic, tactile, visual and auditory sensations. *Quarterly Journal of Experimental Psychology, 19,* 344-349.

Monsell, S. & Sternberg, S. (1981). *Speech programming: A critical review, a new experimental approach, and a model of the timing of rapid utterances. Part 1.* Internal report.

Peters, H.F.M. & Hulstijn, W. (1987). Programming and initiation of speech utterances in stuttering. In H.F.M. Peters & W. Hulstijn (Eds.), *Speech Motor Dynamics in Stuttering.* Wien: Springer Verlag.

Raibert, M.H. (1977). *Motor control and learning by the state space model.* Unpublished doctoral dissertation. Massachusetts Institute of Technology.

Rosenbaum, D.A., Inhoff, A.W. & Gordon, A.M. (1984). Choosing between movement sequences: A hierarchical editor model. *Journal of Experimental Psychology: General, 113,* 372-393.

Schmidt, R.A. (1975). A schema theory of discrete motor skill learning. *Psychological Review, 82,* 225-260.

Schmidt, R.A. (1976). The schema as a solution to some persistent problems in motor learning theory. In G.E. Stelmach (Ed.), *Motor control: Issues and trends* (pp. 41-65). New York: Academic Press.

Schmidt, R.A. (1982a). More on motor programs. In J.A.S. Kelso (Ed.), *Human motor behavior: An introduction* (pp. 189-217). Hillsdale, NJ: Lawrence Erlbaum Associates.

Schmidt, R.A. (1982b). *Motor control and learning: A behavioral emphasis.* Champaign, IL: Human Kinetics.

Schmidt, R.A., Zelaznik, H.N. & Frank, J.S. (1978). Sources of inaccuracy in rapid movement. In G.E. Stelmach (Ed.), *Information processing in motor control and learning* (pp. 183-203). New York: Academic Press.

Schmidt, R.A., Zelaznik, H.N., Hawkins, B., Frank, J.S. & Quinn, J.T., Jr. (1979). Motor-output variability: A theory for the accuracy of rapid motor acts. *Psychological Review, 86,* 415-451.

Sheridan, M. (1984). Planning and controlling simple movements. In M.M. Smyth & A.M. Wing (Eds.), *The psychology of human movement* (pp. 47-82). London: Academic Press.

Sternberg, S., Monsell, S., Knoll, R.L. & Wright, C.E. (1978). The latency and duration of rapid movement sequences: Comparisons of speech and typewriting. In G.E. Stelmach (Ed.), *Information processing in motor control and learning* (pp. 117-152). New York: Academic Press.

Sternberg, S., Wright, C.E., Knoll, R.L. & Monsell, S. (1980). Motor programs in rapid speech: Additional evidence. In R.A. Cole (Ed.), *Perception and production of fluent speech* (pp. 507-534). Hillsdale, NJ: Lawrence Erlbaum Associates.

Teulings, H.L., Mullins, P.A. & Stelmach, G.E. (1986). The elementary units of programming in handwriting. In H.S.R. Kao, G.P. van Galen & R. Hoosain (Eds.), *Graphonomics: Contemporary research in handwriting* (pp. 21-32). Amsterdam: North-Holland.

Tuller, B.H., Turvey, M.T. & Fitch, H.L. (1982). The Bernstein perspective: II. The concept of muscle linkage or coordinative structure. In J.A.S. Kelso (Ed.), *Human motor behavior: An introduction* (pp. 253-270). Hillsdale, NJ: Lawrence Erlbaum Associates.

Viviani, P. & Terzuolo, C. (1980). Space-time invariance in learned motor skills. In G.E. Stelmach & J. Requin (Eds.), *Tutorials in motor behavior* (pp. 525-533). Amsterdam: North-Holland.

Van Galen, G. & Wing, A.M. (1984). The sequencing of movements. In M.M. Smyth & A.M. Wing (Eds.), *The psychology of human movement* (pp. 153-181). London: Academic Press.

Chapter **4**

Multilevel Control Model for Speech Motor Activity

Vincent L. Gracco

It has been suggested that a current limitation in our understanding of the mechanisms of motor control is the limited knowledge regarding the structure of the central nervous system as a multivariable controller (Ito, 1982). In attempting to understand the control of speech movements and the aberrations associated with speech movement disorders, the problem is compounded because the multiple movements of this motor act are subordinate to an overall communication goal. This is illustrated by the presence of motor equivalence in which speech motor actions are implemented in a complex, but systematically variable manner (cf. Abbs, 1986; Gracco & Abbs, in press, b; Hughes & Abbs, 1976; MacNeilage, 1970). In response to the apparent variability in the movements and muscle activities associated with speech production, experimental effort has been directed toward the identification of invariant relations in the speech production process. The search for invariance is based on the assumption that stereotypic or invariant motor actions reduce the control complexity of a motor task. While the search for movement invariance has provided some general insight into motor control considerations, many issues remain unresolved (cf. Perkell, 1986; Stein, 1982 for reviews).

A major factor often overlooked in the search for and identification of invariant or simplifying relations is the mechanisms by which such relations are mediated. For example, one hypothesized invariant relation for limb and speech movements involves the scaling of a base velocity profile which accounts for the kinematic changes associated with movements of different amplitudes and durations (Atkeson & Hollerbach, 1985; Munhall, Ostry & Parush, 1985; Ostry & Cooke, in press). One consequence of focused attempts to uncover underlying control principles reflected in invariant relations has been in the limited consideration of sensory information in the motor control process. It is often overlooked that scalar adjustments could not be accomplished without sensory information regarding the relative position of the structures prior to movement as well as an estimation of the distance to be moved.

In this chapter, it will be suggested that sensory information is used in multiple ways during the planning, programming, and execution of speech movements. Without considering the influence of sensory information and the underlying dynamic process, invariance may be relegated to an interesting observation. Variance, on the other hand, provides information on the underlying task-specific goals as well as insight into the mechanism underlying hypothesized invariant relations. Perhaps more can be gained in our understanding of the speech motor process if we attempt to account for the sources of variability as well as continue the search for invariant articulatory relations. In the next section, a perspective will be presented which briefly considers the importance of sensory information in the control of speech movements. More detailed considerations have been presented elsewhere (Borden, 1979; Gracco, 1984; Gracco & Abbs, in press, a).

THE IMPORTANCE OF SENSORS

The ability of an organism to carry out certain motor tasks with reduced or absent sensory information has been used to argue against the role of sensors in the guidance of movement (Fentress, 1973; Polit & Bizzi, 1979; Taub & Berman, 1968). However, as has been shown repeatedly, movements carried out in such states are often only grossly normal and require rather simple or stereotypic tasks (Bossom, 1974; Polit & Bizzi, 1979; Rothwell, Traub, Day, Obeso, Thomas & Marsden, 1982; Sanes & Evarts, 1983).

For the control of speech movements, it has been shown that sensorimotor mechanisms have the requisite characteristics to be used in the control and coordination of speech (Abbs & Gracco, 1984; Folkins & Abbs, 1975; Gracco & Abbs, 1985; Kelso, Tuller, Bateson, & Fowler, 1984; Shaiman, Abbs & Gracco, 1985). These studies have demonstrated that the motor control processes underlying speech production are afferent-dependent, task specific, functionally organized, and can operate at short latencies. Further, given the multiple paths through which different sensory modalities may access motor centers, it is doubtful that all sensory information is ever really eliminated. Even for highly patterned and automatic behaviors such as locomotion, sensory information has been shown to interact with neural pattern generators providing the necessary adjustments in motor output to accommodate moment-to-moment environmental (terrain) changes (cf. Grillner, 1981; Grillner & Wallen, 1985). The important finding from sensory reduction or deafferentiation studies is that motor tasks can, and probably do, rely on some internal (stored) motor relations; however, normal motor actions are never carried out in the absence of continuous sensory information.

In addition to the experimental results summarized above, the importance of sensory information in the control of speech movements is suggested by anatomic considerations related to orofacial sensory receptor density and expanded thalamic and cortical orofacial representations. For example, Munger and Halata (1983) and Halata and Munger (1983) examined the sensory innervation of primate facial skin finding dense sensory innervation in the perioral and intraoral regions. These authors reported multiple innervation of cutaneous receptor sites suggesting that stimulation of any site is capable of activating multiple ascending pathways. Numerous investigations have demonstrated multiple ascending pathways from peripheral orofacial structures to the thalamus, multiple sensory and motor cortical areas, the basal ganglia, and cerebellum (cf. Gracco & Abbs, in press, a (for review). For example, there are at least four orofacial representations within the parietal lobe (Leinonen & Nyman, 1979; McKenna, Whitsel & Dreyer, 1982; Sur, Nelson & Kaas, 1982) and at least five orofacial representations within the primary and nonprimary motor areas in the frontal lobe (Muakkassa & Strick, 1979; Rizzolatti, Scandolara, Gentilucci & Camarda, 1981; Schell & Strick, 1984; Sessle & Wiesendanger, 1982). In addition, there are orofacial representations in the "motor" portion of the basal ganglia (Crutcher & DeLong, 1984; DeLong & Georgopoulos, 1981), the deep cerebellar nuclei (Schell & Strick, 1984; Stanton, 1980), and multiple nuclear regions of the thalamus (Carpenter, Nakano & Kim, 1976; Kaas, Nelson, Sur, Dykes & Merzenich, 1984; Smith, 1975). Furthermore, somatic sensory information is known to project, directly or indirectly, from peripheral orofacial sensory nuclei to all of these cortical and subcortical areas. It appears, as with other motor systems, that multiple afferent innervation and parallel sensorimotor processing is a characteristic of the orofacial system (cf. Merzenich & Kaas, 1980; Mountcastle, 1979). The presence of multiple pathways providing sensory information directly and indirectly to the multiple cortical and subcortical orofacial areas underscores the potential sensorimotor processing and reflects on the importance of the orofacial sensorimotor system.

In addition to the multiple afferent channels and extensive cortical and subcortical representation, other indirect evidence underscores the potential importance of sensory information in the control of orofacial actions. It has been observed in numerous experiments that the orofacial region, consisting of both perioral and intraoral regions, is one of the most sensitive of the human body (Schmidt, 1978). Psychophysical studies of tactile discrimination have shown that the lips and the tongue tip are extremely sensitive skin regions, second only to the finger tips. While psychophysical studies do not reflect motor control capabilities, they nevertheless indicate that the dense somatic sensory information is finely-tuned and utilized in "higher level" sensorimotor processes. When considering the classic motor and sensory homunculus found in any neurological text, one is struck by the massive amounts of cortical tissue representing the orofacial structures. It has been suggested that the expansive cortical *motor* representation of the speech structures reflects the importance of speech and verbal communication in the phylogenetic development of the species (Phillips & Porter, 1977; Young, 1950). Similarly, what is the importance of the expansive orofacial representation within the somatic *sensory* cortex? It seems illogical that the extensive, multiple sensory representation is used solely for the psychophysical identification of objects placed on and around the lips, jaw, or tongue. It also seems inconceivable that the sensory representation of orofacial structures reflects swallowing or mastication processes exclusively since lesions to the orofacial areas of the parietal cortices do not produce significant dysphagia or related problems. Considering the orofacial sensory receptor density, sensitivity, and the extensive cortical orofacial representation, it is suggested that peripheral orofacial sensors and the somatic sensory information transduced are an integral component in the modification of speech motor output.

In the following sections, this conceptualization will be elaborated by considering speech physiology investigations which support a speech motor control hierarchy involving goal-level planning, temporal specification of individual movements, predictive sensorimotor parameterization, and on-line coordination within and among the articulators. These stages are similar in many respects to the traditional motor behavior concepts of motor planning, motor programming, and motor execution. However, the present model will be defined with specific emphasis on the role of sensory information during each stage to ultimately produce the observable motor output. It is suggested that sensory information is an essential component of each of the levels in the motor control hierarchy, although the sensory information extracted may be used in different ways throughout the unfolding motor act.

GOAL-DIRECTED MOTOR PLANNING

Attempting to understand the nervous system actions involved in the coordination of movement, Bernstein (1967) suggested it was important to determine what was represented within the central nervous system. Bernstein hypothesized that it was not the individual movements themselves, but the actual goal of the individual movements represented as an abstract entity, later becoming realized through the motor execution process. For a certain class of speech movements (bilabial closing), we have recently suggested that it is the *combined* actions of the articulators which may be represented as the motor plan for oral closure (Gracco & Abbs, in press, b; see also Saltzman, 1979; Saltzman, in press). That is, at an early stage in the speech production process, the movement plan reflects an abstract representation of the subsequent movement goal (e.g., oral closure).
The individual articulators are considered as a single entity and the goal of the subsequent motor act is established. The movement plan essentially links the goal with the physical reality of establishing and subsequently executing the appropriate motor patterns to accomplish the task. This hierarchical structure involving the goal and subsequent specification of the individual components is a general characteristic of the communication process. That is, speech involves the conveyance of a message to a listener. The individual

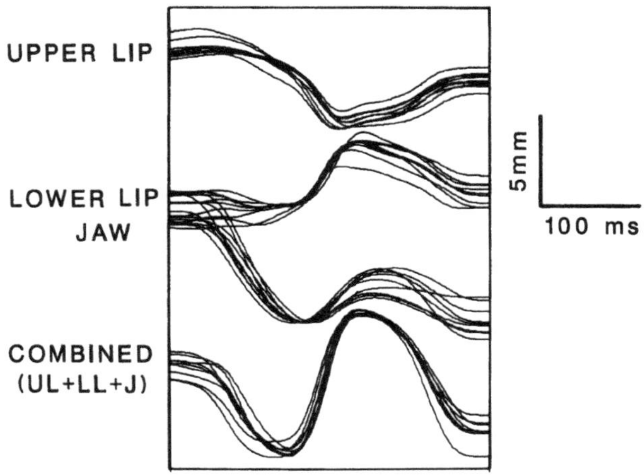

Figure 1. Nine superimposed closing movements of the upper lip, lower lip, and jaw for the first /p/ in sapapple. The bottom trace is a derived signal obtained by adding the separate displacements.

muscle contractions and resulting movements producing the acoustic cues are subordinate to the goal of communication. In the present chapter, goal-directed speech motor planning is only evaluated within the context of the movement goal, although such movements are always subordinate to the acoustic consequences they produce and ultimately to the listeners' perception.

As mentioned previously and illustrated in Figure 1, it appears that the motor plan for speech, at least during oral closure, is formulated in terms of the combined action of the articulators. Presented in Figure 1 are superimposed closing movements of the upper lip (UL), lower lip (LL), and jaw (J) during multiple repetition of the utterance "sapapple". The bottom trace is a derived displacement signal representing the instantaneous sum of the individual lip and jaw movements over the same time interval. As can be seen, while the action of individual articulators is variable with regard to their final displacements, the combined action, illustrated at the bottom of Figure 1, remains relatively invariant. This can be seen qualitatively in this figure and has been shown quantitatively (Gracco & Abbs, in press, b). The apparent goal of oral closure may reflect a tendency to produce an invariant vowel formant trajectory or may simply reflect a movement goal of closing the acoustic tube in preparation for the upcoming implosion of air for the /p/ these two possibilities are not mutually exclusive. However, it does appear that the invariant movement characteristic for this speech gesture is the combined oppositional action of the articulators. As such, speech movement invariance reflects an abstraction not obvious from the actions of the individual articulators.

The role of sensory information at this stage of the motor control process is not obvious. However, if one considers the oral closing movements within a broader time frame, a hypothetical

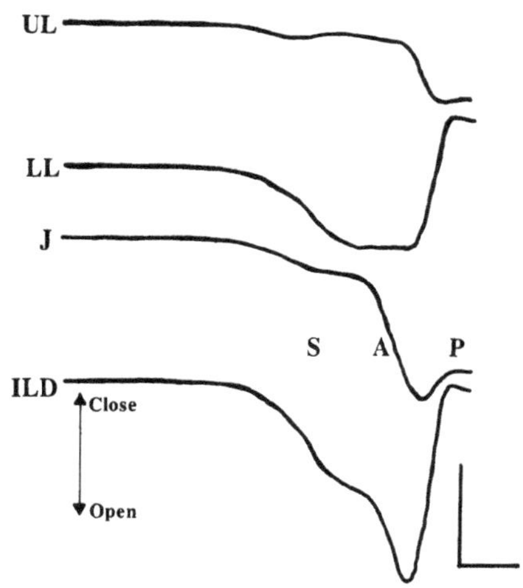

Figure 2. Subject's production of "sapapple" starting with lips closed at rest. The four traces from top to bottom are movements of the upper lip (UL), lower lip (LL), jaw (J), and interlip distance (ILD) obtained by calculating the distance between the lips during the utterance. Calibrations are 5 mm (vertical) and 50 ms (horizontal).

function of sensory information may be formulated. The superimposed movements displayed in Figure 1 represent the closing actions of the UL, LL, and J from maximum opening for the vowel to peak closing displacement. The behavior of the articulators, considered prior to the onset of movement, reveals another aspect of the goal-level motor plan. Figure 2 illustrates a single kinematic profile from a subject repeating 'sapapple'; the subject began this trial with lips together at rest. As with the previous figure, the bottom trace is a representation of the interlip distance during the entire utterance. As can be seen, the lips and jaw displacements prior to closure reflect not just the vowel opening, but the total oral opening with reference to the lips at rest. That is, the total closing movement must incorporate the immediate goal of closing the oral cavity based on the opening for the vowel /ae/ as well as the distance previously opened for the /s/. Therefore, the total movement goal can be thought of as moving the lips and jaw back to their original position (closure) following maximal oral opening. However, as we have recently shown, the positions of the articulators at opening and closing and their moment-to-moment trajectories are not invariant, but vary substantially (Gracco & Abbs, in press, b). Rather than each articulator returning to some prespecified spatial target, the overall goal-level movement plan may be to generate the appropriate amount of total sensory input resulting in a condition similar to that attained at rest. That is, the referent for oral closure in terms of the lips and jaw movement may be a somatic-sensory based pattern reflecting a combined level of sensory input. This conceptualization suggests that many combinations of UL, LL, and J final positions will result in the same total sensory "experience". This speculation is consistent with the systematic spatial variability observed experimentally. Thus, speech motor planning may reflect an abstract relational state among all articulators involving a predetermined sensory-based referent. The ongoing sensory information most likely involves immediate somatic sensory as well as later occurring auditory information extracted from the kinematic and acoustic signals, respectively.

Once the plan is specified, the remaining processes involve the programming of the appropriate motor actions, including coordinating the multiple articulators, and subsequently, motor execution. Prior to considering the programming and execution processes, it will first be helpful to review some results from speech physiology studies which provide some insight into these hypothesized sensorimotor processes.

SPEECH MOTOR PROGRAMMING

Folkins and Abbs (1975) were the first to demonstrate that the speech system had the capability to respond at short latencies to sensory input resulting from unanticipated mechanical disruptions. Subsequent reinterpretation of those data by Abbs and Cole (1982) led to another important characteristic of the speech system. When a speech structure is perturbed or impeded during its goal-directed movement, adjustments are made in the perturbed and unperturbed articulators. Such functional autogenic and nonautogenic adjustments have been observed for many of the speech articulators, apparently reflecting a general characteristic of all speech movements (cf. Abbs & Gracco, 1984; Folkins & Zimmermann, 1982; Kelso et al., 1984; Riordan, 1977; Shaiman, Abbs & Gracco, 1985). Similar observations have been made for postural adjustments (Marsden, Merton & Morton, 1981; Nashner & Cordo, 1981; Nashner, Woollacott & Tuma, 1979), compensatory eye-head movements (Bizzi, Kalil & Tagliasco, 1971; Morasso, Bizzi & Dichgans, 1973), wrist-thumb interactions (Traub, Rothwell & Marsden, 1980), and thumb-finger actions (Cole, Gracco & Abbs, 1984). The implication from these findings is that sensory information is an integral component in the control of movement. More importantly, the presence of sensorimotor interactions reflects the existence of specific anatomical pathways within as well as across motor structures. These connections provide convergence and divergence of sensory information onto various, synergistically-related motor structures. However, these pathways are not obligatory or "hard-wired" as in a stereotypic reflex pathway. Rather, these connections can be flexibly and specifically activated or inactivated depending on task requirements (cf. Abbs et al., 1984; Kelso et al., 1984). It appears that a distinction can be made between the anatomical connections for voluntary motor behaviors and a more functional process used to activate and route the relevant sensory signals.

One way of conceptualizing such processes is through the construct of a motor program. It is reasonable to suggest that motor programs may reflect the specific anatomical connections and synaptic interactions between various and related body regions, and the (internal) activation of the relevant pathways prior to movement. The programming process would consist of the subsequent (external) sensory parameterization or scaling of these connections in a functionally task-specific manner. The distinction between an internal program and an external parameterization process synthesizes the concepts of movements as stored motor programs and movements generated afresh through ongoing sensory information. Without doubt, there must be some type of stored motor patterns or synergistic relations which then rely on updated sensory information to specify movement characteristics. The cortical activity preceding voluntary movement recorded through the intact human scalp (e.g., Bereitschaftspotential or BP potential) and the subsequent premotion positivity (cf. Deecke, Becker, Grozinger, Schied & Kornhuber, 1973) may be a direct reflection of the internal activation of a motor program or sequence of motor programs. Without extensive anatomical investigations, the extent and details of the anatomical connections or interconnections underlying motor programs within the orofacial system can only be implied. However, recent physiological studies provide some insight into the characteristics of the motor programming process.

Considering the dynamically changing peripheral conditions (e.g., time-varying articulator positions and highly specific articulator interactions), the underlying control process must be extremely flexible. The flexibility and concomitant complexity of the speech motor control process is reflected in results of perturbation studies demonstrating multiple time dependent sensorimotor mechanisms operating during ongoing speech production (Gracco, 1984; Gracco & Abbs, 1982; Gracco & Abbs, 1985). The compensatory movement and EMG response patterns and variable compensatory response latencies demonstrated in these studies appear to reflect systematically variable sensorimotor actions. For example, lower lip perturbations introduced prior to the onset of muscle contraction result in long latency compensatory responses in all the synergistic muscles of the labial complex (Gracco & Abbs, 1982). These displacement perturbations result in proportional increases in the EMG activity and subsequent movements to almost totally readjust to the altered peripheral conditions (Gracco, 1984; Gracco & Abbs, 1985). These results suggest that prior to *motor activation* (EMG onset) for a particular movement, sensory signals can rapidly access and significantly modify motor output. Further, these sensory signals can be used to reparameterize or reprogram the previously programmed response. The latency and functionality of these compensatory responses suggest that for normal unperturbed speech movements, sensory information related to articulatory position could be used to compute the necessary forces required to generally specify or program the articulators. From this perspective, speech motor programming reflects the general physiological "tuning" of the hard-wired neural circuitry with later execution adjustments providing the details (cf. Abbs et al., 1984; Gracco & Abbs, 1985 for further elaboration).

However, the exact mechanism to accomplish such a task has not been specified and leads to a major consideration for the utilizing of sensory information during the ongoing control of speech movements. For speech motor programming, the time required for such processing becomes a limiting factor. For example, consider

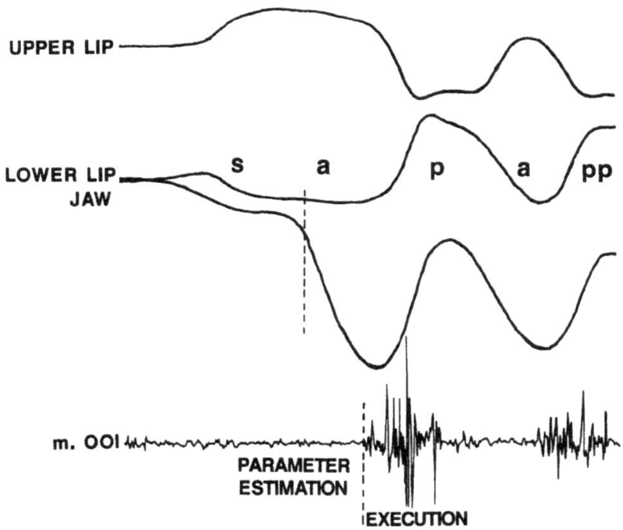

Figure 3. The upper lip, lower lip, and jaw movements for sapapple and the corresponding muscle activity from Orbicularis oris inferior (OOI). Also illustrated is the time interval for the hypothesized parameter estimation (parameterization) and subsequent motor execution processes.

the simple speech gesture shown in Figure 3. From the previous conceptualization, the parameterization of the first 'p' in "sapapple" requires that the nervous system know or estimate the amount of oral opening for the /ae/ in order to issue the appropriate commands to achieve oral closure. As can be seen, however, the jaw is the major structure in determining interlip distance and is never really in a static state. The problem of parameterization becomes one of available time. For bilabial sounds, for example, the dynamics of oral closure are based on the amount of oral opening. If sensory information is to be used in the programming process, based on the position of the articulators at peak oral opening, there does not appear to be enough time available between maximum oral opening and the onset of EMG activity for oral closure. That is, at the time of maximum oral opening, the EMG signals associated with lip closing are initated within approximately 10 to 15 msec. This is probably not sufficient time to scale and certainly not to compute the necessary labial and mandibular forces and subsequently generate the appropriate neural signals to the synergistic muscles.

One possibility which we are exploring is that certain sensory receptors can provide predictive information on the extent of the oral opening prior to completion of oral opening. As mentioned, the jaw is the primary articulator specifying the extent of oral opening. The jaw closing muscles are heavily endowed with muscle spindles which have been shown to have a velocity sensitive component and discharge in relation to muscle stretch (Cody, Harrison & Taylor, 1975; Goodwin & Luschei, 1975; Larson, Smith & Luschei, 1981).

During opening, the jaw closing muscles (specifically masseter) would be stretching and the muscle spindles would be discharging with a signal proportional to jaw velocity. Given the consistent velocity/amplitude relationship characteristic of all movements, the jaw velocity information could be used to estimate jaw opening magnitude. From the jaw opening signal, along with the sensory information from the static lip positions prior to closing, the nervous system would have enough information to generally determine the task dynamics (i.e., how much force will be required to achieve oral closure). In support of this speculation are data illustrating the relationship between the magnitude of jaw opening velocity and total closing displacement of the upper lip, lower lip, and jaw for the first "p" in sapapple (Figure 4). As can be seen, the total closing displacement is highly related to the jaw opening velocity indicating that as the jaw opens farther, its velocity is higher and the amount of total displacement required of the combined articulators increases. Similar results are obtained when the individual articulators are plotted as a function of jaw opening velocity.

These data provide some support for the hypothesis that sensory signals arising from jaw opening may be used in a predictive manner to parameterize the motor program for subsequent oral closure. However, it is necessary to consider the time course of the jaw opening velocity and its relationship to the muscle actions generating the lip and jaw movements. Presented in Figure 5 is a single trial example illustrating the temporal relationship between jaw opening velocity and the EMG activity of OOI.

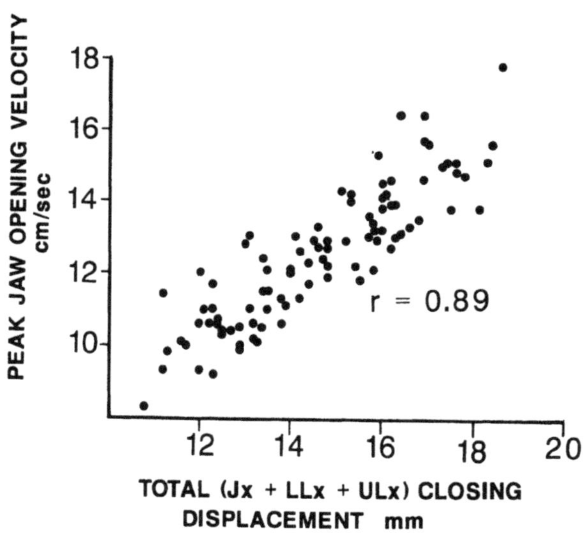

Figure 4. Peak jaw opening velocity (Jx) plotted as a function of the total combined oral closing displacements obtained by summing the peak displacement of the upper lip, lower lip, and jaw (ULx, LLx, Jx). Also shown is the correlation coefficient obtained for the multiple trials.

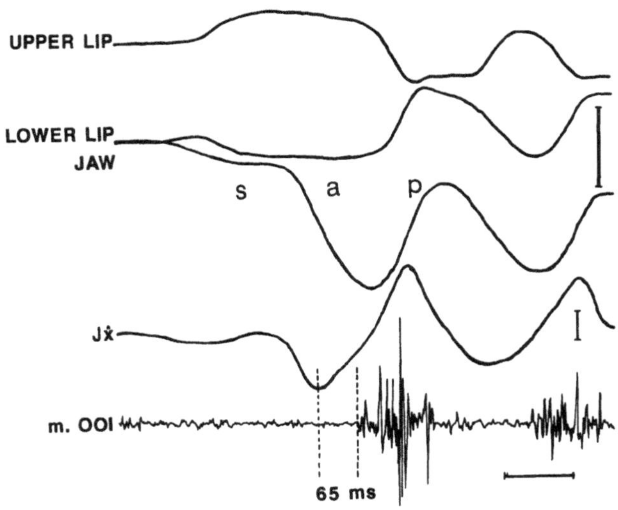

Figure 5. Illustration of the time course of jaw opening velocity (Jx) and the relationship between peak opening velocity and the onset of OOI activity for the first closing movement. Calibration is 100 ms.

It appears that there is approximately 65 msec between the peak jaw opening velocity and the onset of the labial EMG (this does not take into account the actual burst duration which is on the order of 100 msec). Previous studies have shown that compensatory responses to perturbations occur at latencies between 25 - 75 msec (Abbs & Gracco, 1984; Gracco & Abbs, 1982; Kelso et al., 1984), making 65 msec sufficient time to parameterize the articulators. It appears that the time is available for sensory information from the preceding speech movement to be used in the programming of the following speech movement. Experiments are currently under way to address the hypothesis that sensory signals arising from the stretching of jaw closing muscles are critical in the programming of orofacial closing movements.

In the preceding discussion, it has been suggested that speech movements are constructed, prior to execution, through the interaction of two processes, each relying on different amounts of stored and incoming sensory information. The motor program may be considered the more hard-wired process, relying on both synaptic connections and stored internal activation patterns for the appropriate muscles. The programming process, in contrast, is the more dynamic process relying heavily on sensory information to adjust the timing and magnitude of the motor program patterns underlying movements. This distinction between the program and the programming process is currently a heuristic one; however, it is worth considering in that it is a recognition that motor behavior relies on the anatomical connections that must exist as well as the internal (CNS) and external (sensory receptors) interactions necessary to activate and adjust these connections in a functionally task-specific manner.

SPEECH MOTOR EXECUTION

Motor execution, the final stage of the motor control process, can perhaps be considered an extension of the programming process. Motor execution is the actual implementation of the programmed motor plan consisting of the EMG output and any motor adjustments which occur during the initial phases of the resulting movement. Speech motor adjustments have been observed up to approximately 40 msec following EMG onset associated with bilabial closure (Gracco & Abbs, 1985). After this time, the system gain drops to almost nothing indicating a phasing out of sensory influences on the programmed speech motor output. It is interesting to note that the movement acceleration peaks at about this same time suggesting that only the very early sensory input from the actual movement may affect the final execution process. It is possible, however, that the sensory input generated during the movement may be used to modify the antagonist muscle (for closure, depressor labii inferior) to adjust the terminal movement characteristics. Overall, it appears that the early stages of speech motor programming may be sufficiently precise to require only minimal adjustments of the synergistic actions. While the characteristics of speech motor execution are limited, it appears that these adjustments apparently travel by way of short latency neural pathways in which the metrics of the transfer function between afferent input and motor output have been preset (cf. Gracco & Abbs, in press, a, for further elaboration). Furthermore, sensorimotor characteristics during speech motor execution possibly suggest different neural centers mediating these responses than those underlying speech motor programming (Gracco & Abbs, 1985). While somewhat speculative, the suggestion that speech production reflects a time-dependent modulation of multiple cortical and subcortical areas is consistent with numerous behaving animal investigations (Brinkman & Porter, 1979; Crutcher & DeLong, 1984; DeLong, Crutcher & Georgopoulos, 1981; Evarts & Tanji, 1976; Godschalk, Lemon, Nijs & Kuypers, 1981; Halsband & Passingham, 1982; Horak & Anderson, 1984a, 1984b; Lemon & van der Burg, 1979; Thach, 1975, 1978; Wise & Tanji, 1981). Collectively, such studies have demonstrated a dynamic and differential involvement of cerebellar, basal ganglia, supplementary motor area, premotor area, and sensorimotor cortical regions during different phases of the motor implementation process.

Another sensorimotor mechanism which appears to have significant influence on speech motor execution is the gating or modulation of sensory input during the initial phases of movement. That is, the reduced gain evidenced by the limited compensatory capability of the perioral system immediately preceding EMG onset (Gracco & Abbs, 1985) appears to reflect a modulation or reduction in the influence of sensory information immediately prior to and during the actual movement. It has been shown that the sensory transmission via most ascending pathways is reduced prior to movement onset (Coulter, 1974; Dubner & Sessle, 1971; Ghez & Pisa, 1972; Kuypers & Tuerk, 1964). This modulation results in a reduction in the amount of sensory information reaching thalamic and cortical centers

(Chapin & Woodward, 1982a, 1982b; Starr & Cohen, 1985). Such modulation has been shown to originate, in part, from projections of sensorimotor cortical neurons onto brainstem or spinal nuclei resulting in primary afferent depolarization. Such modulation would minimize (not eliminate) the influence of sensory input generated during the later phases of the movement. It is interesting that at the time when sensory influences on motor output would be greatest, much of the effect is minimized by the sensory gating. One possible explanation is that given the finely-tuned predictive capability of the nervous system, only minor adjustments need to be accomplished as the actual movement unfolds. Additionally, the sensory gating of afferent influences may be used to diminish or eliminate the interaction of reflexes with the voluntary motor commands. Whatever the explanation, it appears that speech motor execution involves multiple sensorimotor adjustments to coordinate the multiple degrees of movement freedom and achieve the multiarticulate movement goal.

SUMMARY

The preceding chapter has attempted to speculate on the nervous system control of speech with explicit consideration of sensory information and the underlying sensorimotor processes. Shown in Figure 6 is a schematic representation of the hypothesized levels of the speech motor control process. The movement plan involves the establishment of the movement goal incorporating the necessary acoustic consequences of the combined articulator actions.

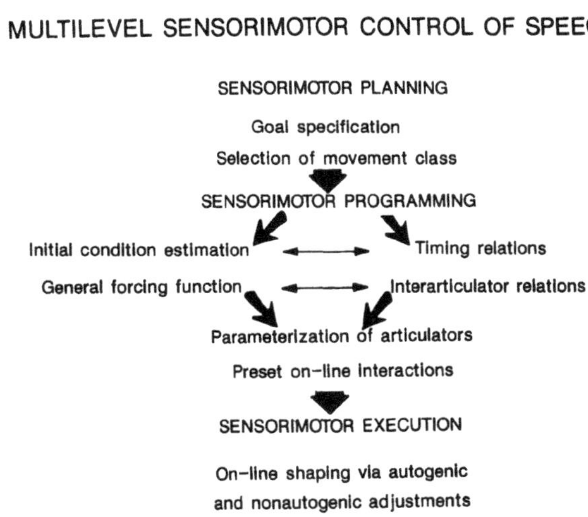

Figure 6. Schematic representation of the multilevel sensorimotor control processes hypothesized to underlie speech production.

As a way to generalize this conceptualization of speech movement planning to different speech sounds, it is suggested that within the planning process there is a general specification of a movement class. That is, the speech movement plan would involve specification of a general action (closing the acoustic tube) and the selection of the appropriate muscles. This general movement action could apply to all closing movements whether they involve the lips, jaw, or tongue and need only be adjusted for different preceding vowels. The acoustic-encoded movement goal of bilabial, lingual alveolar, and lingual velar stops would be to produce a terminal vowel formant trajectory appropriate to the specific vowel and ultimately close the acoustic tube through the combined articulator actions.

During the programming process, the first consideration is articulator timing. In the present representation, the temporal specification of movement timing is included within the programming process; however, it could easily be considered part of the movement plan and may reflect a separate nervous system process. One important aspect of the timing specification is that the underlying mechanism takes into account the different biomechanical characteristics of the lips, jaw, tongue, etc. to produce the orderly and consistent invariant timing patterns observed within (Gracco & Abbs, in press, b) and across (Tuller, Kelso & Harris, 1982) speech movements.

Within the invariant temporal framework, the relevant articulators are parameterized based on incoming sensory information. The parameterization involves the estimation of initial conditions (e.g., magnitude of oral opening) via predictive mechanisms, resulting in the establishment of general forcing functions and the resultant scaling of the individual articulator actions. The final stage in the motor control process is the actual implementation of the motor plan based on the previously programmed articulator adjustments, executed through flexible sensorimotor mechanisms.

The conceptualization of the speech motor control process presented above reflects a number of considerations that are crucial in developing a complete understanding of normal and disordered speech motor behavior. First, sensory information is an integral part of movement control and coordination and is potentially available throughout the movement planning/execution process. It appears that ongoing sensory information can influence both the spatial and temporal adjustments within and across articulatory subsystems. This suggests that observations of a single system (e.g., larynx, tongue, etc.) or a single variable may not provide a clear picture of the complex sensorimotor adjustments underlying speech production. Second, it is important that we consider the underlying neurophysiological substrate in any hypothetical process. The constructs of planning, programming, coordinative structures, synergies, etc. are only simplifying analogies to help understand the actions of the central nervous system. Attempts must continue to uncover the detailed characteristics of these constructs as well as to synthesize human behavioral studies with relevant nonhuman research which can deal directly with the potential functions of certain neural centers. While not elaborated in the present chapter, the potential neural processes underlying the planning, programming, and execution of speech and movement in general have been presented elsewhere (cf. Abbs, 1986; Brooks, 1979; Gracco & Abbs, in press, b). Finally, the hierarchical control process provides a structured task level of analysis that may be helpful in characterizing normal speech motor behavior and, subsequently, understanding speech movement disorders.

ACKNOWLEDGEMENTS

The author would like to express gratitude to Deborah Hoffman for her excellent editorial assistance and patience with this manuscript. This research was supported by NIH grants NS-20668-03, NS-13274, and HD-03352.

REFERENCES

Abbs, J.H. (1986). Invariance and variability in speech production: A distinction between linguistic intent and its neuromotor implementation. In J.S. Perkell & D.H. Klatt (Eds.), *Invariance and variability in speech processes.* Hillsdale, New Jersey: Lawrence Erlbaum Associates, Inc. 202-219.

Abbs, J.H. & Cole, K.J. (1982). Consideration of bulbar and suprabulbar afferent influences upon speech motor coordination and programming. In S. Grillner, B. Lindblom, J. Lubker & A. Persson (Eds.), *Speech motor control.* Oxford: Pergamon Press. 159-186.

Abbs, J.H. & Gracco, V.L. (1984). Control of complex motor gestures: Orofacial muscle responses to load perturbations of lip during speech. *Journal of Neurophysiology, 51,* 705-723.

Abbs, J.H., Gracco, V.L. & Cole, K.J. (1984). Control of multimovement coordination: Sensorimotor mechanisms in speech motor programming. *Journal of Motor Behavior, 16,* 195-231.

Atkeson, C.G. & Hollerbach, J.M. (1985) Kinematic features of unrestrained vertical arm movements. *The Journal of Neuroscience, 5* (9), 2318-2330.

Bernstein, N. (1967). *The Co-ordination and Regulation of Movements.* New York: Pergamon Press.

Bizzi, E., Kalil, R. & Tagliasco, V. (1971). Eye-head coordination in monkeys: Evidence for centrally patterned organization. *Science, 173,* 452-454.

Borden, G.J. (1979). An interpretation of research on feedback interruption in speech. *Brain and Language, 7,* 307-319.

Bossom, J. (1974). Movement without proprioception. *Brain Research, 71,* 285-296.

Brinkman, C. & Porter, R. (1979). Supplementary motor area in the monkey: Activity of neurons during performance of a learned motor task. *Journal of Neurophysiology, 42,* 681-709.

Brooks, V.B. (1979). Motor programs revisited. In R.E. Talbott & D.R. Humphrey (Eds.), *Posture and movement.* New York: Raven Press. 13-49.

Carpenter, M.B., Nakano, K., Kim, R. (1976). Nigrothalamic projections in the monkey demonstrated by autoradiographic techniques. *Journal of Comparative Neurology, 165,* 401-416.

Chapin, J.K. & Woodward, D.J. (1982a). Somatic sensory transmission to the cortex during movement: Gating of single cells to touch. *Experimental Neurology, 78,* 654-684.

Chapin, J.K. & Woodward, D.J. (1982b). Somatic sensory transmission to the cortex during movement: Phasic modulation over the locomotor step cycle. *Experimental Neurology, 78,* 670-684.

Cody, F.W.J., Harrison, L.M. & Taylor, A. (1975). Analysis of the activity of muscle spindles of the jaw-closing muscles during normal movements in the cat. *Journal of Physiology (London), 253,* 565-582.

Cole, K.J. & Abbs, J.H. (1986). Coordination of three-joint digit movements for rapid, finger-thumb grasp. *Journal of Neurophysiology, 55* (6), 1407-1423.

Cole, K.J., Gracco, V.L. & Abbs, J.H. (1984). Autogenic and nonautogenic sensorimotor actions in the control of multiarticulate hand movements. *Experimental Brain Research, 56,* 582-585.

Coulter, J.D. (1974). Effects of stimulation of sensorimotor cortex on primate spinothalamic neurons. *Brain Research, 65,* 351-356.

Crutcher, M.D. & DeLong, M.R. (1984a). Single cell studies of the primate putamen. I. Functional organization. *Experimental Brain Research, 53,* 233-243.

Deecke, L., Becker, W., Grozinger, B., Schied, P. & Kornhuber, H.H. (1973). Human brain potentials preceding voluntary limb movements. *Electroencephalography and Clinical Neurophysiology. Supplement (Amsterdam), 33,* 67-94.

DeLong, M.R., Crutcher, M.D. & Georgopoulos, A.P. (1981). Relations between movement and single cell discharge in the substantia nigra of the behaving monkey. *Journal of Neuroscience, 3,* 1599-1606.

DeLong, M.R. & Georgopoulos, A.P. (1981). Motor functions of the basal ganglia. In V.B. Brooks (Ed.), *Handbook of physiology: Section 1. The nervous system: Vol. 2. Motor control, Part 2.* Bethesda, Maryland: American Physiological Society. 1017-1061.

Dubner, R. & Sessle, B.J. (1971). Presynaptic excitability changes of primary afferent and corticofugal fibers projecting to trigeminal brain stem nuclei. *Experimental Neurology, 30,* 223-238.

Evarts, E.G. & Tanji, J. (1976). Reflex and intended responses in motor cortex pyramidal tract neurons of monkey. *Journal of Neurophysiology, 39,* 1069-1080.

Fentress, J.C. (1979). Development of grooming in mice with amputated forelimbs. *Science, 179,* 704-705.

Folkins, J.W. & Abbs, J.H. (1975). Lip and jaw motor control during speech: Responses to resistive loading of the jaw. *Journal of Speech and Hearing Research, 18,* 207-220.

Folkins, J.W. & Zimmermann, G. (1982). Lip and jaw interaction during speech: Responses to perturbation of lower-lip movement prior to bilabial closure. *Journal of the Acoustical Society of America, 71,* 1225-1233.

Ghez, C. & Pisa, M. (1972). Inhibition of afferent transmission in cuneate nucleus during voluntary movement in the cat. *Brain Research, 40,* 145-151.

Godschalk, M., Lemon, R.N., Nijs, H.G.T. & Kuypers, H.G.J.M. (1981). Behavior of neurons in monkey peri-arcuate and precentral cortex before and during visually guided arm and hand movements. *Experimental Brain Research, 44,* 113-116.

Goodwin, G.M. & Luschei, E.S. (1975). Discharge of spindle afferents from jaw-closing muscles during chewing in alert monkeys. *Journal of Neurophysiology, 38,* 560-571.

Gracco, V.L. (1984). *Time varying sensorimotor processes of the perioral system during speech.* Unpublished doctoral dissertation, University of Wisconsin-Madison.

Gracco, V.L. & Abbs, J.H. (1982). Temporal response characteristics of the perioral system to load perturbations. *Society for Neuroscience Abstracts, 8,* 282.

Gracco, V.L. & Abbs, J.H. (1985). Dynamic control of the perioral system during speech: Kinematic analyses of autogenic and nonautogenic sensorimotor processes. *Journal of Neurophysiology, 54* (2), 418-432.

Gracco, V.L. & Abbs, J.H. (in press, a). Programming and execution processes of speech movement control: Potential neural correlates. In E. Keller & M. Gopnik (Eds.), *Motor and sensory processes in language.* Hillsdale, New Jersey: Lawrence Erlbaum Associates, Inc.

Gracco, V.L. & Abbs, J.H. (in press, b). Variant and invariant characteristics of speech movements. *Experimental Brain Research.*

Grillner, S. (1981). Control of locomotion in bipeds, tetrapods, and fish. In V.B. Brooks (Ed.), *Handbook of physiology: Section 1. The nervous system: Vol. 2. Motor control, Part 1.* Bethesda, Maryland: American Physiological Society. 1179-1236.

Grillner, S. & Wallen, P. (1985). Central pattern generators for locomotion, with special reference to vertebrates. *Annual Review of Neurosciences, 8,* 233-261.

Halata, Z. & Munger, B.L. (1983). The sensory innervation of primate facial skin. II. Vermilion border and mucosa of lip. *Brain Research Reviews, 5,* 81-107.

Halsband, U. & Passingham, R. (1982). The role of premotor and parietal cortex in the direction of action. *Brain Research, 240,* 368-372.

Horak, F.B. & Anderson, M.E. (1984a). Influence of globus pallidus on arm movements in monkeys. I. Effects of kainic acid-induced lesions. *Journal of Neurophysiology, 52,* 290-304.

Horak, F.B. & Anderson, M.E. (1984b). Influence of globus pallidus on arm movements in monkeys. II. Effects of stimulation. *Journal of Neurophysiology, 52,* 305-322.

Hughes, O.M. & Abbs, J.H. (1976). Labial-mandibular coordination in the production of speech: Implications for the operation of motor equivalence. *Phonetica, 33,* 199-221.

Ito, M. (1982). *The Cerebellum and Neural Control.* New York: Raven Press.

Kaas, J.H., Nelson, R.J., Sur, M., Dykes, R.W. & Merzenich, M.M. (1984). The somatotopic organization of the

vertroposterior thalamus of the squirrel monkey, saimiri sciureus. *Journal of Comparative Neurology, 226,* 111-140.
Kelso, J.A.S., Tuller, B., Bateson, E.V. & Fowler, C.A. (1984). Functionally specific articulatory cooperation following jaw perturbations during speech: Evidence for coordinative structures. *Journal of Experimental Psychology: Human Perception and Performance, 10,* 812-832.
Kuypers, H.G.J.M. & Tuerk, J.D. (1964). The distribution of the cortical fibres within the nucleus cuneatus and gracilus in the cat. *Journal of Anatomy, 98,* 143-162.
Larson, C.R., Smith, A. & Luschei, E.S. (1981). Discharge characteristics and stretch sensitivity of jaw muscle afferents in the monkey during controlled isometric bites. *Journal of Neurophysiology, 46* (1), 130-142.
Leinonen, L. & Nyman, G. (1979). II. Functional properties of cells in anterolateral part of area 7 associative face area of awake monkeys. *Experimental Brain Research, 34,* 321-333.
Lemon, R.N. & Van der Burg, J. (1979). Short-latency peripheral inputs to thalamic neurones projecting to the motor cortex in the monkey. *Experimental Brain Research, 36,* 445-462.
MacNeilage, P.F. (1970). Motor control of serial ordering of speech. *Psychological Review, 77,* 182-196.
Marsden, C.D., Merton, P.A. & Morton, H.B. (1981). Human postural responses. *Brain, 104,* 513-534.
McKenna, T.M., Whitsel, B.L. & Dreyer, D.A. (1982). Anterior parietal cortical topographic organization in macaque monkey: A reevaluation. *Journal of Neurophysiology, 48* (2), 289-317.
Merzenich, M.M. & Kaas, J.H. (1980). Principles of organization of sensory-perceptual systems in mammals. In J.M. Sprague & A.N. Epstein (Eds.), *Progress in Psychobiology and Physiological Psychology, Vol. 9.* New York: Academic Press. 1-42.
Morasso, P., Bizzi, E. & Dichgans, J. (1973). Adjustments of saccade characteristics during head movements. *Experimental Brain Research, 16,* 492-500.
Mountcastle, V.B. (1979). An organizing principle for cerebral function: The unit module and the distributed system. In F.O. Schmitt & F.G. Worden (Eds.), *The neurosciences. Fourth study program.* Cambridge, Massachusetts: MIT Press. 21-42.
Muakkassa, K.F. & Strick, P.L. (1979). Frontal lobe inputs to primate motor cortex: Evidence for four somatotopically organized 'premotor' areas. *Brain Research, 177,* 176-182.
Munger, B.L. & Halata, Z. (1983). The sensory innervation of primate facial skin. I. Hairy skin. *Brain Research Reviews, 5,* 45-80.
Munhall, K.G., Ostry, D.J. & Parush, A. (1985). Characteristics of velocity profiles in speech movements. *Journal of Experimental Psychology: Human Perception and* Performance, 11, 457-474.
Nashner, L.M. & Cordo, P.J. (1981). Automatic postural responses. *Experimental Brain Research, 36,* 463-476.
Nashner, L.M., Woollacott, M. & Tuma, G. (1979). Organization of rapid responses to postural and locomotor-like perturbation of standing man. *Experimental Brain Research, 36,* 463-476.
Ostry, D.J. & Cooke, J.D. (in press). Kinematic patterns in speech and limb movements. In E. Keller & M. Gopnik (Eds.),

Motor and sensory language processes. Hillsdale, New Jersey: Lawrence Erlbaum Associates, Inc.

Perkell, J.S. & Klatt, D.H. (Eds.) (1986). *The Proceedings of the Symposium on Invariance and Variability of Speech Processes.* Hillsdale, New Jersey: Lawrence Erlbaum Associates, Inc.

Phillips, C.G. & Porter, R. (1977). *Corticospinal neurons. Their role in movement.* London: Academic Press.

Polit, A. & Bizzi, E. (1979). Characteristics of motor programs underlying arm movements in monkeys. *Journal of Neurophysiology, 42,* 183-194.

Rizzolatti, G., Scandolara, C., Gentilucci, M. & Camarda, R. (1981). Response properties and behavioral modulation of 'mouth' neurons of the postarcuate cortex (area 6) in macaque monkeys. *Brain Research, 255,* 421-424.

Rothwell, J.C., Traub, M.M., Day, B., Obeso, J., Thomas, P. & Marsden, C.D. (1982). Manual motor performance in a deafferented man. *Brain, 105,* 515-542.

Saltzman, E.L. (1979). Levels of sensorimotor representation. *Journal of Mathematical Psychology, 20,* 91-163.

Saltzman, E.L. (in press). Task dynamic coordination of the speech articulators: A preliminary model. *Experimental Brain Research (Supplement).*

Sanes, J. & Evarts, E.V. (1983). Regulatory role of proprioceptive input in motor control of phasic or maintained voluntary contractions in man. In J. Desmedt (Ed.), *Advances in neurology, Vol. 39: Motor control mechanisms in health and disease.* New York: Raven Press. 47-59.

Schmidt, R.F. (Ed.) (1978). *Fundamentals of sensory physiology.* New York: Springer.

Schell, G.R. & Strick, P.L. (1984). The origin of thalamic inputs to the arcuate premotor and supplementary motor areas. *Journal of Neuroscience, 4,* 539-560.

Sessle, B.J. & Wiesendanger, M. (1982). Structural and functional definition of the motor cortex in the monkey (Macaca Fascicularis). *Journal of Physiology, 323,* 245-265.

Shaiman, S., Abbs, J.H. & Gracco, V.L. (1985). Sensorimotor contributions to oral-laryngeal coordination for speech. *Society for Neuroscience Abstracts, 15,* 76.

Smith, R.L. (1975). Axonal projections and connections of the principal sensory trigeminal nucleus in the monkey. *Journal of Comparative Neurology, 163,* 347-376.

Stanton, G.B. (1980). Topographical organization of ascending cerebellar projections from the dentate and interposed nuclei in macaca mulatta: An anterograde degeneration study. *Journal of Comparative Neurology, 190,* 699-731.

Starr, A. & Cohen, L.G. (1985). 'Gating' of somatosensory evoked potentials begins before the onset of voluntary movement in man. *Brain Research, 348,* 183-186.

Stein, R.B. (1982). What muscle variable(s) does the nervous system control in limb movements? *Behavioral and Brain Sciences, 5,* 535-577.

Sur, M., Nelson, R.J. & Kaas, J.H. (1982). Representations of the body surface in cortical areas 3b and 1 of Squirrel monkeys: Comparisons with other primates. *Journal of Comparative Neurology, 211,* 177-192.

Taub, E. & Berman, A.J. (1968). Movement and learning in the absence of sensory feedback. In S.J. Freedman (Ed.), *The neurophysiology of spatially oriented behavior.* Homewood, Illinois: Dorsey Press.

Thach, W.T. (1975). Timing of activity in cerebellar dentate nucleus and cerebral motor cortex during prompt volitional movement. *Brain Research, 88,* 233-241.

Thach, W.T. (1978). Correlation of neural discharge with pattern and force of muscular activity, joint position, and direction of intended next movement in motor cortex and cerebellum. *Journal of Neurophysiology, 41,* 654-676.

Traub, M.M., Rothwell, J.C. & Marsden, C.D. (1980). A grab reflex in the human hand. *Brain, 103,* 869-884.

Tuller, B., Kelso, J.A.S. & Harris, K.S. (1982). Interarticulator phasing as an index of temporal regularity in speech. *Journal of Experimental Psychology: Human Perception and* Performance, 8 (3), 460-472.

Wise, S.P. & Tanji, J. (1981). Supplementary and precentral motor cortex: Contrast in responsiveness to peripheral input in the hindlimb area of the unanesthetized monkey. *Journal of Comparative Neurology, 195,* 433-451.

Young, J.Z. (1950). *Doubt and Certainty in Science: A Biologist's Reflections on the Brain.* London: Oxford University Press.

Part Three

Methods in Research in Speech Motor Production

Overview

A section on methods usually bridges the gap between theory and data. In this book it is inserted between Part Two on models and Part Four and Five on stuttering research. However, the reason that a section with methodological considerations is included in a book like this, is not just to meet conventions but to expose a few interesting developments in methodology that recently have taken place.

One of these has already been signalled by Starkweather in Chapter 1, i.e. the remarkable increase of research in which simultaneous measurements are used. Overviewing a number of studies that are described in Part Four conveys the impression that studies that rely on single response measures often provide too restricted information about the underlying processes in stuttering. Given the complexity of the relationships between the muscle systems involved in articulation, voicing and respiration, and our presently limited understanding of these relationships, it seems impossible to use single measurements at one level to infer properties of activities at another level. The most convincing arguments for the recording of multiple physiological responses however, come from theories that place coordination and timing as the core issues in motor research. The earlier chapters on speech motor models all used data from multiple recordings to make their point and Chapter 5, by Borden and Watson, presents this argument in more detail.

The second development that necessitates a section on methods is that major improvements in a technical domain have been achieved. Research on the coordination of respiratory functions, laryngeal adjustments and articulatory activities, although increasing in number, still has been limited for technical reasons. The last ten years, however, a good deal of progress has been made in the development of improved techniques for analysing, storing and displaying these signals, and although studies on the coordination of speech mechanisms still are to be categorized under the more time consuming ones and still ask for rather expensive equipment, they are becoming more feasible. Moreover, the recording of certain activities, like subglottal airpressure, articulatory behavior and electroencephalographic signals, has seen interesting developments, which are described in this section.

This Part (three) in fact consists of two subparts. The first subpart is made up of three broad review chapters. These are followed by three chapters that each go into one specific measurement technique or method of analysis.

The first review, Chapter 5 by Borden and Watson, discusses at length the advantages and disadvantages of various measurement techniques. Respiratory kinematics are covered by a discussion of inductance plethysmography, laryngeal function is dealt with by describing a fiberoptic transillumination system and by giving the pro's and con's of electroglottography. Finally, some supralaryngeal measurement techniques are mentioned and an (infrared LED) optical tracking system is considered in detail. The best approach of stuttering is to combine these techniques into simultaneous measurements, and Borden and Watson advocate this approach by providing beautifull examples of the precise relative timing and coordination of the various simultaneously recorded components of speech. At the end of their chapter the authors address the issue of the number of subjects. The strategy they suggest is to perform noninvasive measurements on a large number of subjects and to follow this up by more invasive, multidimensional physiological measurements on only a few subjects.

The issue of the minimum number of subjects that have to be used in stuttering research has been the subject of much debate both before and during the conference from which this book arose. The history of stuttering research has seen too many studies on only a very few subjects. This practice often stretches inductive inferences beyond reasonable limits. Using a very small research group is already a hazardous affair if normal subjects are used, but if stutterers are the research subjects the risk may be too great. The variations among stutterers is so great that studies relying on a small number of cases simply can not encompass the diversity actually observed across stutterers. A diversity which possibly will be higher if multiple recordings are made.

Borden and Watson's plea for multiple measurements should not be used as an argument to do away with all acoustic analyses. As Boves, in Chapter 6, points out, acoustic analyses often function as a means for inferring information on physiological processes that underly the production of speech. The detour via the acoustic signal is often necessitated by the fact that the direct physiological measurements are impossible to carry out, or can only be performed at the cost of some discomfort done to the subjects. Also, practically all physiological measurements more or less interfere with uninhibited spontaneous speech production.

As discussed by Boves in Chapter 6, attempts to infer physiological processes from the results of acoustic analyses have to rely heavily on models of speech production. The power and limitations of these production models form the larger part of the chapter. First, acoustic models and Linear Prediction analysis are discussed. Most of the chapter is devoted to models that try to specify the relation between acoustic measurement and physiological recordings. Electroglottographic recording of laryngeal function is dealt with first, but most room is made for modelling glottal airflow. Simultaneous recordings of glottal airflow at two points below and two points above the larynx, as well as the registration of glottographic activity by impedance measurements and by photoelectric recording, demonstrate that these signals do not always provide compatible information. The chapter ends with a short discussion of a better alternative for production models: analysis models. The possibility to devise these models, as well as their possible application in large scale studies is reflected upon.

The third review, Chapter 7 by Conture, views the simultaneous recording of physiological and acoustic measures from quite a different point of view: from the standpoint of the subject, in particular from a child-subject. Most speech motor research in stuttering concerns stuttering in adults. This is most unfortunate since children are closer to the onset of stuttering than adults and may present a less complicated picture of the disorder. The objective study of speech production in young children, however, is much more difficult than in adults and always requires a compromise between employing ideal methods for the collection of data and the realities of what youngsters can and will do in an experimental setting. Conture's chapter addresses the numerous problems encountered when studying young stutterers' speech production. He stresses the necessity of providing basic demographic data and an objective definition of stuttering as a methodological precaution with young children. He then describes instrumentation and data analysis suited for research with children and discusses a number of procedural concerns and often encountered errors. Conture is careful to make the point that children are not "little adults" and he therefore directs considerable attention toward practical considerations in research with surface electromyography, inductive respiratory plethysmography, electroglottography and acoustic microphones.

The second part of the following section on methods is formed by chapters introducing new special techniques in stuttering research.

The first of these techniques is the X-ray microbeam pellet-tracking, described by Alfonso, Watson and Baer in Chapter 8, which seems to be a powerful method for gathering kinematic data on supralaryngeal articulatory behavior. The advantage of this technique over traditional cineradiography is that the allowable exposure times can be increased to about 45 to 60 minutes, while subject safety is also increased by virtue of lower radiation levels. In the experiment described in this chapter, the X-ray microbeam technique is used with a simultaneous recording of respiratory inductance plethysmography and electroglottography. The stutterer in this experiment showed a greater variability in the positioning of the tongue and jaw than the normal speaker, and the experiment nicely illustrates the importance of monitoring tongue position in relation to the behavior of other structures.

In Chapter 9, Pool, Freeman and Finitzo describe a technique to display electroencephalographic (EEG) data, called the brain electrical activity mapping technique. This method was recently developed for examining both EEG and evoked potential data. In the chapter by Pool et al. the technology of this method is described and findings with this technique from preliminary studies with two 'vocal motor control disorders' - spasmodic dysphonia (13 subjects) and stuttering (3 subjects) - are presented. A large number of abnormalities in the fronto-temporal regions of both groups of patients was found.

The last chapter in this section (Chapter 10, by Nudelman, Herbrich, Hoyt and Rosenfield) stands more or less apart since it does not describe a new recording technique but offers an unusual approach to the investigation of stuttering. Stuttering, according to the authors, can be conceived as an instability in the speech motor control system. The causes of such an instability may be understood by applying an engineering approach: Systems Analysis. Although the speech motor control system is a complex nonlinear system it can be adequately described, according to the authors by the linear term of the dynamic relationship between its input and output. The evidence for this was found in an experiment in which four stutterers and three nonstutterers had to follow, by humming, a tone which frequency was modulated by ramps, sine and square waves. The stutterers followed the changes in the tone with longer delays than the nonstutterers which, in the language of Systems Analysis means that their phase shift was closer to the point where, theoretically, the system becomes unstable.

Chapter 5

Methodological Aspects of Simultaneous Measurements: Limitations and Possibilities

Gloria J. Borden and Ben C. Watson

Research on the physiology of stuttering has reached the point where single factor studies, such as investigations of only one dimension of speech production (i.e., air pressure alone or muscle activity alone) are inadequate to fully characterize the disorder. Instead, advances in our understanding of stuttering necessitate a multidimensional research approach. This multidimensional research is designed either to record from different systems of the speech mechanism simultaneously or to record at different physiological levels within a single system (Baer & Alfonso, 1984). Research that cuts across systems might concurrently sample respiratory, laryngeal, and supralaryngeal activity. Research that cuts across several levels within a single system might simultaneously record muscle activity, structure movements, and aerodynamic changes in parallel with the acoustic signal. The problem with this new emphasis on simultaneous measurement is that it puts added strain on the subjects, on the instrumentation needed to collect and process the data, and on the experimenter to discover the method of analysis that will best uncover the dynamic principles underlying fluent and disfluent speech. However, the possibilities may be worth our taking on the problems.

Our view that normal speech is a dynamic coordinated event requires that we pursue multidimensional measurements that can reveal the interactions that define the coordination. Studies of relative timing and relative activity across components of the speech system may prove to be the keys needed to unlock the dynamic principles underlying well coordinated speech as well as the changes in coordination that are inherent in stuttering.

Before discussing the particulars of physiological research methods that can be applied to the investigation of stuttering, we wish to make a general observation on such laboratory experiments. Specifically, the laboratory may serve as a fluency enhancing setting to the detriment of the research. We are often interested in recording both stuttered and fluent speech samples from stutterers, but have found that the act of bringing stutterers into the laboratory and attaching several instruments to them for a recording session seems to effect a temporary abatement of stuttering. To counteract the lab effect, we have had to modify the materials to be spoken and to place temporal and social pressures upon the speaker. By presenting difficult speech tasks to stutterers and asking them to respond as quickly as possible without sacrificing accuracy we endeavor to capture the habituated patterns of discoordinated speech during stuttered utterances and the habituated patterns of relatively coordinated speech during fluent utterances.

In this chapter we will touch upon some studies in which simultaneous measurements were made. Our goal is not to report on the results of these studies, but rather to discuss the instrumentation involved, highlighting the possibilities and limitations of each instrument. Beginning with some instrumentation used to record respiration, we shall then select some methods used to record laryngeal function, and finally discuss some measures of vocal tract dynamics. Instruments that are non-invasive will be emphasized and we will not discuss the more invasive techniques of electromyography and cineradiography.

RESPIRATORY FUNCTION

With respect to investigations of respiratory kinematics in stutterers, it is of interest to examine the coordination of thoracic and abdominal movements as well as the coordination between movements of the respiratory and laryngeal systems. Coordination of thoracic and abdominal movements can be evaluated in terms of patterns of cavity wall displacements executed to generate changes in lung volume before and during speech production. For example, displacement patterns may reveal transient interruptions and/or oscillations during expansion or compression gestures. Coordination between movements of the respiratory and laryngeal systems can be evaluated in terms of the temporal relationship between changes in lung volume and vocal fold position. For example, onset of respiratory expansion gestures before the onset of vocal fold opening could indicate discoordination between the respiratory and laryngeal systems during attempted inspiration.

Respiratory kinematics have been investigated by monitoring changes in three dimensions of the thoracic and abdominal cavities. First, Hixon, Goldman, and Mead (1973) monitor changes in the anteroposterior diameter of the cavities by use of a magnetometer system. Second, Baken (1977) monitors changes in the anterior hemi-circumference of the cavities by use of a Whitney strain-gauge system. Finally, Cohn, Watson, Weisshaut, Stott, and Sackner (1977) monitor changes in the total circumference of the cavities by use of an inductance coil system. Although differing with respect to their specific principles of operation and to the dimension of cavity wall displacement monitored, all three systems provide information regarding the coordination between the thoracic and abdominal cavities as well as changes in absolute or relative lung volume.

At our laboratory, we use the inductance plethysmograph, or Respitrace, system developed by Cohn et al. (1977) to monitor circumferential changes of the thoracic and abdominal cavities. Consequently, this discussion of the advantages and disadvantages of monitoring respiratory kinematics is drawn from our experience with this system. However, with few exceptions, these disadvantages and advantages are common to all three monitoring systems.

Table 1. Inductance plethysmography

Disadvantages:	
1.	Requires Calibration.
2.	Cross-talk between Thoracic & Abdominal Bands.
3.	Movement Artifacts.
Advantages:	
1.	No Interference with Speech Production.
2.	Absolute or Relative Measures of Lung Volume.
3.	Unique Contributions of Thoracic & Abdominal Cavities to Lung Volume Change.
4.	Functional and Temporal Measures.

Table 1 summarizes disadvantages and advantages of the Respitrace system. We consider first the disadvantages. First, valid measures of absolute or relative lung volume exchange require the recording of calibration maneuvers before and after the experimental session. These maneuvers are recorded while the subject is sitting, standing, and supine. For measures of relative volume change, calibration maneuvers involve repeated exchange of a known, constant volume of air. For measures of absolute volume change, calibration maneuvers involve air exchange through a respirometer with simultaneous recording of respirometer output. In either case, calibration procedures prolong the experimental session and may contribute to subject fatigue. The second disadvantage of inductance plethysmography is that the reliability of displacement signals is dependent upon accurate placement of the elastic bands carrying the inductance coils. That is, bands must be positioned so that the abdominal band does not respond to movements of the thoracic cavity or vice versa. Failure to achieve sufficient separation will invalidate displacement data and prevent determination of changes in relative or absolute lung volume. The third disadvantage reflects the sensitivity of the inductance coils to movement artifacts. For example, changes in body posture can move the bands and result in the imposition of a D.C. shift on output signals. As another example, muscular connections between the sternum and humerus can introduce signal artifacts due to arm movements. Both sources of artifact are minimized with a magnetometer system.

We now consider the advantage of inductance plethysmography as a measure of respiratory kinematics. First, unlike conventional respirometry, this procedure monitors changes in lung volume without interfering with speech production. Second, calibrated and summed thoracic and abdominal signals can provide information regarding the absolute or relative magnitude of total lung volume change. Third, analysis of separate calibrated thoracic and abdominal displacement signals can reveal the unique contributions of changes in these cavity volumes to changes in total lung volume. These data can be informative in evaluating the coordination between the two components of the respiratory system. Finally, temporal analysis of these signals can reveal the onset latency and duration of cavity wall displacements.

To summarize, three systems were described that monitor respiratory kinematics during speech production. All three systems have several advantages. First, they do not interfere with speech production. Second, all three systems can provide information regarding functional and temporal parameters of thoracic and abdominal wall displacements. Finally, calibrated signals can reveal absolute or relative changes in lung volume. These data can be informative in evaluating the coordination and timing of respiratory events in stutterers. A marked disadvantage of the Respitrace and Whitney strain-gauge systems is that arm movements and gross changes in posture can introduce artifacts in the output signals.

LARYNGEAL FUNCTION

Two questions are of interest in the study of laryngeal kinematics in stutterers. As mentioned above, the first question addresses the coordination of vocal fold abduction and adduction with dynamic changes in the respiratory system. The second question addresses the coordination of vocal fold vibration within the laryngeal system as revealed in details of the vibratory cycle. Two different technologies are appropriate to investigate these questions. Vocal fold abduction and adduction are best monitored using transillumination procedures with simultaneous filming or videotaping of the vocal folds. Details of the vibratory cycle are best monitored using electroglottographic procedures. We will begin with a discussion of advantages and disadvantages of transillumination procedures, followed by an example of simultaneous respiratory and laryngeal kinematic data that demonstrate the coordination between these systems. Next, we will discuss advantages and disadvantages of electroglottographic procedures.

Transillumination procedures monitor the relative degree of vocal fold separation in terms of the amount of light, emitted from a supraglottal source, detected by a photoreceptor located superficially on the anterior midline of the neck at the level of the cricoid cartilage. In our laboratory, the supraglottal light source is provided by a fiberoptic endoscope inserted pernasally and positioned approximately 5 cm above the glottis. The distal end of the fiberscope is coupled to a video camera to permit filming of the vocal

Table 2. Transillumination

Disadvantages:	
1.	Invasive Procedure.
2.	Tolerance of Fiberscope Insertion.
3.	Expensive Equipment.
Advantages:	
1.	No Calibration Procedures Required.
2.	Observation of Prephonatory Vocal Fold Movements.

folds. Videotape records are reviewed to determine whether posterior movements of the epiglottis may have introduced artifacts in the transillumination signal. Output voltages produced at the photo transducer correspond to the amount of light passing through the glottis. For example, completely abducted folds produce a maximum voltage output while completely adducted folds produce a baseline voltage output.

Table 2 summarizes disadvantages and advantages of a fiberoptic/transillumination system for monitoring vocal fold movements. The first disadvantage of this system is that insertion of the fiberoptic bundle is an invasive procedure and the participation of a physician is required in most research settings. The second disadvantage is that not all subjects are able, or willing, to tolerate insertion of the fiberoptic bundle. The third disadvantage is that the expense of a fiberoptic system, including a cold light source, high resolution video camera/recording unit, and video monitor, may be prohibitive for small laboratories and clinics.

We now consider the advantages of a fiberoptic/transillumination system. First, no calibration procedures are required, or indeed possible, for transillumination. However, to avoid signal clipping we ask subjects to execute sequences of deep inspiration followed by phonation for production of a voiced vowel. This maneuver insures that maximum and minimum voltage output levels are within the range of our recording system. Second, the transillumination signal provides a direct measure of relative vocal fold position before phonation onset. Since stutterers are frequently characterized as having difficulty initiating phonation, this information is of particular interest in investigations of the disorder.

We now consider the possibilities and limitations of using data obtained from simultaneous recordings of Respitrace and transillumination signals to understand the coordination within the respiratory system as well as between the respiratory and laryngeal systems in stutterers. Figure 1 displays respiratory and laryngeal kinematic data and the acoustic signal recorded from a mild stutterer during a reaction time task. The top record shows the reaction signal. Onset of this signal serves as a warning cue and offset serves as a phonate cue. That is, subjects are instructed to prepare to produce the isolated vowel /i/ following presentation of the warning cue and to initiate this vowel as rapidly as possible following presentation of the phonate cue. The second record shows the transillumination signal. Upward displacement of this signal corresponds to vocal fold opening and downward displacement corresponds to vocal fold closing. The third and fourth records show calibrated Respitrace signals for the thoracic and abdominal cavities, respectively. We should note here that the magnification factor for display of the abdominal signal was twice that used for the thoracic signal. That is, the vertical scale is not the same for these records. The fifth record shows the sum of the thoracic and abdominal signals and reflects the total change in relative lung volume. Upward displacement of all Respitrace signals corresponds to increasing lung volume and downward displacement corresponds to decreasing lung volume. Finally, the sixth record shows the speech signal.

Both quantitative and qualitative characteristics of respiratory and laryngeal coordination can be extracted from these data. Quantitative characteristics include the onset latency and relative timing of respiratory and laryngeal movements as well as changes in relative lung volume. Qualitative characteristics include patterns of movement trajectories. We first consider coordination of movements of the thoracic and abdominal systems.

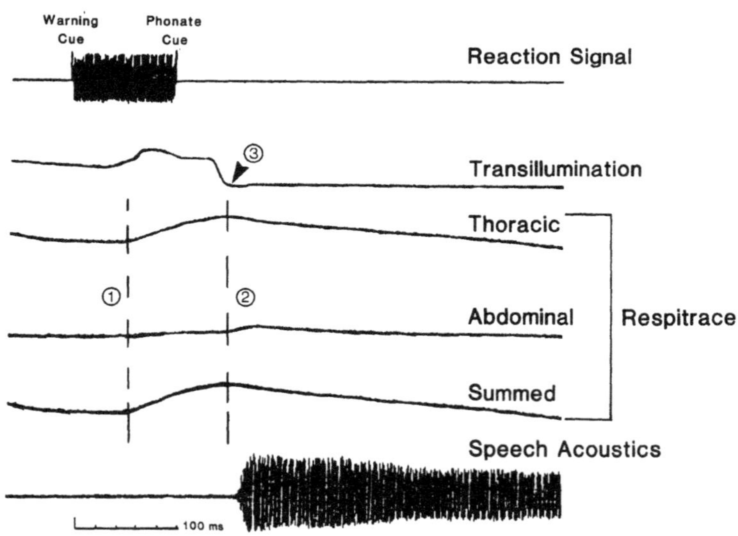

Figure 1. Simultaneous Transillumination, Respitrace, and acoustic data channels.

Relative contributions of thoracic and abdominal wall displacements to changes in relative lung volume are indicated by the three Respitrace signals. Since these signals were not calibrated against a respirometer, measures of volume change are relative. For this response, the three calibrated Respitrace signals clearly show that the thoracic cavity makes a greater contribution to changes in lung volume than does the abdominal cavity. For example, between the dashed lines labelled 1 and 2, total lung volume increases 333 cc, thoracic cavity volume increases 307 cc, and abdominal cavity volume increases 26 cc. Qualitative analysis of the Respitrace signals reveals oppositional displacements of the thoracic and abdominal walls, at the line labelled 2, before phonation onset. That is, the thoracic cavity demonstrates a compression gesture while the abdominal cavity demonstrates an expansion gesture. However, the summed signal shows that the net effect of these displacements is the respiratory compression necessary for phonation onset.

Coordination between the respiratory and laryngeal systems is revealed by analysis of the relative timing relationship of movement trajectories for these two systems. Note that the arrow labelled 3 represents the moment of vocal fold closure before phonation onset while the line labelled 2 represents onset of respiratory compression. The relative timing relationship between these two points reveals that, for this response, respiratory compression began nearly simultaneously with the moment of vocal fold closure. That is, the relative timing of respiratory and laryngeal movements was appropriate for the soft mode of vocal attack produced by this subject.

There are certain limitations, however, to the interpretation of these data. First, the transillumination signal does not indicate absolute degree of vocal fold opening. Consequently, information provided by this procedure is useful only in identifying the onsets and offsets of vocal fold abductory and adductory gestures and of vocal fold closure. Second, unless calibrated with a respirometer, Respitrace signals do not indicate percent of vital capacity from which lung volume either increases or decreases. That is, failure to observe prephonatory inspiratory gestures cannot be reliably attributed to either a breakdown in respiratory coordination or the existence of an already adequate lung volume for phonation onset. Finally, kinematic data are a relatively superficial means of observing the speech production system in that they only indirectly reflect underlying neuromotor activities. For example, abnormally long delays in movement onsets could be a consequence of several different neuromotor events. This information is clearly not available in the kinematic data.

The second instrument for recording vocal fold activity that we will consider is the electroglottograph or EGG. Developed by Fourcin (1974) who prefers the term laryngograph, this instrument records the transmission of a high frequency low intensity signal passing between electrodes placed on each side of the thyroid prominence. To the degree that the vocal folds increase contact with one another, impedance to the transmission of the signal decreases, while glottal opening increases impedance. Thus, vocal fold movements may be inferred from changes in signal amplitude. In addition to the Fourcin model, there are at least two other electroglottographs available: the F-J Electronics ApS and Synchrovoice Inc. models.

The disadvantages and advantages of an electroglottographic system are summarized in Table 3. The first disadvantage is that it offers no information on vocal fold position, such as the configuration of the glottal opening, the vertical or horizontal phase differences in vocal fold tissue displacement during vibration, or the degree of abduction or adduction of the folds. Second, it is impos-

Table 3. Electroglottography

Disadvantages:
1. No Information Regarding Vocal Fold Position.
2. Cannot be Calibrated.
3. Movement Artifacts.
4. Subject Variability.

Advantages:
1. Noninvasive and Inexpensive.
2. Slow (articulatory) and Fast (vibratory) Signals.
3. Compute FO Changes.
4. Reliable Measure of Maximum Vocal Fold Contact.
5. Analysis of Details of the Vibratory Cycle.

sible to calibrate the system. Like the transillumination system, one can determine the dynamic range for each subject by having the speaker alternate productions of [s] with [ʌ] to identify impedance maxima and minima. During speech, however, impedance changes may result from sources other than adductory-abductory gestures, so that one cannot infer a linear relationship between the impedance signal and vocal fold position. In addition, a mucousal bridge across the vocal folds can alter the magnitude of the signal. It has been found by directly viewing the vocal folds simultaneously with EGG recordings that less confidence can be placed in the relationship between the EGG signal and glottal opening than in that for glottal closure (Baer, Löfqvist & McGarr, 1983; Childers, Naik, Larar, Krishnamurthy & Moore, 1983). The third disadvantage, related to the second, is the presence of movement artifacts. Tongue movements for /i/, as an example, will elevate the hyoid bone and the larynx resulting in a change in the electroglottographic signal. Laryngeal lowering will have a similar effect. A fourth disadvantage is that EGG recordings are not equally good across subjects. Recordings from people with more fat around the neck or those with a less acutely angled thyroid cartilage may be inferior to recordings made from thin people with relatively sharply angled thyroid cartilages. In our experience, women are generally poorer candidates for electroglottographic recordings than are men.

The advantages of electroglottography, however, make it an attractive instrument for research and clinical uses. First, the fact that it is noninvasive and relatively inexpensive makes it appropriate for clinical and research applications with children as well as adults. Second, one can use electroglottography to measure relative timing of slow articulatory positioning of the vocal folds (from the low frequency impedance shifts of the unfiltered signal) as well as of the fast vibratory cycles (from the high pass filtered signal). In addition, changes in fundamental frequency can be derived from the higher frequency voicing cycles for analysis of intonation contours. Third, the EGG gives a highly reliable signal of maximum vocal fold contact which can be used in studies of relative timing of voice onset with other speech events. Finally, the fast vibratory changes in impedance that indicate voicing can be analyzed at closer range for detailed analysis of the glottal cycle such as computation of the closed or open quotients.

In Figure 2, the EGG waveform is displayed so that upward deflection indicates increased vocal fold contact (decreased impedance). The EGG waveform is normally characterized by a steep rise (a) in 'vocal fold contact' followed by slower 'opening,' (b) and 'open phase' (c). Amplitude of the first EGG pulses, in this instance, build rapidly (d), compared with the acoustic waveform (e) for the onset of voicing in the word 'four'.

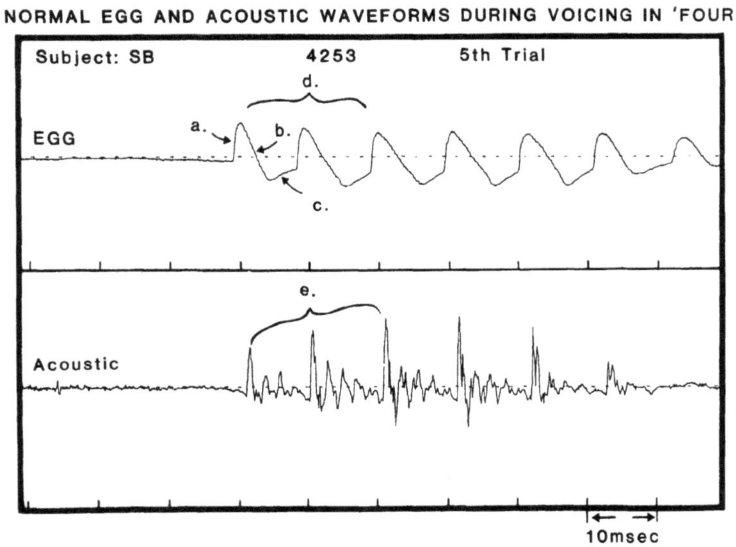

Figure 2. Simultaneous electroglottographic and acoustic recordings of the initial pulses for voicing of the segment /r/.

SUPRALARYNGEAL FUNCTION

In tracking activity of the supralaryngeal articulators during speech, researchers have turned to cineradiography, ultrasound, palatography, and optical tracking systems. The problem of radiation exposure has shifted attention away from standard cineradiographic techniques to the relatively safe X-ray microbeam system (Alfonso, Watson & Baer, 1985). Ultrasound holds promise for obtaining tongue configuration images but is not generally available in laboratories and clinics. Dynamic electropalatography currently depends upon fashioning a speaker- specific palatal prothesis with imbedded transducers to record changing patterns of tongue-palate contact during speech. In the future, when palatal forms are developed that can be easily adapted to different palate shapes and sizes, the dynamic electropalatograph should prove to be useful clinically as well as in research.

Table 4. Infrared LED tracking

Disadvantages:
1. Observation of Only Visible Articulators.
2. Nonlinearity at Edge of Scanning Field.
3. Expensive.
4. Movement Artifacts.

Advantages:
1. Noninvasive.
2. Unique Contributions of Horizontal & Vertical Displacements to Articulator Trajectories.
3. Contributions of Lip & Jaw Displacements to Bilabial Articulations.
4. Temporal and Kinematic Measures.

A noninvasive instrument for recording articulatory speech movements that we will discuss further here is an optical tracking system. Visible flesh points such as the lip and jaw can be tracked by attaching small infrared light emitting diodes (LEDs) to the points of interest. Modulated light from these LEDs is viewed by a camera equipped with photosensors and transmitted to circuits that decompose LED movements into their vertical and horizontal displacement components.

Table 4 summarizes disadvantages and advantages of an infrared LED tracking system. The obvious disadvantage of such a system is that it limits investigation of supralaryngeal activity to visible articulators. A second disadvantage is that although it can be calibrated by moving a diode a known distance in the field of view, the relationship between distance moved and voltage produced is linear only in the center of the field. Distortions occur toward the periphery of the field of view. The third disadvantage is that the instrument is relatively expensive. Fourth, and finally, it is susceptible to artifacts produced by non-speech movements. Consequently, the subject's head should be stabilized or held relatively motionless.

Besides being noninvasive, the possibilities afforded by optical tracking include the advantage of direct recording of movement information (rather than indirect measures of impedance changes). That is, one can record the individual contributions of vertical and horizontal movement components to the summed trajectory observed. In addition, the individual contributions of lip and jaw movements to labial speech sound production can be determined. Finally, this system facilitates measurement of the relative timing and displacement of lip/jaw movements as well as derived properties of these movements (i.e., velocity and acceleration).

An example of simultaneous recordings of respiratory, laryngeal, and supralaryngeal activity during speech is presented in Figure 3. The top trace represents the summed displacement waveform of the lip/jaw system as recorded by the optical tracking system. In this instance, the vertical and horizontal displacements were summed to yield the actual trajectory of the lip/jaw system. The second trace shows the slow impedance changes recorded from the electroglottograph and illustrates the maximum and minimum

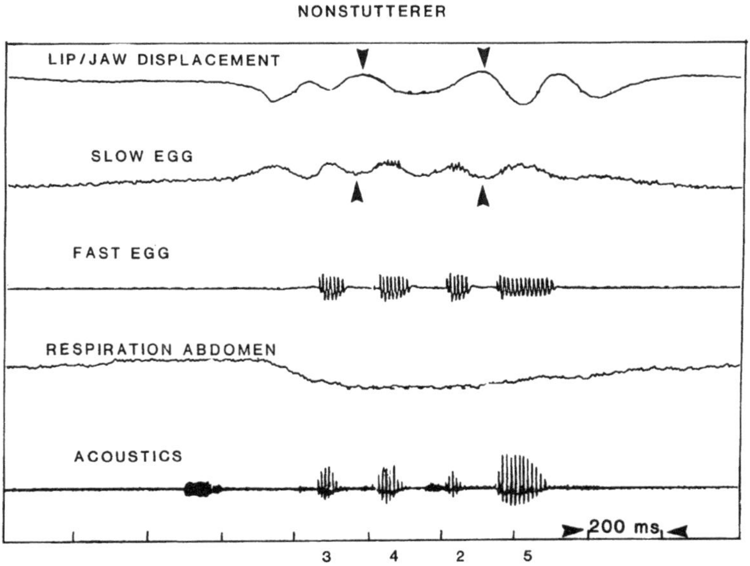

Figure 3. Simultaneous recordings from the supralaryngeal, laryngeal, and respiratory systems during a counting task.

vocal fold contact. The polarity is set here so that upward deflection reflects the maximum contact that accompanies vocal fold adduction for voicing and downward deflection corresponds to vocal fold opening. The rapid impedance changes corresponding to the vibratory cycles of voicing can be seen in the filtered EGG trace labelled 'Fast EGG'. The fourth trace represents abdominal expansion and compression recorded by use of a semihemispheric Whitney gauge. Finally, the acoustic signal appears at the bottom of the figure. These movement trajectories are well suited to analyses of the relative timing of displacement onset latencies and durations, of peak displacements, and of phase relationships among articulators. For example, the arrows in this figure show that during utterance of the numbers 'four' and 'five' for which lip/jaw movement is relatively pronounced, the onset of lip/jaw lowering corresponds with peak vocal fold opening as inferred from the slow electroglottographic signal. It can also be seen that voice onset is more clearly defined in the fast EGG signal than in the acoustic signal.

In addition to measuring relative timing from movement records, it is informative to compute the first- and second-order derivatives of these trajectories for analysis of movement velocity and acceleration characteristics. Movement trajectories and associated velocity traces for the lip/jaw LED and the slow EGG signals during production of the utterance '3425' are displayed in Figure 4. These traces illustrate the relationship between supralaryngeal and laryngeal displacements in the top two traces and the relationship between their respective velocities in the bottom two traces. The middle trace displays the fast EGG signal representing periods of voicing during the utterance. Peak velocity for lip/jaw closing

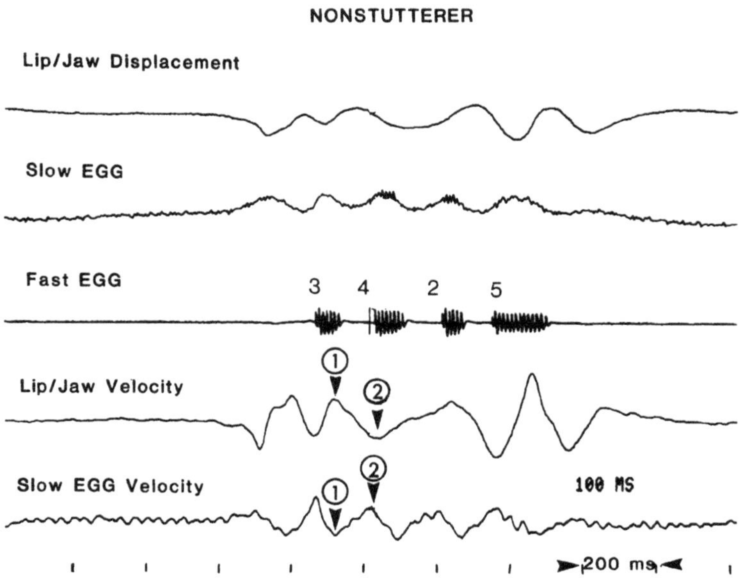

Figure 4. Displacement and velocity records from the supralaryngeal and laryngeal systems.

gestures and for vocal fold adduction are represented by positive maxima while peak velocity for lip/jaw opening gestures and for vocal fold abduction are represented by negative maxima. In this example, before production of the initial /f/ in the word 'four', peak velocity for lip/jaw closing corresponds to peak velocity for vocal fold abduction. This is indicated by the arrows labelled 1. The opposite relationship is observed for production of the following vocalic segment. That is, peak velocity of lip/jaw opening corresponds to peak velocity for vocal fold adduction. This is indicated by the arrows labelled 2.

In conclusion, we would like to suggest a general methodological principle. Specifically, application of instrumentation for the investigation of stuttering may be guided by a two-pronged approach. First, clinical and research settings equipped with relatively noninvasive instrumentation would be appropriate sites in which experiments with large numbers of subjects could be undertaken. Second, laboratories equipped with more invasive instrumentation might of necessity run experiments on smaller numbers of subjects but gather a large amount of multidimensional physiological data from each subject. For example, a relatively large study of laryngeal-supralaryngeal coordination in stutterers using noninvasive recordings of acoustics and articulator movement indices might reveal a significant difference between the fluent utterances of mild and severe stutterers. A parallel study could be then conducted on a smaller sample of severe and mild stutterers, along with nonstutterers as controls, using more invasive techniques such as electromyography along with the recording of kinematic and acoustic data. Taken together, studies of large numbers of subjects using fewer and less invasive measures and studies of smaller numbers of subjects using multiple and more invasive measures should yield maximum information with minimum strain on subjects, experimenters, and equipment.

REFERENCES

Alfonso, P.J., Watson, B.C. & Baer, T. (1985). *Measuring stutterers dynamical vocal tract characteristics with x-ray microbeam pellet tracking.* Paper presented at the International Conference on Speech Motor Dynamics in Stuttering, Nijmegen, The Netherlands.

Baer, T. & Alfonso, P.J. (1984). On simultaneous neuromuscular, movement, and acoustic measures of speech articulation. In R.G. Daniloff (Ed.), *Articulation Assessment and Treatment Issues.* San Diego: College Hill Press. 195-214.

Baer, T. Löfqvist, A. & McGarr, N.S. (1983). Laryngeal vibrations: A comparison between high-speed filming and glottographic techniques. *Journal of the Acoustical Society of America, 73,* 1304-1308.

Baken, R.J. (1977). Estimation of lung volume change from torso hemicircumferences. *Journal of Speech and Hearing Research, 20,* 808-812.

Childers, D.G., Naik, J.M., Larar, J.N., Krishnamurthy, A.K. & Moore, G.P. (1983). Electroglottography, speech, and ultra-high speed cinematography. In I.R. Titze & R.C. Scherer (Eds.), *Vocal Fold Physiology: Biomechanics, Acoustics, and Phonatory Control.* Denver: The Denver Center for the Performing Arts. 202-220.

Cohn, D.E., Watson, H., Weisshaut, R., Stott, F. & Sackner, M.A. (1977). *A transducer for noninvasive monitoring of respiration.* Paper presented at the 2nd International Symposium on Ambulatory Monitoring, Harrow, Middlesex, U.K.

Fourcin, A. (1974). Laryngograph examination of vocal fold vibration. In B. Wyke (Ed.), *Ventilatory and phonatory control mechanism.* London: Oxford University Press. 315-333.

Hixon, T., Goldman, M. & Mead, J. (1973). Kinematics of the chest wall during speech production: Volume displacements of the rib cage, abdomen, and lung. *Journal of Speech and Hearing Research, 16,* 78-115.

Chapter 6

Acoustical Analysis and Physiological Parameters

Louis Boves

INTRODUCTION

Speech is produced by complex movements of the articulators, which are known to be extremely complex structures themselves. Moreover, many articulators are not accessible for direct observation of their behavior. Some articulators can be monitored in principle, but only by means of invasive recording techniques like photoglottography or hooked wire EMG electrodes, or by other possibly dangerous techniques like cineradiography. For these reasons speech researchers have got used to the necessity to try to infer behaviors of articulators that cannot be observed directly from indirect measurements. Such inferences are crucially dependent on the way in which we think that underlying behaviors and measurable phenomena are related. An other, somewhat more formal way to formulate this dependence is to say that the inferences are based on models.

Models come in many different forms, ranging from differential equations via electronic circuits to diagrams on paper in which boxes labelled with words are connected by arrows. In fact, every construct that allows us to make statements like 'if this structure here moves in this way, than we will there observe a signal with those properties' is a model. Yet, of course, not all models are created equal; some have greater predictive power than other. Also, some models describe a small number of events very precisely, whereas other models cover a wider range of events in more approximate terms.

It is of considerable importance to distinguish two essentially different ways of using models. Perhaps one might even say that we must distinguish two fundamentally different classes of models. The models discussed in the previous paragraph can be characterized as production models. They predict the output of a given system when we know its inner workings. In speech production research, however, the situation is usually quite different: we know the output of the system and we would like to infer the inner workings. Browsing the speech research literature one might get the impression that the familiar models, that are usually production models, can also be used for the inference task. Yet, on second thought it becomes evident that predicting the output of a model we know and control completely may be very different from inferring the parameters of a model from its output. The single most instructive example is the phenomenon known as 'compensatory articulation': it is not too difficult to produce completely acceptable tokens of an open vowel with the teeth firmly set. This fact, which indeed is common knowledge in speech science, was formalized by Atal, Chang, Mathews & Tukey (1978), who showed thad very different configurations of their vocal tract model produced sounds with indistinguishable spectra. Consequently, there is no unique way for inferring the vocal tract shape from the spectrum of the speech signal. Unfortunately, the one-to-many mapping of acoustic signal to vocal tract configurations is not an accident; after all, it occurs in the field of acoustic theory of speech production, one of the best researched domains of speech science. It is not too difficult to see why such a many-to-one relation should be considered the rule rather than an exception. Realistic models, even very simple ones, of a process as complex as speech production must necessarily contain a considerable number of parameters. If the number of model parameters exceeds the number of independent characteristics (e.g. formants and bandwidths) that can be established in the output signal, a unique solution of the model parameters is clearly impossible. Even if the model has less parameters than the signal, a unique way for inferring model parameters from the characteristics of the output signal is not guaranteed, for very often the relation between model parameters and output signal characteristics is highly non-linear.

The message that this somewhat abstract introduction attempts to convey is that we need a second class of models in speech science, viz. analysis models. The second class of models, that would allow us to automatically infer information about speech processes that cannot be observed directly, just begins to be developed. Yet, for research in speech pathology this kind of models may become of crucial importance, probably even more so than in speech technology research, where detailed knowledge about the behavior of the articulators is not too often called for.

The single most prominent difference between production models and analysis models is that the former are deterministic, i.e. their output can be predicted with a high degree of precision, whereas the latter are non-deterministic, i.e. the result of their application may be ambiguous in the sense that they do not allow a final choice to be made between a number of alternatives (that do not need to be equally likely).

In the remaining part of this chapter we will first look into the prospects and limitations of acoustic models of speech production. Next we will discuss models that allow to combine acoustic measurements and physiological recordings. We wil conclude with a short discussion of the possibility to devise analysis models for multidimensional registrations of speech production processes and their application in large scale studies.

ACOUSTIC MODELS OF SPEECH PRODUCTION

The acoustic speech signal is attractive to work with for a number of reasons. Perhaps the most compelling, though not frequently mentioned advantage of the acoustic signal is that it is the only speech signal that can be recorded in an unobtrusive manner. Therefore, the acoustic speech wave is virtually the only signal that may be recorded in a situation that approaches normal speech communication. If a stuttering therapy is to fulfill its claim that will render clients' speech normal in every day communication the acoustic speech signal is the only viable means of assessment. Another reason why the acoustic wave is attractive to work with is that researchers from many disciplines, including speech coding and speech transmission engineering, take an interest in this signal. As a result numerous powerful techniques for processing the speech wave have become available, and although most of those techniques have been developed with technical applications in mind they are widely employed in speech pathology research. Implicitly or explicitly all analysis techniques rely in one way or another on some model of the acoustics of speech production.

It is instructive to summarize the steps that must be taken to go from a schematic picture of the speech production mechanism to the prevalent model of acoustic speech production underlying frequently used analysis techniques like Linear Prediction (LP) and its derivatives (Fant, 1960; Flanagan, 1972; Markel & Gray, 1976). Figure 1.a shows such a schematic drawing; part b of that figure shows that, from an acoustic point of view, the speech production mechanism can be viewed as consisting of a number of tubes and valves. The form and area of the tubes depend on the distance from the lips. As far as the cross sectional area is concerned this dependence can be seen from Figure 1.b, but no attempt has been made to visualize changes in the form of the cross sections. This is in accord with the usual assumption that the tubes can be assumed to be cylindrical. The next step is the approximation of the continuously changing area by a series of (cylindrical) tubes of constant cross sectional area and equal length. The walls of the tubes are supposed to be so hard that they will in no way be affected by the sound pressure changes in the tubes. Such a tube model is equivalent to the electrical network shown in Figure 1.c, where each tube element is represented by a T-network. Here we have already lost much of the detail of the original schematic of the human speech production mechanism, but we still are far removed from our goal, the model underlying LP analysis. In calculating the acoustic behavior of the network in Figure 1.c the parallel connection of the

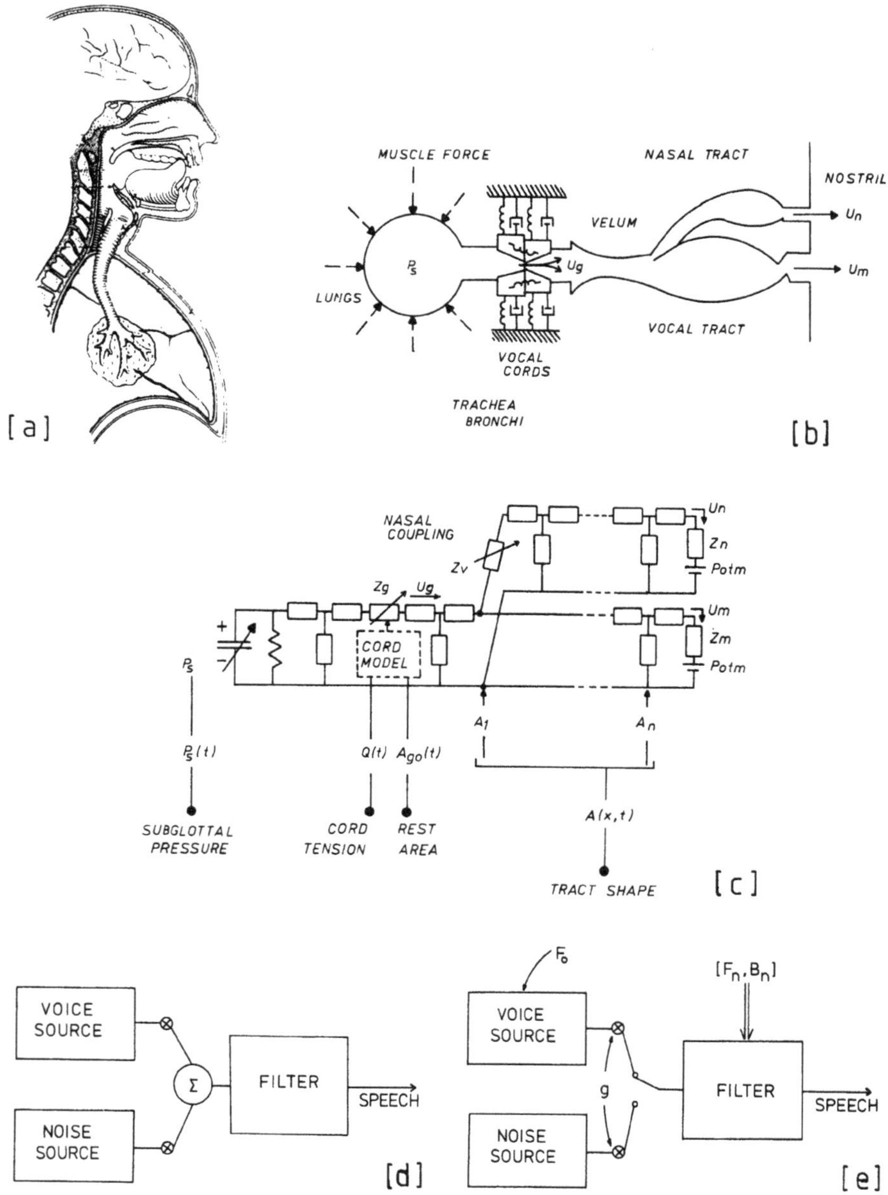

Figure 1. Construction of an acoustic model of speech production.
a: A schematic drawing of the anatomical structures involved in speech production.
b: The anatomy reduced to the acoustic essentials, viz. a complex system of tubes and valves.
c: An electrical analogon of the system of tubes and valves.
d: Further reduction of the electrical analogon to a linear system of sources and an all-pole system.
e: The model underlying Linear Prediction and most other speech analysis techniques.

nasal and oral tracts appears to complicate things considerably. Therefore, the nasal tract is eliminated, which does no harm for vowels nor for most consonants, but which prevents any physiological interpretation of the analysis results for nasal sounds. The next simplification is the removal of the subglottal system and the exchange of the vocal fold model by an ideal current source. If we assume that this current source can produce a periodic signal and a white noise in any combination of power levels, we arrive at the model in Figure 1.d, where the box labelled 'Filter' is a system that only contains resonances; this is what is meant with the term 'all pole'. In order to arrive at the usual Linear Prediction model we need one further simplification in the source section of the model. In LP analysis it is assumed that the source produces either white noise or a periodic series of unit impulses. The usual LP analysis model is shown in Figure 1.e. It will be obvious that the LP model is a so severely stripped representation of the real speech production mechanism that any attempt to interpret the results of an LP analysis in terms of vocal tract configurations necessarily runs the rise of being very far off. Note that we do not say that every such interpretation must necessarily lead to nonsense; it may be correct but chances are that it will not. The fact that Wakita (1973) shows that under certain (very restrictive) conditions LP analysis results can be related to a series of uniform cylindrical tubes, nor the fact that one popular representation of LP parameters is known under the name 'log area ratios' can do away with the danger of making misinterpretations. In realistic research conditions we have no means of ascertaining that all conditions for an articulatory interpretation of the LP parameters are fulfilled.

Linear Prediction analysis may be the most popular technique for processing speech these days, it is certainly not the only one (Rabiner & Schafer, 1978). However, most of the alternative techniques appear to be based on the same simplistic model in Figure 1.e. The detailed discussion of the limitations of that model is by no means meant to suggest that the customary signal processing techniques should not be used in speech pathology research in general or stuttering research in particular. The high quality of the output of vocoders based on this model for a large number of talkers irrefutably shows that the model is able to capture much of the perceptually significant characteristics of somebody's voice. The very notable degradation of the output quality for other voices, however, should make us aware of the fact that the model certainly does not account for all aspects of the speech signal that may be relevant. And even if the analysis retains most of the perceptually relevant information, this does by no means warrant an interpretation in articulatory terms. What this discussion should convey is that a thorough understanding of the restrictions of the model underlying an analysis technique is needed before an interpretation of the results is attempted.

Usually researchers in speech pathology favour the use of ready made instruments or software packages for acoustic signal processing. If those commodities are used for parameter tracking, for instance pitch (Fo) or formant tracking, one should realize that more often than not the model underlying the parameter extraction contains an important additional restriction besides those discussed

so far. After the foregoing discussion it should not come as a surprise that an analyser will have great difficulty in relating the parameters of the simplistic model to real live phenomena like the frequency with which the vocal folds vibrate or the natural frequencies of the vocal tract. The results of the first stage of the analysis may indeed be highly ambiguous. Because for all practical applications an unambiguous output is necessary, the device or subroutine must contain some strategy for choosing one (the most likely) alternative. The by far most frequently used decision criterion is that physical phenomena are supposed to change slowly and in a continuous way. Thus the alternatives resulting for a given part of the speech wave are compared with the ones in a number of preceding (and possibly also following) parts and a choice is made that guarantees maximal smoothness or continuity.
The continuity criterion certainly makes a great deal of sense. Yet it should not be considered as universally applicable, because in some cases it may imply an idealization.

An unusually clear example of the detrimental effect of the continuity criterion is the clinical application of voice pitch trackers developed for use in vocoders. Clinicians are often interested in the presence and seriousness of period-to-period fluctuations in the vibration of the vocal folds. There are essentially three different principles that can be used for tracking pitch in quasi periodic signals, viz. autocorrelation techniques, techniques that search the spectrum for harmonics, and peak detection in the time domain waveform. The techniques that operate in the frequency (spectral) and autocorrelation domains always entail the analysis of a signal segment comprising at least two complete pitch periods. Consequently, the result is an estimate of the pitch period that conforms to the average of the periods in the analysis window. If the raw output of such a pitch tracker is processed by a decision logic designed to remove outliers from the pitch track (because outliers violate the continuity criterion) the eventual output is of no use in a situation where one has to obtain information on period-to-period fluctuations. Clearly, for this type of application the most appropriate measurement technique is a time domain peak picking strategy that produces estimates of the duration of all individual periods. However, using such a technique in a situation where wild fluctuations of the pitch periods may occur, it is extremely difficult to distinguish actual irregularities in vocal fold vibration from measurement errors.

SIMULTANEOUS RECORDINGS OF PHYSIOLOGICAL AND ACOUSTIC SIGNALS

In the preceding discussion of the relation between vocal tract configurations and measurable properties of the acoustic speech signal it has been pointed out that a given set of acoustic properties can be produced by a number of quite different tract configurations. If the acoustic speech wave is the only source of information there is no way to disambiguate the one-to-many mapping. However, if we would have additional and independent information, it might well be possible to eliminate at least some of the alternatives. A simple example is the case where we can observe the speaker's face. If the sound under analysis is known to have been produced with a large lip opening, all tract configurations with small lip opening can immediately be discarded. Similarly, every independent indication that the simplifying assumptions underlying the customary speech production model do indeed apply will facilitate the articulatory interpretation of the outcomes of an anlysis of the speech wave.

Unfortunately, in actual practice the situation is not always as straightforward as in the previous example. Usually we can at best record more or less indirect indications of what we would like to know. Even the case of lip opnening is not trivial if we need absolute data that then must be calculated in some way from a picture. If we are to extract useful information from physiological recordings we need again models that allow us to understand and interpret the data. These models may be extremely simple, so simple perhaps that the term 'model' seems to be slightly overdone. Sometimes it seems to be sufficient to know and observe the limitations of the measurement procedure, as e.g. with measuring lip opening from pictures. Even in those cases, however, in a formal sense there is an underlying model.

Measurement of Laryngeal Function

Recent years have witnessed considerable interest in (quasi) non invasive techniques for measuring laryngeal function. By far the most popular non invasive instrument for recording laryngeal function is the electroglottograph (EGG). Developed in the early fifties by Fabre as a device that clearly reflected the opening and closing movements of the vocal folds, it was not until 1975 that Lecluse was able to establish the exact relation between the phase of the EGG signal and the actual movements of the folds (Lecluse, Brocaar & Verschuure, 1975; Childers & Krishnamurthy, 1985). Actually, Lecluse and his coworkers showed that the measurement model underlying the EGG represents the glottis as a variable resistor, the value of which is determined by the area over which the folds touch each other. Their model, in which the variable glottis resistor is only one element in an electrical analogon consisting of several (fixed) resistors and capacitors, can explain both the rapid pitch synchronous and the slow non pitch synchronous variations in the EGG. The EGG measurement model of Lecluse et al. can readily be 'translated' into natural language by saying that the EGG reflects the variation of the contact area between the vocal folds. Careful study of the model helps in interpreting and detailing that statement. A constant EGG does indeed indicate that the contact area does not change. However, it may not change either because the folds remain constantly adducted, or because they remain constantly abducted. To make things even worse, if the folds are constantly abducted they need not be motionless; on the contrary, they may be vibrating in a regular way, but as long as they do not touch their motion will not be visible in the EGG. Thus it appears that the EGG cannot be used to detect the absence or presence of vocal fold vibration proper; the only thing that one can

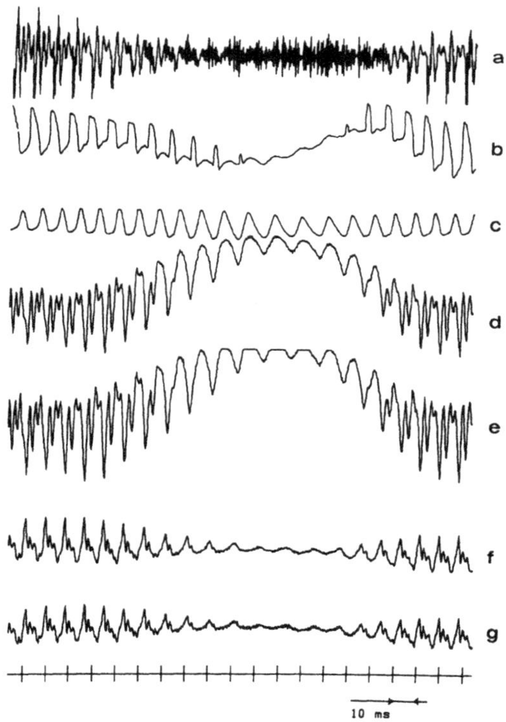

Figure 2. Simultaneous registrations of the acoustic speech wave (a) and a number of physiological signals, viz. the EGG (b), the PGG (c), subglottal pressure at 7.5 cm and 2.5 cm distance from the glottis (d) and (e) respectively, and mouth pressure at 2.5 cm and 7.5 cm from the glottis (f) and (g). Note the discrepancy between the acoustic signal and the EGG that do not show fricative voicing and the other signals that show period behavior throughout the complete utterance /aza/.

ascertain with the EGG is whether the folds vibrate in such a way that they do touch during part of a glottal period. Also, the vocal fold contact area can only be measured in relative terms. The EGG cannot provide absolute data on the area of contact, nor is it possible to determine from the EGG whether the glottis does or does not close completely.

Although the restrictions on the possible ways to interpret the EGG can be derived from the model underlying the measurement, they tend to be easily forgotten. However, they become readily apparent if the EGG recordings are combined with recordings of the Photoelectroglottogram (PGG), that records the area changes of the glottis by means of a measurement of the intensity of the light that shines through the glottis. Figure 2 shows recordings of (among others) the acoustic speech wave, the EGG and the PGG for a vowel-consonant-vowel transition. From that figure it can be seen that during the consonant the glottal area, as represented by the PGG, keeps varying in a regular way and with about the same frequency as in the surrounding vowels. Yet, the EGG and the

PGG, keeps varying in a regular way and with about the same frequency as in the surrounding vowels. Yet, the EGG and the acoustic speech wave do not show any periodic behavior during the consonant. The discrepancy between voicing information in the speech signal, the EGG and the PGG gives rise to a number of warnings. First of all it emphasizes the need for very precise definitions of all aspects of speech production, like in the present example 'voicing'. Secondly, it shows the need for separate definitions of each phenomenon on all relevant levels; also, there does not need to be a one-to-one relation between the definitions on several levels. Thirdly, the example shows that, although physiological recordings may be a useful aid in interpreting the acoustic speech signal, their use should not be stretched beyond the limits of the model underlying the physiological signal itself, even if it tends to corroborate what one thinks to observe in the speech wave.

Measurement of Glottal Air Flow

From the acoustic point of view the single most important phenomenon for describing phonation is the time varying transglottal airflow which forms the excitation source for the vocal tract filter. It is quite obvious that there must be some relation between the airflow through the glottis and the glottal area (Van den Berg, Zantema & Doornenbal, 1957; Flanagan, 1972). Thus it seems that the PGG should make for an excellent indicator of the voicing source. One should realize, however, that there is more to the transglottal flow than glottal area.

For stationary flow the relation between flow and area was determined empirically by Van den Berg et al. (1957) as

$$U_g = A_g \cdot \sqrt{2P_{tr}/k_\rho} \qquad (1)$$

where U_g is transglottal flow
A_g is glottal area
P_{tr} is transglottal pressure
k is the kinetic resistance factor
ρ is the mass density of air saturated with vapor

Flanagan (1958) convincingly argued that the Van den Berg equation can also be used for describing glottal flow in the non-stationary conditions that prevail during phonation, when the flow is periodically interrupted. He also showed that there is good reason to believe that the transglottal pressure is essentially constant over a complete glottal cycle. Therefore, there seemed to be everybreason to suppose that the glottal area and the glottal flow shouls be essentially congruent. This result would only support the assumption that the PGG might perhaps contain sufficient information for describing the voice source.
Direct measurement of the glottal air flow during phonation is impossible. Therefore, one has to rely on indirect measurement

techniques, among which inverse filtering of the air flow at the lips (Rothenberg & Zahorian, 1977) or the acoustic speech signal (Boves, 1984) are by far the most popular. Inverse filtering, however, is crucially dependent on the assumption that source and filter in the speech production model in Figure 1e are linearly separable; most implementations of the technique also assume that the filter is all-pole.

Although the early inverse filter experiments did not entail an explicit comparison of the glottal area as obtained from the PGG and the glottal air at the output of the inverse filter, there were reasons to cast some doubt upon the hypothesis that area and flow were congruent. Rothenberg & Zahorian (1977) were among the firsts to observe that the overall shapes of the area and flow waveforms tend to be significantly different. They showed that, whereas glottal area waveforms seem to be essentially symmetric, flow pulses tend to be skewed to the left, i.e., the closing phase of the flow pulses seems to be more abrupt than the opening phase. Rothenberg (1983) made a reasonable case for the assumption that the discongruence of area and flow waveforms is due to nonlinear interaction between the voice source and the vocal tract filter.
Now if the source-filter coupling is essentially nonlinear, one of the crucial assumptions underlying the inverse filtering technique breaks down. Therefore, other techniques for estimating glottal air flow would be most welcome. In our own laboratory we have made an attempt to develop such an alternative technique, that makes as few assumptions as possible with respect to the acoustic theory of speech production (Cranen & Boves, 1983; 1985).

Of the many techniques that have been developed for measuring flow only two can be implemented in such a way that they may be used for recording air flow in the direct neighbourhood of the glottis during phonation. Teager & Teager (1983) describe the use of hot-wire anemometry; although they seem to be able to measure flow in the vocal tract, hot-wire anemometry has a number of serious drawbacks. For one thing, hot-wire anemometers are extremely difficult to calibrate at flow levels as low as those prevailing near the glottis. Also, due to technical problems, hot-wire anemometers cannot be constructed in such a way that they can be inserted pernasally; thus their use seems to be limited to the measurement of air flow in the production of sustained vowels.

The technique employed in the work of Cranen and Boves (1985, 1987) is based on the principle that, under fairly general conditions, flow through a tube is proportional to the pressure difference between its entry and exit. The set up for making the measurements is shown in Figure 3. Pressure is recorded at two points in the trachea and at two points in the pharynx, using a Millar PC-784K Micro Tip catheter with four semiconductor strain gauge miniature pressure transducers mounted at equal distances of 5 cm. These transducers allow the recording of pressure variations in a frequency band extending well beyond 5 kHz. Along with the pressure signals EGG, PGG, and the acoustic speech wave were recorded simultaneously. EGG and PGG contain information that is useful for checking the validity of the flow estimates. The EGG was recorded using a slightly modified Laryngograph (Boves, 1984); the PGG was recorded by means of a Frokjaer-Jensen LG600 photo-

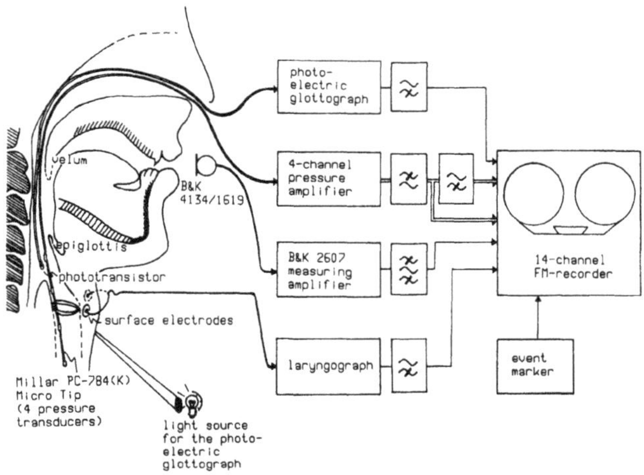

Figure 3. Schematic view of the situation during the recording of the signals displayed in Figure 2.

electric glottograph in connection with a photo-detector mounted at the distal end of a flexible plastic tube. The position of the photo-detector was not fixed. Note that this way of recording the amount of light passing the glottis has the positions of light source and sensor exchanged compared with the technique described by Borden and Watson (cf. Chapter 5). The principles underlying the measurement technique are, however, identical in both implementations.

The proportionality relation between pressure difference and flow is easy to prove for steady flow. During phonation the flow in the neighbourhood of the glottis is all but steady; the pressure in the trachea and pharynx varies also very rapidly, as can be seen from the registrations in Figure 2. If we are willing to make a number of assumptions, it can be shown that the proportionality relation remains valid in the case of pulsatile flow. The assumptions that must be made are (1) that the flow is uni-directional (i.e., there is no flow perpendicular to the axis of the tube), (2) that the flow is laminar (i.e., the particle velocity is constant at a constant distance from the axis of the tube), (3) that the air is incompressible (which it obviously is not, but which is still a viable asumption as long as the pressure variations are much smaller than atmospheric pressure, a requirement that is certainly fulfilled), and (4) that the temperature of the air (and consequently its viscosity) can be considered as constant. These assumptions may seem to be quite restrictive, but is must be realized that they are but a subset of the assumptions underlying the customary models of acoustic speech production.

Because neither flow nor pressure are constant in the pulsatile flow during phonation, the relation between pressure and flow must be expressed in the form of the (partial) differential equation (2),

$$\rho \frac{\partial u(x,t)}{\partial t} = - \frac{\partial p(x,t)}{\partial x} \qquad (2)$$

where u(x,t) is the particle velocity at time t and at distance x from the glottis and p(x,t) the pressure at the same point and moment. Equation (2) describes a relation between the time derivative of the particle velocity and pressure gradient. In order to otain the particle velocity proper (2) must be integrated with respect to time, giving equation (3).

$$u(x,t) = - \frac{1}{\rho} \cdot \int_{-\infty}^{t} \frac{\partial p(x,\tau)}{\partial x} \partial\tau \qquad (3)$$

As a last step, one must convert particle velocity into volume flow this is easily done by multiplying the particle velocity and cross-sectional area A(x,t):

$$U(x,t) = A(x,t).u(x,t) \qquad (4)$$

Writing particle velocity, pressure, flow, and cross-sectional area as functions of both the distance x to the glottis and the time t enables us to account for changes due to articulatory maneouvres that may displace the larynx relative to the pessure transducers or that may cause the pharynx to contract or dilate.
The pressure gradient $dp(x,t)_x dx$ cannot be measured directly. In our set up it is approximated by the pressure differential of (5).

$$\frac{\partial p}{\partial x} = \lim_{\Delta x \to 0} \frac{p(x + \Delta x/2) - p(x - \Delta x/2)}{\Delta x} \qquad (5)$$

The approximation of the pressure gradient given in (5) applies to the point halfway between the two pressure transducers in either cavity. From Figure 3 it can be inferred that this means that we have estimates of the pressure gradients (and therefore, hopefully, eventually estimates of flow) at two points which lie approximately 5 cm below (upstream) and above (downstream) the glottis. Thus it is clear that our technique measures flow close to the glottis, but not exactly at the glottis. The flow 5 cm upstream of the glottis does not need to be identical to the flow at the glottis, because (a small) part may (temporarily) get stuck in the cavity between the point of measurement and the glottis. In a similar vein, the flow in the glottis may have changed its shape somewhat when it finally reaches the position 5 cm downstream where the second measurement location is, because part of the flow may have been absorbed by the cavity between the glottis and the point of measurement. Obviously, we have to obtain some estimate of the flow that is taken up by the cavities between the points of measurement and the glottis.

In order to obtain such an estimate it is necessary to develop a model of the behavior of a section of a tube. For the sake of simplicity we assume the tube to be cylindrical. For a large number of reasons it is more convenient to discuss the behavior of the electrical analogon of such a tube section shown in Figure 4.

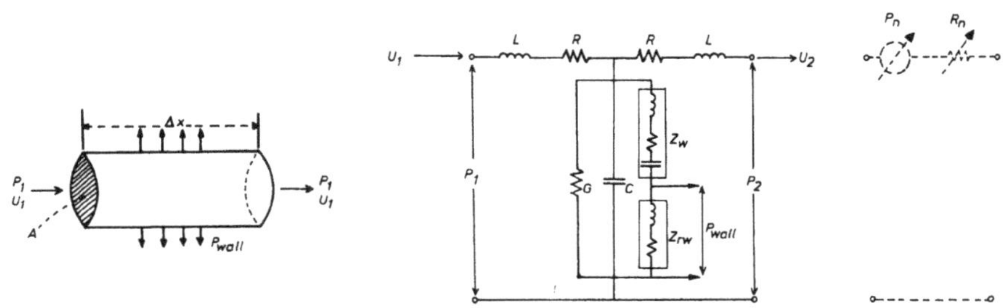

Figure 4. Electrical analogon of the acoustic behavior of a section of a cylindrical tube.

The general model in Figure 4 does not only account for the behavior of the air in the tube, but also for the walls of the tube. The behavior of the air is modelled by the resistance and inductance in the serial branch, together with the conductance and capacitance in the shunting branch. The inductance L represents the inertance of the maas of air, the resistance R accounts for the viscous losses, the conductance G for the heat conduction losses, and the capacitance C represents the compliance of the air mass contained in the tube section. The mechanical impedance of the wall of the tube is modelled by the RLC circuit Z_w. in the shunting branch; the RL circuit in that branch, finally, represents the radiation losses through the wall of the vocal tract. The acoustic behavior of a cascade of circuits like the one in Figure 4 is extremely difficult to calculate. Also, it is not trivial to obtain sensible values for the circuit elements that represent the effects of the vocal tract walls. Therefore, it is customary to simplify the model by first removing the effects of the vocal tract wall. In practice, this amounts to adopting the assumption that the walls are completely rigid. Heat conduction losses are also virtually always neglected. It appears that one can even omit the viscous losses and still remain with a model that describes the essentials of the acoustics of speech production.

Starting with the basic model in Figure 4 we have developed three different models of the situation that applies to our attempts to measure glottal flow. These models are shown in Figure 5. All three models show the four locations where pressure is measured, the two points, halfway between the transducers in a cavity, where

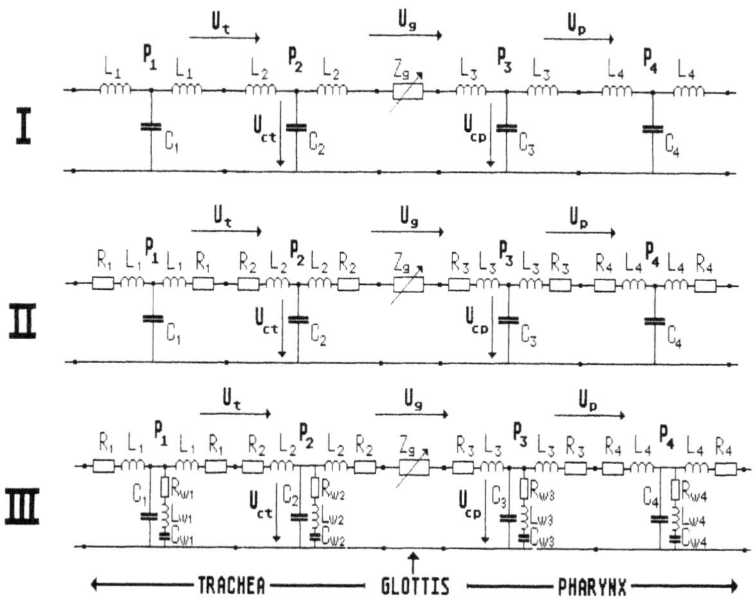

Figure 5. Measurement models for the estimation of transglottal flow from pressure recordings in the trachea and pharynx.

measurement positions and the glottis. The difference between the models lies in the way in which the behavior of the tube sections (or cavities) is represented. Model I assumes that the walls of the tubes are completely rigid; it also assumes that no flow energy is converted into heat because of viscous drag. Model II retains the assumption of completely rigid walls, but viscous losses are accounted for by means of the resistances in the serial path. Model III, the most complex one, can account for both non-rigid walls and viscous losses. The values of the circuit elements in models I and II can be obtained directly from the physical dimensions of the tube sections (Flanagan, 1972). 'Correct' values for the elements representing the elastic properties of non-rigid walls in model III are far more difficult to come by; the best approximation is probably still Ishizaka, French and Flanagan (1975).

If all assumptions underlying the measurement technique hold, and if model I applies, all elements in the measurement model can be measured or calculated directly, except for the capacitances C_2 and C_3. Capacitances form an exception because it is not possible to ascertain the exact position of the glottis relative to the pressure transducers. We know, however, that the tube between transducers #2 and #3 has a total length of 5 cm. If we are willing to assume that the estimate of glottal flow obtained from the flow 5 cm upstream of the glottis should be identical to the estimate obtained from the flow 5 cm downstream, we have a means for optimizing the values of C_2 and C_3. Clearly, if the length of the cavity between the upstream measurement location and the glottis is n cm, then the length of the supraglottal cavity should equal 10-n cm. Assuming reasonable values for the cross sectional areas of the cavities it is then possible to calculate C_2 and C_3 simultaneaously from the value of n. Actually, the task is to find the value of n for which the sub- and supraglottal estimates of the glottal flow are maximally similar. Figure 6 shows the results of two different vowels produced by the same talker. For the open vowel (/a/) the two estimates of the glottal flow are almost identical. For the closed vowel (/u/), on the other hand, the two estimates hardly show any resemblance. Thus it seems that for open vowels the assumptions (simplifications) in the underlying measurement model are warranted, whereas in the case of the closed vowel they are clearly not. Extensive experiments with a production model corresponding to the models II and III in Figure 5 have shown that only the most complete one (viz. III), which incorporates vocal tract wall impedance, is adequate for all types of vowels. Thus we have another example of a situation where physiological signals that are difficult to obtain need a model for their interpretation. Worse even, the correct interpretation appears to be crucially dependent on the correct choice of the model (which happens to be more complicated than the customary lossless model of the vocal tract).

PRODUCTION MODELS VERSUS ANALYSIS MODELS

Conceptually, speech production models (which often are called speech synthesis models if they are sufficiently explicit and detailed to make for useful research tools) have very little in common with automatic techniques for speech analysis. The most characteristic feature of the well-known automatic speech analysis techniques is that they yield optimal estimates for one or more parameters. From the section on acoustic models of speech production it should be clear that these techniques do not so much provide estimates of parameters of the speech signal proper, but rather of the parameters of some model that is assumed to have generated the signals under analysis. Compared with real speech production mechanism the model underlying the analysis may be extremely simplified. Indeed, we have seen that the parameters of the most frequently used analysis model cannot always safely be interpreted in terms of a realistic speech production system. For a large number of interesting applications, particularly in speech technology, such an interpretation is not needed. Moreover, the usefulness of these extremely simplified models in many applications derives from the simplification, because it permits one to develop straightforward techniques for the estimation of unique optimal values for all parameters in the model. From a mathematical point of view this can be stated by saying that additional simplifications are introduced in the model until it becomes possible to formulate the parameter estimation problem in the form of linear equations for which analytic (closed form) solution techniques are known to exist. The non-uniqueness stressed in the previous sections only arises if one attempts to interpret the model parameters in terms of a physiologically realistic speech production apparatus.

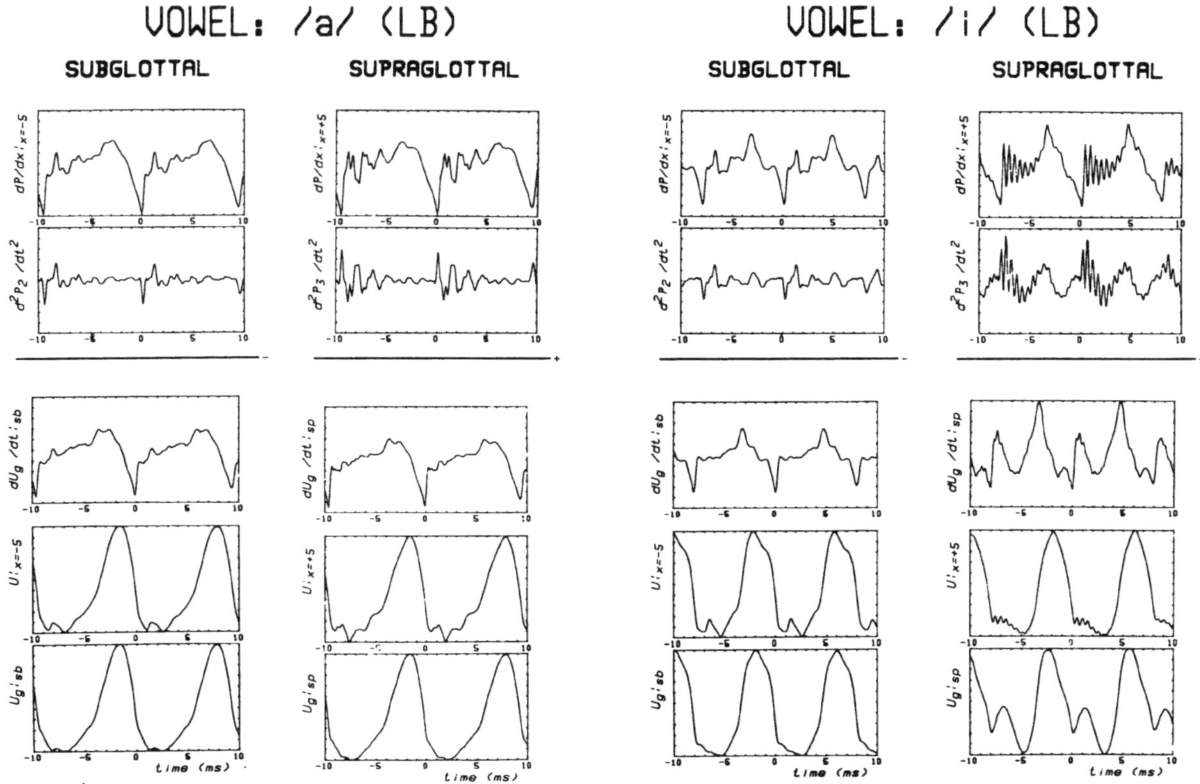

Figure 6. Results of attempts to estimate glottal flow from pressure differentials in the trachea and pharynx for the vowels/a/ and /i/ using the simplest electrical analogon of the acoustic behavior of cylindrical tubes.

Perhaps the most salient characteristic of the production models is the way in which they are normally used. Because they tend to comprise large numbers of parameters and because the effect of changes of parameter values on the output of the model is usually extremely difficult to predict with a high degree of accuracy, production models seem to be used primarily in studies where a competent scientist interactively adjusts the values of all parameters until some desired form of output is obtained. This type of research can lead to considerable insight in the influence of a single parameter or combinations of parameters. Here too it must be realized, however, that the dependability of the results is limited by the realism of the model. A major drawback of the research paradigm based on interactive simulations with production models is that this kind of experiments is extremely time consuming. Consequently, the increased level of physiological reality is obtained at the cost of a (severe) limitation of the number of cases that can be studied in detail. This makes it only natural that from time to time the question arises to what extent the results obtained in model simulations may be generalized to other situations than those studied in a particular experiment.

The critical remarks in the preceding paragraph are in no way meant to diminish the importance of this type of studies. On the contrary: often it is the best one can accomplish. Also, careful simulation studies can accumulate a knowledge base and the attendant experience that allows one to build up a framework in which it is possible to make intelligent interpretations of the results of large scale analyses using simpler models. A good case in point are glottographic signals, particularly the EGG. The large number of detailed model studies carried out during the last decade have led to such deepening of our understanding of the details of the phonation process that EGG signals now may be interpreted to such an extent that the EGG, some thirty years after its invention, could mature into a viable research tool. There is even a promise that further studies will allow the EGG to develop into an instrument that can be used in routie clinical work.

Up to now the differences between (simplified) analysis models and (complex but hopefully physiologically interpretable) production models has been emphasized. Yet, the discrepancy between the two kinds of models needs not be as unbridgeable as it may seem. If in a simulation experiment the parameter values are updated until the output signal optimally resembles some previously recorded signal (which may be a natural speech signal) the difference between analysis and simulation seems not so great anymore. What remains different compared with the usual analysis procedures is that the eventual parameter values are not obtained automatically and that there is no guarantee that the resemblance between the recorded and simulated signals is optimal in some rigorous mathematical sense. Incidentally, analysis-by-simulation is nothing new; under the slightly different heading "analysis-by-synthesis" it has been around for quite some time. The work of Paul, House & Stevens (1964) is just one example, and certainly not the first. Also, it should be realized that there is an increasing number of automatic signal analysis procedures that do not produce parameters values that are guaranteed to be optimal in a rigorous mathematical sense.

This applies to all procedures that involve some form of non-linear (iterative) optimization. Foremost among these techniques is pole-zero (ARMA) analysis of speech signals, i.e., an analysis technique in which the assumption that the vocal tract filter can adequately be described by its resonances only has been mitigated in such a way that anti- resonances are also accounted for. Pole-zero models would give realistic descriptions of e.g. nasal consonants and nasalized vowels. If one adopts a model in which anti-resonances may appear it is no longer possible to formulate the parameter estimation problem in the form of a set of equations that are guaranteed to have a unique solution. On the contrary, one is obliged to take recourse to iterative procedures, at least if one is interested in more than a sub-optimal solution; in most cases it is not possible to prove that the iterative procedure will converge, nor that the solution it provides when it does converge is the global optimum instead of one of a set of local optima. Despite of their non-linear character most ARMA analysis techniques still can only be applied to one-dimensional signals, like for instance the acoustic speech signal. In speech pathology research there is a real need for analysis procedures that allow for the simultaneous analysis and interpretation of multiple signals, like for instance the speech signal and glottographic signals or EMG signals. With the promise of ever more powerful computers these analysis techniques might come within reach during the next decade. One foreshadow of a feasible way to analyse multiple speech signals simultaneously is the multi-dimensional ARMA analysis technique described in Pandit & Wu (1983), even if none of the examples given in their text refer to speech. An even more interesting and promising example is perhaps the work reported by Flanagan, Ishizaka & Shipley (1981) in which they describe an attempt to have a digital computer atomatically adjust the parameters of a very detailed speech production model (including a self- oscillating two-mass model of the vocal folds) in order to approximate a natural speech signal. Their paper also gives a good idea of the difficulties that still must be solved and of the enormous computational complexity of the problem. Awaiting the advent of low-cost supercomputers speech scientists have still an enormous amount of work to do that can be (and perhaps should be) carried out by less powerful equipment, for there remains very much to be learned about basic physiological signals that must be understood before new models can be sensibly constructed and used in experiments like the one of Flanagan and his co-workers.

REFERENCES

Atal, B.S., Chang, J.J., Mathews, M.V. & Tukey, J.W. (1978). Inversion of articulatory-to-acoustic transformation in the vocal tract by a computer sorting technique. *Journal of the Acoustical Society of America, Volume 67*, 1535-1555.

Boves, L. (1984). *The phonetic basis of perceptual ratings of running speech.* Foris Publications, Dordrecht-Cinnaminson.

Childers, D.G. & Krishnamurthy, A.K. (1985). *A critical review of electroglottography.* CRC Critical Reviews in Biomedical Engineering, Volume 12, 131-161.

Cranen, B. & Boves, L. (1983). A set-up for testing the validity of the two-mass model of the vocal folds. In: I.R. Titze & R.C. Scherer (Eds.) *Vocal Fold Physiology* Biomechanics, Acoustics and Phonatory Control. The Denver Center for the Perfoming Arts, Denver, 500-513.

Cranen, B. & Boves, L. (1985). Pressure measurements during speech production using semiconductor miniature pressure transducers: Impact on models of speech production. *Journal of the Acoustical Society of America, Volume 77,* 1543-1551.

Fant, G. (1960). *Acoustic theory of speech production.* Mouton, The Hague.

Flanagan, J.L. (1958). Some properties of the glottal sound source. *Journal of Speech and Hearing Research, Volume 1,* 99-116.

Flanagan, J.L. (1972). *Speech analysis, synthesis, and perception.* Springer Verlag, Berlin, New York.

Ishizaka, K., French, J.L. & Flanagan, J.L. (1975). Direct determination of vocal tract wall impedance. *IEEE Transactions Acoustics, Speech, Signal Processing, Volume ASSP-23,* 370-373.

Lecluse, F.L.E., Brocaar, M.P. & Verschuure, J. (1975). The electroglottograph and its relation to glottal activity. *Folia Phoniatrica, Vol. 27,* 215-224.

Markel, J.D. & Gray, A.H. (1976). *Linear prediction of speech.* Springer Verlag, Berlin, New York.

Rabiner, L.R. & Schafer, R.W. (1978). *Digital processing of speech signals.* Prentice-Hall, Englewood-Cliffs, N.J.

Rothenberg, M. (1983). An interactive model for the voice source. In: *D.M. Bless & J.H. Abbs (Eds.) Vocal Fold Physiology* Contemporary Research & Clinical Issues. College-Hill Press, San Diego, 155-165.

Rothenberg, M. & Zahorian, S. (1977). Nonlinear inverse filtering technique for estimating the glottal area waveform. *Journal of the Acoustical Society of America, Volume 61,* 1063-1071.

Teager, H. & Teager, S. (1983). Active Fluid Dynamics Voice Production, or There Is a Unicorn in the Garden. In: *I.R. Titze & R.C. Scherer (Eds.)* Vocal Fold Physiology; Biomechanics, Acoustics and Phonatory Control. The Denver Center for the Performing Arts, Denver, 387-403.

Van den Berg, J.W., Zantema, J.T. & Doornenbal, P. (1957). On the air resistance and Bernoulli effect of the human larynx. *Journal of the Acoustical Society of America, Volume 29,* 626-631.

Wakita, H. (1973). Direct determination of the vocal tract shape by inverse filtering of acoustic speech waveforms. *IEEE Transactions Audio Electroacoustics, Vol AU-21,* 417-427.

Chapter 7

Studying Young Stutterers' Speech Productions: a Procedural Challenge

Edward G. Conture

There are many things researchers would like to know about young stutterers' speech behavior but are afraid to ask. Actually, that statement is not exactly correct. Most researchers are not as much afraid to ask the question as they may be to seek the answer. In this chapter, a variety of issues and concerns will be addressed which relate to the objective study of young stutterers' speech production. These youngsters' participation in speech research will be discussed in terms of three different but related topics: (1) Behavioral and Subject Definitions/Specifications; (2) Methodological and Procedural Issues and (3) Instrumental Considerations.

Before beginning this discussion, some general remarks will be made. While perhaps apparent, young stutterers' speech productive can be studied by one of two different means: (1) descriptive investigations or (2) theory-driven experiments. Differences between these two types of investigations make little difference, however, in terms of the instrumental procedures involved. Surface electromyographic electrodes, for example, must be employed in the same way with the same cautions regardless of the researcher's intent. Although some experimental paradigms, for example, reaction time experiments, may entail additional equipment and procedures than those employed in a descriptive investigation, such experimental paradigms may be inappropriate for subjects under 7 years of age. Thus, the differences that make a difference, at least in terms of the present chapter, is the fact that the subjects currently being discussed are children between 3 and 7 years of age. Ironically, it is these youngsters - the ones between 3 and 7 years of age - that researchers and clinicians alike need to know much more about. To do so, the experimenter must be willing to adapt and

Table 1. Some "subject-induced" experimental difficulties or errors encountered during the recording of youngsters acoustic speech signal and–or speech physiology. Some of these concerns can be *a priori* controlled and–or mitigated while some must be factored out, if possible, during data analysis. After Caruso (1983).

Subject induced errors
1. Child speaks in an extremely soft (low intensity) voice
2. Child's saliva "drool" causes surface EMG electrodes to fall off or become loose on child's skin
3. Child physically "squirms" in chair causing sensors to fall off or become loose
4. Child becomes fatigued–uncooperative and–or has trouble performing because of short attention span.
5. Child is not sufficiently "electrically quiet" during recording so that surface EMG has very high "noise" floor making determination of muscle activity during particular speech act very difficult if not impossible.
6. Child unable to correctly and–or reliably articulate speech sounds under study.
7. Child able to say target words or syllable but not when embedded in carrier phrase; related to this is the child who consistently truncates carrier phrase and–or seemingly can't produce the phrase.

modify his or her methodologies to suit the abilities and behaviors of these small children.

If stuttering is a "disorder of childhood," then why is there apparently so little known about young stutterers' speech production? As Wall and Myers (1984, p. vii) point out, the research literature are replete with descriptive as well as experimental studies of the speech behavior of older, adult stutterers. Consequently, this same literature contains very little factual information regarding young stutterers' speech production. This is most unfortunate because these children are more apt than adults to be closer to the onset of their stuttering problem and thus exhibiting behavior which is relatively less "contaminated" by the learned reactions and adjustments typically developed by adult stutterers. Why, it might ask, isn't the speech behavior of young stutterers more frequently studied? One partial answer is contained in Table 1 which shows only a few of the *specific* "subject-induced errors" or problems encountered when studying young stutterers' speech production. A cursory review of this table suggests that the answer is quite simple, but further study indicates that the situation is quite complex. To begin illustrating such complexity, one of the more common difficulties encountered with stuttering research will be discussed: Behavioral and Subject Definition/Specification.

BEHAVIORAL AND SUBJECT DEFINITIONS

As will be described in further detail below, Table 2 shows four issues which have as much application to research with adult stutterers as they do to that with children who stutter. What seems to matter, in this writer's opinion, is that the researcher pays as much attention to subject specification as to procedural and instrumental detail. It can't be stressed enough: defining who is a stutterer and what is a stuttering is fundamental for empirical replication of a study, descriptive or otherwise. So often, we encounter in the literature studies that are excellent in terms of methodology, instrumentation and analysis but whose subject description is so vague or incomplete as to make replication all but impossible. What happens? Typically, the next researcher tries to perform the same study using the "same subjects" (after all, isn't any stutterer as good as any other?) then reports different or contradictory findings. There is a growing body of information to suggest that differences among stutterers themselves may be as significant as differences observed between normally fluent speakers and stutterers (for example, Andrews and Harris, 1964; Conture and Schwartz, 1984; Daly, 1981; Gregory, 1973; Preus, 1982; Prins and Lohr, 1972; Rentschler, 1984; Schwartz, 1984; Schwartz et al., 1982; St. Onge, 1963). Obviously, therefore, such *a priori* within-group differences in the stuttering population should be considered when comparing the results of similar studies or when trying to replicate same.

Table 2. Some behavioral and subject definitions and specifications germane to empirical investigations of children and adults who stutter. Such variables are every bit as relevant to stuttering research as careful delineation of procedural and instructional detail.

Behavioral and subject definitions/specifications
1. Basic demographic data, for example, mean age and its range
2. Objective definition of stuttering, for example, frequency and type of disfluency
3. Objective definition of stutterer, for example, criterion measures
4. Length, nature and clinical site of subjects' therapy

What we are leading to is this: researchers are encouraged to try to change their usual approach toward behavioral and subject definition and specifications in stuttering research. We all have some stake in trying to alter the current state of affairs. Researchers can no longer round up the stuttering subjects *after* the study has been developed. Instead, they should be encouraged to establish their subject and behavioral definitions *before* they begin collecting data. Such descriptors as "severe" or "mild" or "primary" or "secondary" are all but useless to readers and researchers interested in replication. So are such descriptors as "blocks" or "evidence of struggle behavior". Simply put, the referents for these nebulous words are unclear at best and impossible to get agreement on at worst. At the risk of delivering a polemic (if one hasn't been delivered already); provided below are some suggestions that should help experimenters give their interested readers as well as fellow researchers enough detail to evaluate who their subjects were, what they produced and the means to replicate same.

First, the experimenter should provide *basic demographic data:* (1) there should be a description of the number of males and female subjects in the sample; (2) there should be a description of the subjects' mean age and range (in years and months or at least months); (3) there should be explication regarding the number of subjects who have had or are presently having therapy (as well as therapy site); (4) there should be description of how the subjects came to be part of study as well as their knowledge of same, for example, (un)paid volunteers naive to method and purpose of experiment, etc. and (5) the experimenter should enumerate the number of subjects, if any, who were rejected from the study, the reason(s) for their rejection as well as something about the general population from which subjects were drawn, for example, the first trough six grades of the public and parochial schools within the Central New York school district(s). It would also help if the experimenter tells whether subjects were screened for other (non)speech, hearing or language problems and indicate if concomitant "problems" exist for any or all subjects (see Blood and Seider, 1981; Merits-Patterson and Reed, 1981), for example, developmental articulation concerns.

Second, the experimenter should try to provide an *objective definition of stuttering:* (1) describe the specific disfluencies types that were and were not "called" stuttering (cf., Table 1, Conture, 1982a); (2) explain whether the frequency of these stutterings were tabulated per 100 words, syllables or some other "normalizing" procedure (for data regarding frequency of youngsters' "normal" disfluencies, see Branscom et al., 1955); (3) make clear whether judgements of stuttering were based on auditory and/or visual information and whether these judgements were based on "on-line" assessment versus previously recorded audio or audiovideo tapes; and (4) indicate whether the sample was obtained during reading or speaking and specify the nature of both, for example, single-word lists, conversations, short stories, etc. If duration and/or units of repetitions are part of the behaviors used to determine an instance of stuttering, the experimenter should provide criterion measures for both.

Third, the experimenter should provide a *definition of stutterer:* (1) explicate the criterion measures used to include and exclude a subject from being considered a stutterer, for example, number and type of disfluencies, expressed concerns of family, relatives and associates, etc.; (2) if the experimenter uses a formalized test or scale to define subjects as normal or stutterer, then the experimenter should report each subject's actual score (plus group mean and dispersion of scores) on such scales as the Iowa Scale of Stuttering Severity (Johnson et al., 1963; Williams, 1978), Stuttering Severity Instrument (Riley, 1972; Riley, 1980), Stuttering Prediction Instrument (Riley and Riley, 1982) or Stocker Probe Test (Stocker, 1976; Conture and Caruso, 1978); and (4) the experimenter should indicate the number and nature of associated behaviors such as head jerking, eye blinking (see, Barr, 1940; Brutten, 1975; Prins and Lohr, 1974; Schwartz, 1984) and so forth if they were part of subject selection criteria.

Fourth, the experimenter should, if at all possible, indicate the *length, nature and clinical site of subjects' therapy.* At the very least, the experimenter should make every attempt to explicate the number of stutterers who have had or are having therapy at time of study. It would be nice if the nature of such therapy was included but since different clinics may use the same *name* to refer to therapy procedures which may actually vary in some subtle and some not so subtle ways, it presently seems prudent to consider providing such information as optional.

As mentioned above, if researchers in the area of stuttering would attend to subject and behavioral as much as they do procedural and instrumental detail, research in this area would be much better served. Until we can replicate ALL aspects of each other's research, the subject and behavioral parts as much as the rest of the method, we can continue to expect to find divergent and inconsistent findings. This is particularly true with children, who are neither little adults nor little adult stutterers. That is, because children are so rapidly and constantly developing in so many different areas, careful, objective matching of subjects is a must if replication is going to stand a chance of confirming previous findings. We submit that results obtained from apparently identical studies of stutterers can be significantly influenced by differences in subjects studied. However, until researchers make such differences more apparent in their subject descriptions, their colleagues will continue to find it difficult to sort out the numerous reasons for contradictory findings among various studies.

GENERAL PROCEDURAL CONSIDERATIONS

As mentioned above, the main difference that appears to make a difference between studying children versus adult stutterers is age. While obvious, this difference has profound implications for what procedures can and/or should be used with these younger subjects. Table 3 shows some *specific* procedural concerns typically encountered in the study of young stutterers' speech behavior. In the following space, we'd like to highlight some of the more important general issues that bear consideration when studying these young subjects (Table 4).

First, some methodologies are, by their very nature, invasive, for example, intramuscular, hooked-wire electromyography, flexible fiber optic naso-laryngoscopy, and so forth. That is, these procedures involve inserting some device into a bodily orifice or under the skin. Clearly, with an "elective", voluntary procedure like research, the researcher may find it difficult to justify to him or herself, the child, his/her parents and society the necessity of such procedures. Likewise, human subject protection committees (cf., Metz and Folkins, 1985) are ever watchful for procedures which might involve short-, medium- or long-term injury. Since invasive procedures appear, at least on the surface, to have a high likelihood for causing "sudden pain or loss of blood," mental, psycho-social trauma and anguish, these committees are particularly skeptical of their use with youngsters 18 years old and younger.

Second, children themselves have healthy concerns regarding, shall we say, the sanctity of their bodies. It really makes little difference whether the procedure involves *real* versus *perceived* danger to the child. Once the child decides him or herself that "it's

Table 3. Some specific procedural concerns and errors encountered in the instrumental study of human speech production, particularly that of young children.

Procedural errors	
1.	Loose contact of surface EMG or EGG electrodes resulting in weak, no or irregular signal; this problem may also relate to inappropriate electrode placement on skin surface
2.	Loose contact of EMG system ground whereby all EMG signals (even those electrodes which are securely fastened) are poorly recorded
3.	Inducive phethsmographic "straps" of "bands" ("respibands") used for recording chest wall and abdominal movement during speech are too loose fitting for a particular child; sometimes the chest and abdominal respibands overlap one another causing inappropriate–inaccurate readings of respiratory deflation patterns
4.	"Skin bond" (a liquid electrode-to-skin adhesive) for surface EMG electrodes temporary irritates child's skin; sometimes very difficult to make sufficient electrode-to-skin contact for purposes of recording electrical interference patterns associated with muscle activity
5.	Record levels of FM or other recording devices too low ("too noisy") or too high ("peak clipping") for signals, EMG and acoustic in particular
6.	Failure to electrically power all instrumentation necessary for the sensing and recording of speech acoustic–physiologic signals
7.	Failure to engage all recording devices at point in experiment when child actually begins to speak
8.	Difficulty in visually determining on multi-channel oscilloscope the best placement (highest amplitude, most "noise-free" signal) for EGG electrodes because of size of child's larynx, its placement in neck relative to skin surface or untoward vertical displacements of larynx and–or contraction of laryngeal strap muscles; as with surface EMG electrodes, correct placement of EGG electrodes is necessary for accurate, reliable recordings

Table 4. General procedural considerations relative to the objective study of young stutterers' speech and related behavior.

General procedural considerations	
1.	(Non)Invasive procedures
2.	Child's real versus perceived danger
3.	Child's need to be in control of situation
4.	Influence of child's parents, prior as well as during experiment
5.	Children fatigue quickly when they give concentrated attention
6.	Child has *active* role in speech production research
7.	Communicate with and reinforce child's efforts and behaviors

gonna hurt," the experiment is essentially over. When we say "over," we mean that there are very few experiments involving the study of speech physiology whose data can be considered "clean" if it was obtained from a child during or directly after a 20 to 30 minute crying jag or from a child who has "frozen" his oral musculature as he maintains his body as rigid as a board due to fright! Of course, the child is more apt to react inappropriately to some procedures than others. Procedures that involve insertion of wires, needles, tubes and the like into the child or under his or her skin are almost invariably going to cause the child and/or his or her parents some degree of concern.

Third, children like to feel in control of the situation. If they want to move, they want to be able to move. If they want to sit or stand, they want to sit or stand! They'll cooperate a good deal with the adult but they have to feel some degree of control over the situation. Therefore, any procedure which either in reality or in the child's perception diminishes their control, makes them sit or move *when they don't want to* will not be well received by the child. Simply put, they must feel like participating partners rather than a captive audience of one. This is an important variable and one we'll discuss further.

Fourth, the child's parent(s) exerts a powerful influence on the child's (un)willingness to cooperate. If the parent expresses, by word or deed, fears, doubts, worries or concerns about an experimental procedure, then the child will surely do likewise. The parents are the researcher's biggest ally in the attempt to study the small child. They are, of course, also the biggest foe if their concerns and fears are disregarded or left unattended by the researcher. Leaving the parent outside the examination or testing room may work for the very experienced experimenter - some seasoned pediatric dentists do the same - but for the rest of us, having the parents in the same room as the child and "involved" in the experiment is a must.

Fifth, children fatigue sooner than adults when they must give a task their "undivided" attention. Certainly, speaking with the examiner while various wires and gadgets are hanging on or around constitutes such a task. The child must not only sit *still* while recording sensors are placed on or about him, he or she must *cooperate* through a variety of calibration procedures and *wait* for the experimenters to make sure all is running and recording smoothly. And then, after all that, he has to *talk*! The child's degree and level of concentration, cooperation and activity involvement has to be observed to be truly appreciated. None of this says that these children can't or shouldn't so participate, but their relatively short attention span and low threshold of fatigue for concentrated "mental" effort must be appreciated and taken into account if the experimenter wants to meaningfully study their speech production behavior.

Sixth, the experimenter must remember that the subject is going to actively *do* something during the experiment, that is, talk. Thus, in speech research the child is an active participant. Such experiments should not be viewed as analogous to taking a blood sample from the child or filling a cavity in one of his or her teeth. With the study of stuttered speech production, in particular, the child must be an active participant while orally communicating during a (un)structured speaking task. The experimenter must insure that the child will not only cooperate in a physical sense but in a cognitive and communicative sense as well. To enlist such cooperation the experimenter must communicate and reinforce the child's behavior.

Seventh, communication with the child and reinforcement of the child's behaviors are one of the better ways to keep the child involved and cooperative (cf., Chapter 3, Conture, 1982). Let the child and the child's parents actually *handle* the recording electrodes. Let them turn some of the knobs or push some of the buttons on the tape recorder or the oscilloscope. Let them view some of the child's behavior *before* the experiment begins to run, for example, tidal exhalation/inhalation on the oscilloscope. Explain each facet of the equipment to the child and his or her parents *in terms they'll understand*. Small surface EMG electrodes become "little blue buttons" for seeing "how you move and use your mouth when you talk". EGG recording disks become "little cymbals...to see how your voice box works". Lightweight microphones "are just like the ones the astronauts wear...or the airplane pilots...or the TV newsman...so you can talk to us and we can hear you". Cloth bands that circle the thorax and stomach to study speech breathing become "little vests or belts that go around your tummy and chest" so we can see "...what you do when you take air in and blow it out". And so forth. Our point is simply this: communicate with the child on a level they can understand and relate to. Talk to his or her need to feel in control and concern that "it's gonna hurt". Frequently reinforce the child with verbal praise and pats on the shoulder or arm for any and all of their attempts to cooperate as well as their expressed attempts to understand what is going on. Likewise, frequently praise the child for his or her patience and willingness to perform what is asked of him or her. Approached correctly, 80 to 90 % of all children will cooperate with this sort of research and nearly 75% of them will provide some form of analysable data. Simply put, the speech production behavior of these children, if the methodology and approach is tailored to their needs, can and should be meaningfully studied.

Given the foregoing, it is apparent that objectively studying youngsters' speech physiology is different from that of adults! Once again, these remarks are directed to research involving youngsters between 3 and 7 years of age. We've examined a few children slightly under 2 years of age, but for most of what we are presently discussing today, the lower age cut-off is about 36 months or three years of age. Once the typical child gets to be about 7 years of age he or she gets a bit easier to examine, but as we said at the beginning, we are interested in studying young stutterers as close to onset of stuttering as possible. This means, for 90% of all stutterers (Bloodstein, 1981), that we have to study children between 3 and 7 years of age.

INSTRUMENTAL CONSIDERATIONS

The speech physiology of young children involves the same three "speech" systems studied with adults: respiration, phonation, and articulation. The examiner's intent as well as nature of his or her study obviously determines what aspects of these three systems will be studied. While some studies will focus on only one aspect of speech production, for example, the laryngeal aspect (Conture, Rothenberg and Molitor, 1986), others will concentrate on the interactions between systems, for example, onset of phonatory vibration relative to supra-glottal articulatory adjustment (for example, Baken, McManus, and Cavallo, 1984). Still other studies will want to focus on the output of the system and infer "backwards", for example, an acoustic study of temporal parameters of laryngeal and articulatory behaviors and their relations to one another (for example, Metz, Conture, and Caruso, 1979; Watson and Alfonso, 1982; Zebrowski, Conture and Cudahy, 1985) while other studies will focus on relations between muscular activity and structural movement, for example, temporal relations during speech between lip muscle activity and labial displacement (elevation/depression) and movement (for example, Caruso, Gracco and Abbs, 1987). For simplicity, we will discuss each of the three systems (respiration, phonation, and articulation) as they might be studied separately; however, as we will briefly describe, all three systems can be simultaneously studied in relation to one another.

Since stuttering has been hypothesized as being a disorder of timing (Van Riper, 1971, 1982) or as being related to temporal discoordinations among various components of speech production (Perkins, Rudas, Johnson and Bell, 1976), we chose to concentrate on temporal measurements of young stutterers' speech production. For purposes of this discussion, we will avoid the many theoretical controversies regarding the temporal parameters of speech production, for example, whether temporal parameters of speech movements are best accounted for within a dynamically specified model (cf., Kelso, Tuller, and Harris, 1984) versus the more traditional measures of duration and latency (see Dossey, 1982 for overview of temporal/spatial influences on human health and behavior). Instead, we will concentrate on instrumental procedures seemingly most appropriate for use with small children.

Figure 1 is an example of the kinds of data generated by using such instrumentation to study young stutterers' speech production (Zebrowski, Conture, and Colton, 1984). This pilot research, investigating the relative sequence of onsets of respiratory, phonatory and articulatory behaviors during the fluency of young stutterers and that of their normally fluent peers, resulted from implementation of the type of instrumentation we're about to discuss. As we can see, this instrumentation can be used to objectively study temporal events within and relations between the three "major" aspects of speech production: ventilatory activity, laryngeal activity and articulatory activity. For sake of this discussion, we will briefly discuss each activity in terms of available instrumentation and those instrumental approaches seemingly best suited for use with small children. It must be made apparent from the outset, however, that instrumental study of young children who stutter is a compromise between the real and the ideal. The "real" is the child and his or her behaviors and abilities, as previously discussed. The "ideal" is the state-of-the-art instrumentation which provides the most detailed, absolute quantitative information available regarding speech production (for excellent reviews of such instrumentation, see Abbs and Watkin, 1976; Folkins and Kuehn, 1982). Because of the former (the child), however, certain of the latter (instrumentation) many times cannot be applied.

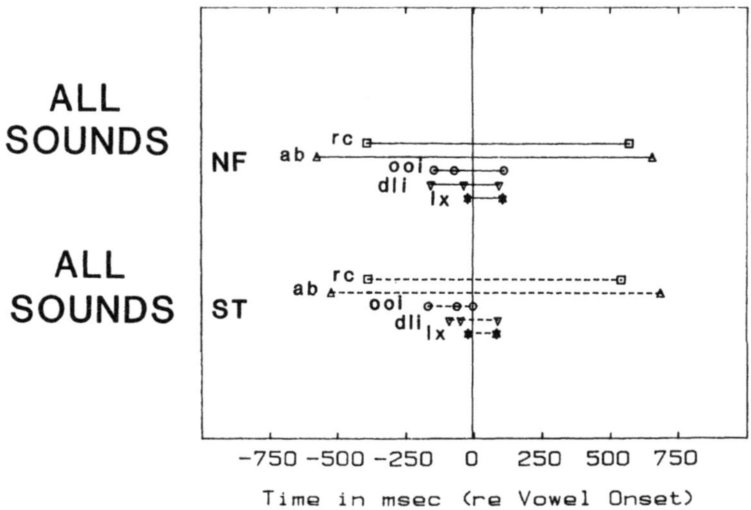

Figure 1. Example of relative temporal sequences of onset and offsets of respiratory, laryngeal and supraglottal behavior during the FLUENT speech productions of five young stutterers (ST) and five young normally fluent (NF) speakers, All sounds= -B p v f m w-, RC = rib cage, AB = abdomen, OOI = orbicularis oris inferior (labial muscle), DLI = depressor labii inferior (labial muscle), and LX = electroglottographic signal, O = acoustic onset of vowel following "target" consonant, for example, the vowel "ee" in after "b" on word "beet." After Zebrowski, Conture and Colton (1984).

RESPIRATION

At present, the speech breathing behaviors of children may be studied in several related, but different ways, for example, (1) electromagnetic devices (magnetometers) (Hixon et al. 1973; 1976) (2) whitney or mercury strain gauges (for example, Baken, 1977, Baken et al., 1979; 1984) or (3) inductive plethsmyography (for example, Caruso, Conture, and Colton, in press, 1986). Each procedure has its pluses and minuses with the magnetometer approach probably resulting in the most accurate, most absolute measures of speech breathing behavior. However, it must be remembered that we are currently considering the objective study of the speech production associated with the (non)fluency of small children. Such youngsters' ability and willingness to cooperate with a therapy session, let alone an experimental procedure, runs between 20 to 45 minutes (60 minutes at the outside). Further, we are working with children who many times find it difficult to provide absolute or accurate indexes of vital capacity or isovolume maneuvers - a problem for any respiratory methodology that requires such calibration procedures. We are also working with youngsters who many times vigorously resist us taking off their T-shirts or blouses to attach electrodes to the bare skin on their chest and back, a procedure seemingly necessary when using magnetometers to study speech breathing.

Our work with children and speech breathing suggests that the whitney gauge procedure or the Respitrace (an inductive plethysmograph) procedure are the most suitable to use with these youngsters. Our experience with the Respitrace convinces us that it provides a reasonable reliable indication of the onset, offset and duration of respiratory deflation during (non)speech tasks. Further, most young children seem to tolerate the procedure fairly well. The Respitrace can be used to sense onsets and offsets of respiratory deflation and thus provide a relative index of abdominal versus chest wall contributions to respiratory deflation. Briefly, the Respitrace is a non-invasive inductive plethysmograph (Sackner, 1979; Watson, 1979) designed to measure volume changes within the thoracic cage and abdominal cavity during (non)speech breathing. It consists of two elastic bands (with the age children we studied, these bands had a width = 3.5 inches and a length = 25 inches), within each band are glued and sewn lengths of wire arranged in a zig-zag fashion. These wires form a simple electrical coil whose inductance varies as the wires' length changes. The varying inductance alters the frequency of an oscillator whose output is demodulated by appropriate circuitry within the Respitrace, amplified and appears as a slow varying dc signal proportional to the volume changes within the lungs or abdominal cavity. The sum of the two compartments representing the total respiratory volumes is also available for measurement. Others have shown that once properly calibrated, the Respitrace is relatively artifact-free for a quietly sitting individual (Bless, Hunker, and Weismer, 1983). Although it may be a function of the particular Respitrace unit we own, the instrument appears to provide the most stable recordings once it has been "warmed up" for about 1-2 hours prior to testing. Of course, if percentage of absolute lung volume relative to a particular aspect of speech production is of interest then the Respitrace with children may be problematic; however, we submit that researchers will have trouble obtaining such absolute respiratory measures during the speech production of 3 to 7 year olds regardless of specific instrumental procedure. "Patterns" of respiratory behavior (Metz, Conture, and Colton, 1976) associated with these youngsters' stutterings could also be readily detected by all three procedures but at present the meaning of these patterns relative to the problem of stuttering is less than clear.

One exciting possibility for future work in the area of speech breathing with young stutterers is the use of the Respitrace for biofeedback type therapy (Adams, Guitar and Conture, 1980 for general review of this topic). We say this because our experimental work with these youngsters strongly suggests that these children and their parents quickly and readily "relate" to and understand the rather slowly varying respiratory traces associated with abdominal/chest wall activity as viewed on an oscilloscope. To the extent that a clinician believes that such respiratory behaviors are inappropriate as well as contributory to the child's stuttering, then the Respitrace or its like may eventually become a useful clinical adjunct for certain young stutterers.

LARYNGEAL

The study of laryngeal activity during young stutterers' speech will probably involve non-invasive procedures such as (1) the electroglottograph (for example, Baer et al., 1983; Borden, Baer & Kenney, 1985; Childers & Krishnamurthy, 1984; Childers et al., 1983; Colton et al., 1983; Dejonckere, 1981; Fourcin, 1974, 1981; Fourcin and Abberton, 1971; Gilbert, Potter and Hoodin, 1984; Kitzing, 1982; Lecluse, 1976; Lecluse, Brocaar, and Verschuure, 1975; MacCurtain and Fourcin, 1982; Rothenberg, 1981) or (2) acoustic inferences of glottal activity (for example, Cullinan and Springer, 1980; DiSimoni, 1974a, b, c; Healey, 1982; Hillman and Gilbert, 1977; Metz, Conture and Caruso, 1979; Metz, Samar, and Sacco, 1983; Watson and Alfonso, 1982; Zebrowski, Conture and Cudahy, 1985). Procedures such as fiber optic assessment of laryngeal behavior (for example, Conture, McCall and Brewer, 1977; Conture, Schwartz and Brewer, 1985), intramuscular electromyography (for example, Freeman and Ushijima, 1978) and high-speed cinematography (for example, Metz et al., 1984), while providing excellent, objective information about laryngeal behavior, are either too invasive or requires too much subject participation to be readily used with this age children. One exciting possibility involves the simultaneous recording of glottal volume velocity airflow with the EGG signal (for example, Rothenberg, 1977; 1981), using equipment and procedures specially adapted for children. However, for the present, the EGG, by itself, appears to have the most promise for studying youngsters' laryngeal behavior.

While current versions of the EGG are limited in terms of such "fine-grained" analysis as cycle-to-cycle changes in absolute glottal area, the EGG appears to be a relatively sensitive index of onset and offset of vocal fold vibration (for example, Baer et al., 1983; Childers et al., 1983; Gilbert, Potter and Hoodin, 1984). With appropriate filtering (Ng and Rothenberg, 1982) as well as adjunctive circuitry, the EGG can be used to indicate cycle-to-cycle changes in relative degree of glottal opening (Conture, Rothenberg and Molitor, 1986). With further work, experimenters will be able to quantitatively document the physiological correlates of the EGG's slowly varying, low-frequency aspects in order to make statements about various laryngeal articulatory adjustments, for example, bringing vocal folds into midline in preparation for voicing; already, some preliminary attempts have been made to use the EGG this way (for example, Baken, McManus and Cavallo, 1985).

One crucial distinction must be made apparent between EGG data and the more commonly cited data coming from studies employing EMG, high-speed filming or fiber optic procedures. At present, it is most accurate to say that EGG data reflects vocal fold vibration NOT laryngeal muscle adjustments prior to vibration. In fact, for a sustained vowel, the acoustic and EGG traces look remarkably similar. Further, EGG measurements are typically unit-less or, at best, relative to an arbitrarily chosen referent. At this point in time, it seems rather imprudent to consider EGG data as either *absolute* indexes of glottal area or degree of glottal opening or closing. The EGG is very sensitive to placement of the electrodes on the skin surface - movement up or down, front to back will significantly contribute to changes in the shape and amplitude of the EGG signal. Thus, the placement of the electrodes must be constantly monitored throughout the experiment and readjusted as the need arises. The electrodes can be held in place by the experimenter or foam-rubber strips or elastic bands closed with velcro.

Whatever, most children readily tolerate EGG electrodes on their skin but seem to prefer the experimenter's holding the electrodes in place to the neck-tie feel of foam-rubber strips or velcro-fastened elastic bands. Our experience to date with the electroglottograph (EGG) strongly suggests that it is suitable for studying young stutterers' laryngeal behavior. The EGG senses the variation in transverse electrical impedance created by vocal fold vibration. It can be used to measure onset and offset of vocal fold vibration, the fundamental frequency of vocal fold vibration (plus perturbations in this frequency), and certain aspects of the laryngeal waveform, in particular the waveform associated with vocal fold contact area. Within the band are contained two surface electrodes which transmit a high-frequency current across the larynx. Vocal fold contact increases such current flow and lack of contact reduces current flow. Changes in current flow correspond to changes in the transverse electrical impedance.

Temporal aspects of laryngeal behavior consist of such measurable events as the onset and offset of vocal fold contact and vibration, the duration of each cycle of vocal fold contact and glottal airflow, the duration of closed and open aspects of glottal cycle, transitions between voiced and unvoiced speech sounds and vice versa. Temporal relations between onset and offset of laryngeal activity and supraglottal articulatory and respiratory behavior can also be assessed. We will not, in this space, cover the voluminous literature relative to voice onset time and voice reaction time experiments; such literature has been reviewed elsewhere (cf., Starkweather, 1982; Adams, Freeman and Conture, 1984). Besides, much of this literature deals with adults rather than children who stutter and for reasons previously mentioned, we are unclear how much we can extrapolate backwards from adult speech production to that of young children. Instead we will here focus on other, more direct indexes of laryngeal timing behavior.

One procedure we have not used with children but has potential for studying temporal aspects of their speech production is "inverse-filtering" either the radiated (extra-oral) pressure waveform, the oral velocity waveform, or the oral volume velocity waveform (Rothenberg, 1968, 1977, 1981; Colton, Brewer and Rothenberg, 1983). The basic problem is that such procedures generally require the subject to wear a mask over the mouth and nose and no matter how lightweight such devices are, children are reluctant to put on such a mask (for reasons previously stated). Assuming, however, the child would wear such a device, by using Rothenberg's (1977) circumferentially-vented pneumotachograph mask the experimenter can transduce the volume velocity waveform associated with the subject's speech productions and this waveform can be inverse filtered to "remove" the effect of the supraglottal acoustic system. Thus, by taking the oral volume velocity waveform emanating from the subject's mouth, information can be obtained regarding the glottal pulses or airflow waveform at the vocal folds and compare with a timelocked EGG signal (Rothenberg, 1981). This inverse filter procedure allows the experimenter to look at fundamental frequency, perturbations in that fundamental frequency, duration of each glottal cycle, onset and offset of glottal vibration, peak flow associated with each glottal pulse, the open quotient of the glottal pulse and certain other aspects of the glottal pulse shape. One of our colleagues, Raymond Colton (Colton et al., 1980), has had extensive experience using a simple, throat-contact microphone, affixed to the skin in the area of the clavicular notch for sensing skin/tracheal vibration associated with subglottal pressure vibrations which are related to vocal fundamental frequency and its perturbations (cf., Casper, 1983). Since the throat mike is a relatively simple, minimally intrusive as well as non-invasive procedure, it should be useable, at least in theory, with older children. However, to date, we have had minimal experience using the throat mike with young children. Further, the throat mike cannot sense as many aspects of laryngeal behavior with as much sophistication as can the EGG and the inverse filter.

One last procedure, although more indirect than the aforementioned, is the "raw" acoustic waveform (radiated pressure). Although this acoustic waveform is confounded by vocal tract response(s), it can provide certain information about certain temporal events happened at the larynx, for example, voice onset time, frication and aspiration durations (Klatt, 1975; Metz, Conture, and Caruso, 1979; Watson and Alfonso, 1982). We have recently co-authored (Zebrowski, Conture, and Cudahy, 1985) a fairly extensive acoustic study of temporal aspects of young stutterers' fluency. This acoustic study suggests that there are no gross temporal differences between young stutterers fluent speech and that of their peers but some subtle difficulties in oral/laryngeal adjustments may be present. However, acoustic measures of laryngeal behavior are rather crude when compared to the EGG (Conture, Rothenberg and Molitor, 1986) or inverse filter (Rothenberg, 1977; Rothenberg, 1981) or the flexible fiber optic naso-laryngoscope (Conture, McCall and Brewer, 1977; Conture, Schwartz, and Brewer, 1985) or intramuscular electromyography (Metz, Conture and Colton, 1976; Freeman and Ushijima, 1978).

ARTICULATION

The articulatory behavior of young stutterers could be assessed in a variety of ways: (1) surface and intramuscular electromyography (e.g., Basmajian, 1979; Harris, 1981) (2) still and cinematic photography (e.g., Gay et al., 1974) and radiography (e.g., Kent, 1972; Folkins and Kuehn, 1982), (3) measures of extra- and intra-oral pressure and oral air flow velocity and volume velocity (Rothenberg, 1981), (4) magnetometers (e.g., Hixon, 1971) and strain gauges (Abbs and Gilbert, 1973; Barlow et al., 1983; Muller and Abbs, 1979) (5) ultrasonically (for example, Minifie et al 1971; Watkin et al., 1978) and (6) optoelectrical movement sensors (e.g., Lindblom and Oeberg, 1974; Honda, 1983; Tuller and Kelso, 1984). Most of our work to date with these youngsters suggested that most of them tolerated surface EMG of superficial labial muscles (for discussion of EMG lip placements with adults see Isley and Basmajian, 1973; Kuksht, 1975; Kennedy and Abbs, 1979; Leanderson and Lindblom, 1972; McClean, Goldsmith, and Cerf, 1984; O'Dwyer et al., 1981; Sussman et al., 1973). However, we also found that only "older" youngsters (seven years and older) could be reliably counted on to cooperate sufficiently with the head-mounted strain-gauge procedure. Abbs and his colleagues (Personal Communication, 1985) are currently developing a *springloaded*, more self-adjusting articulatory version of their headmounted device which should be useable with a wider variety as well as younger subjects. When this spring-loaded articulatory transducer system is developed, its resulting data should allow researchers to relate youngsters' EMG signals to associated structural movements/ displacements just as they currently are able to do with adults. One other, related procedure we have not used with children is the optoelectrical movement sensing system ("Selspot") employed by various Haskins' Laboratory researchers (e.g., Tuller and Kelso, 1984); however, the "Selspot" procedure appears non-invasive and in theory should be simple enough to be used with at least children of 7 years and older.

We avoided using video and cinematic fluoroscopic (x-ray) procedures not only because of their obvious requirement that the child be exposed to x-rays and that this exposure limits the length of the experiment, but also because of the tremendously involved data analysis procedure. Simply put, radiographic (still photos as well as cinematic film) procedures present potential health hazards because of x-ray exposure which suggests that they are not the most appropriate to be used with children; however, continuing development of the microbeam x-ray (e.g., Kiritani, 1977; Edward, 1984) holds promise for future work in this area. This is not to say that EMG data analysis procedures are not equally involved but relatively speaking EMG onset and offset of muscle activity is readily analyzable and directly related to most descriptive/ hypothetical questions considered. The flexible fiber optic naso-laryngoscope can also be positioned in the nostril so as to study certain aspects of velar portal activity (e.g., Benguerel et al., 1977); however, this is an invasive procedure which many children, under 7 years of age and their parents, would not readily tolerate. Ultrasonic procedures could also be used to study articulatory behavior (e.g., Minifie et al., 1973; Watkin et al., 1978), but procedural difficulties with "locating" a small moving object like the tongue of a child with the ultrasonic beam makes this procedure of limited use (Hamlet and Reid, 1974). Furthermore, ultrasonic data analysis is quite problematic because the derived data can be noisy and difficult to interpret. Magnetometers and strain gauges have been used and hold promise for use in the study of articulatory structure displacement, especially jaw and lip movement; however, we hesitate to predict success with these methods with children because to our knowledge they have only been used with adults. What experience we have had with the excellent strain gauge transducer system developed by Abbs and colleagues at Wisconsin suggests, as mentioned above, that it (1) is best used with children of 7 years and older and (2) needs special adaptations in terms of weight, size and manner of mounting on head. Photography can provide information regarding lip and jaw movement, but it is a difficult to automate procedure. Methods for measuring intra-oral pressure are necessarily invasive, but for bilabial stop consonants a pressure-measuring probe placed just inside the lips (e.g., Rothenberg, 1981) could conceivably be used with some youngsters and we fully expect in years to come that such a procedure will see wider usage.

The remaining methods - surface electromyography and acoustic analysis - can provide a wide range of information regarding a child's articulatory behavior. We have had extensive, and on the whole, satisfactory experiences with surface electromyography study of youngsters' labial activity (Caruso, Conture and Colton, in press, 1986). Surface EMG provides information regarding the relative level, onset/offset and duration of articulatory muscle activity and extra-oral (acoustic) pressure contains indirect information about articulatory gestures and steady-state positions. We selected these two procedures - surface EMG and speech sound spectrography - because of they are relatively nonintrusive with regard to speech movements, they are non-invasive, and they provide data which can be compared and contrasted to speech acoustic/production data obtained with adult stutterers (for example, Fibiger, 1971; Hutchinson, 1974; Ford and Luper, 1975; Love and Jeffress, 1972; Shapiro, 1980; Stromsta and Fibiger, 1980; Zimmermann, 1980a,b). To date, we have completed two studies (Zebrowski, Conture and Cudahy, 1985; Caruso, Conture and Colton, in press) reporting the successful use of these procedures with small children who stutter.

In summary, our experience with the instrumental study of the temporal aspects of young stutterers' speech production suggests that respiratory behaviors can be adequately and reliably assessed by means of an inductive plethysmograph (Respitrace), that laryngeal behavior can be similarly assessed by an electroglottograph and supraglottal articulatory activity of lip muscles can be meaningfully studied by surface electromyography. Various other procedures are available or are being developed which may also be useful for studying this population, for example, simultaneous EGG and inverse-filtering volume velocity airflow, x-ray microbeam system, spring-loaded headmount strain gauge transducer system, and the "Selspot" or optoelectrical movement sensing system. Whatever the instrumentation, whatever the procedure and whatever the intent of the study, objective assessment of young stutterers' speech production will necessitate a compromise between the *realities* of what these youngsters can and will do and the *ideal* procedures for collecting speech production data.

REFERENCES

Abbs, J.H. & Watkin, K. (1976). Instrumentation for the study of speech physiology. In N. Lass (Ed.), *Contemporary issues in experimental phonetics.* New York: Academic Press.

Abbs, J.H. & Gilbert, B. (1973). A strain gauge transducer system for lip and jaw motion in two dimensions. *Journal of Speech and Hearing Research, 16,* 248-256.

Adams, M.R., Freeman, F. & Conture, E.G. (1984). Laryngeal Dynamics in Stuttering. In W. Perkins & R. Curlee (Eds.), *Nature and Treatment of Stuttering: New Directions.* San Diego, Calif.: College-Hill Press.

Adams, M.R., Guitar, B. & Conture, E.G. (1979). Clinical questions: ask the experts - a review of biofeedback procedures for school-age stutterers. *Journal of Childhood Communication Disorders, 3,* 1-12.

Andrews, G. & Harris, M. (1964). *The Syndrome of Stuttering.* London: Spastics Society Medical Education and Information Unit in association with Wm. Heinemann Medical Books, Ltd.

Baer, T., Lofqvist, A. & McGarr, N. (1983). Laryngeal vibrations: a comparison between high-speed film and glottographic techniques. *Haskins Laboratories Status Report on Speech Research, SR-73,* 283-291.

Baken, R. (1977). Estimation of lung volume change from torso hemicircumferences. *Journal of Speech and Hearing Research, 20,* 808-812.

Baken, R., Cavallo, S. & Weissman, K. (1979). Chest wall movements prior to phonation. *Journal of Speech and Hearing Research, 22,* 862-872.

Baken, R., McManus, D.A. & Cavallo, S. (1984). Prephonatory chest wall posturing in stutterers. *Journal of Speech and Hearing Research, 26,* 444-450.

Barlow, S., Cole, K. & Abbs, J.H. (1983). A new headmounted lip-jaw movement transduction system for the study of motor speech disorders. *Journal of Speech and Hearing Research, 26,* 283-288.

Barr, H. (1940). A quantitative study of the specific phenomena observed in stuttering. *Journal of Speech Disorders, 5,* 277-280.

Basmajian, J. (1979). *Muscles alive-their functions revealed by electromyography.* (4th Ed.) Baltimore, Maryland: Williams and Wilkins.

Benguerel, A., Hirose, H., Sawashima, M. & Ushijima, T. (1977). Velar coarticulation in French: A fiberscopic study. *Journal of Phonetics, 5,* 159-166.

Bless, D., Hunker, C. & Weismer, G. (1981). Comparison of noninvasive methods to obtain chest-wall displacement and aerodynamic measures during speech. *Tenth Symposium: Care of the Professional Voice.* New York: Voice foundation, Inc.

Blood, G. & Seider, R. (1981). The concomitant problems of young stutterers. *Journal of Speech and Hearing Disorders, 46,* 31-33.

Bloodstein, O. (1981). *A Handbook on Stuttering.* Third Edition. Chicago, Ill.: National Easter Seal Society.

Borden, G., Baer, T. & Kenney, M. (1985). Onset of voicing in stuttered fluent utterances. *Journal of Speech and Hearing Research, 21,* 285-294.

Branscom, M., Hughes, J. & Oxtoby, E. (1955). Studies of nonfluency in the speech of preschool children. In W. Johnson & R. Leutenegger (Eds.), *Stuttering in Children and Adults.* Minneapolis, Minn.: University of Minnesota Press.

Brutten, G. (1975). Stuttering: topography, assessment and behavior-change strategies. In J. Eisenson (Ed.), *Stuttering: A Second Symposium.* New York: Harper and Row.

Caruso, A., Conture, E.G. & Colton, R. (in press). Speech physiology associated with young stutterers' stutterings. Manuscript submitted for publication in *Journal of Speech and Hearing Research.*

Caruso, A., Gracco, V.L. & Abbs, J.H. (1987). *A speech motor control perspective on stuttering: preliminary observations.* In H.F.M. Peters & W. Hulstijn (Eds.), *Speech Motor Dynamics in Stuttering.* Wien: Springer Verlag.

Casper, J. (1983). *Frequency perturbation in normal speakers: A descriptive and methodological study.* Unpublished Doctoral dissertation, Syracuse University, Syracuse, NY.

Childers, D.G. & Krishnamurthy, A.K. (1984). A critical review of electroglottography. *CRC Critical Reviews in Biomedical Engineering,* 12, 131-161.

Childers, D.G., Moore, G., Naik, J. Larar, J. & Krishnamurthy, A.K. (1983). Assessment of laryngeal function by simultaneous synchronized measurement of speech, electroglottography and ultra-high speed film. *Eleventh Symposium: Care of the Professional Voice.* New York: Voice Foundation, Inc.

Colton, R., Reed, G., Sagerman, R. & Chung, N. (1982). *Investigation of voice change after radiotherapy.* Final Report to National Cancer Institute, National Institute of Health.

Colton, R., Brewer, D. & Rothenberg, M.A. (1983). *Journal of Otolaryngology, 12,* 291-294.

Conture, E.G. (1982). *Stuttering.* Englewood Cliffs, NJ.: Prentice-Hall, Inc.

Conture, E.G. (1982a). Youngsters who stutter: diagnosis, parent counseling, and referral. *Journal of Developmental Behavioral Pediatrics, 3,* 163-169.

Conture, E.G.& Caruso, A. (1978). A review of the Stocker Probe Technique for diagnosis and treatment of stuttering in young children. *Journal of Fluency Disorders, 3,* 297-298.

Conture, E.G., McCall, G. & Brewer, D. (1977). Laryngeal behavior during stuttering. *Journal of Speech and Hearing Research, 20,* 661-668.

Conture, E.G., Rothenberg, M.A. & Molitor, R. (1986). Electroglottographic observations of young stutterers' fluency. *Journal of Speech and Hearing Research, 29,* 384-393.

Conture, E.G., Schwartz, H.D. & Brewer, D. (1985). A further study of laryngeal behavior during stuttering. *Journal of Speech and Hearing Research, 28,* 233-240.

Conture, E.G.& Schwartz, H.D. (1984). Children who stutter: diagnosis and remediation. *Communicative Disorders, 9,* No. 1.

Cullinan, W. & Springer, M. (1980). Voice initiation and termination times in stuttering and nonstuttering children. *Journal of Speech and Hearing Research, 23,* 344-360.

Daly, D. (1981). Differentiation of stuttering subgroups with Van Riper's developmental tracks: a preliminary study. *Journal of the National Student Speech Hearing Association, 9,* 89-101.

Dejonckere, P. (1981). Comparison of two methods of photoglottography in relation to electroglottography. *Folia Primatol., 33,* 338-347.

DiSimoni, F. (1974a). Effect of vowel environment on the duration of consonants in three-, and nine-year-old children. *Journal of the Acoustical Society of America, 55,* 360-361.

DiSimoni, F. (1974b). Some preliminary observations on temporal compensations in the speech of children. *Journal of the Acoustical Society of America, 56,* 697-699.

DiSimoni, F. (1974c). Preliminary study of certain timing relationships in the speech of stutterers. *Journal of the Acoustical Society of America, 56,* 695-696.

Dossey, L. (1982). *Space, Time and Medicine.* Boulder, Colo.: Shambhala Publications, Inc.

Edward, J. (1984). Contextual effects on lingual-mandibular coordination. *Haskins Laboratories Report on Speech Research, SR 79/80,* 39-48.

Fibiger, S. (1971). Stuttering explained as a physiological tremor. *STL-QPSR,* Stockholm, Sweden: Royal Institute of Technology, *2-3,* 1-23.

Folkins, J. & Kuehn, D.P. (1982). Speech Production. In N. Lass, L. McReynolds, J. Northern & D. Yoder (Eds.), *Speech, Language and Hearing: Normal Processes.* (Vol 1) Philadelphia, Penna: W.B. Saunders. 246-285.

Ford, S. & Luper, H. (1975). *Aerodynamic, phonatory and labial EMG patterns during fluent and stuttered speech.* A paper presented to the Annual Convention of the American Speech and Hearing Association.

Fourcin, A. (1974). Laryngographic examination of vocal fold vibration. In B. Wyke (Ed.), *Ventilatory and Phonatory Control Systems.* London, England: Oxford University Press. 315-333.

Fourcin, A. (1981). Laryngographic assessment of phonatory function. In C. Ludlow & M. Hart (Eds.), *Proceedings of the Conference on the Assessment of Vocal Pathology.* ASHA Reports 11, Danville, Ill.: Interstate Printers.

Fourcin, A. & Abberton, E. (1971). First application of a new laryngograph. *Medical and Biological Illustrations, 23,* 172-183.

Freeman, F. & Ushijima, T. (1978). Laryngeal muscle activity during stuttering. *Journal of Speech and Hearing Research, 21,* 538-562.

Gay, T., Ushijima, T., Hirose, H. & Cooper, F.S. (1974). Effect of speaking rate on labial consonant-vowel articulation. *Journal of Phonetics, 2,* 47-63.

Gilbert, H., Potter, C. & Hoodin, R. (1984). Laryngograph as a measure of vocal fold contact area. *Journal of Speech and Hearing Research, 27,* 178-182.

Gregory, H. (1973). *Stuttering: differential evaluation and therapy.* Indianapolis, Ind.: Bobbs-Merill.

Hamlet, S. & Reid, J. (1974). Transmission of ultrasound through the larynx as a means of determining vocal fold activity. *IEEE Trans. Biomed. Eng., BME-19,* 1073-1077.

Harris, K.S. (1981). Electromyography as a technique for laryngeal investigation. In C. Ludlow & M. Hart (Eds.), *Proceedings of the Conference on the Assessment of Vocal Pathology.* ASHA Reports 11, Danville, Ill.: Interstate Printers.

Healey, E.C. (1982). Speaking fundamental frequency characteristics of stutterers and nonstutterers. *Journal of Communication Disorders, 15,* 21-29.

Hillman, R. & Gilbert, H. (1977). Voice onset time for voiceless stop consonants in the fluent reading of stutterers and nonstutterers. *Journal of the Acoustical Society of America, 61,* 610-611.

Hixon, T. (1971). An electromagnetic method for transducing jaw movements during speech. *Journal of the Acoustical Society of America, 49,* 603-606.

Hixon, T., Goldman, M. & Mead, J. (1973). Kinematics of the chest wall during speech production: Volume displacements of the rib cage, abdomen and lung. *Journal of Speech and Hearing Research, 16,* 78-115.

Hixon, T., Mead, J. & Goldman, M (1976). Dynamics of the chest wall during speech production: Function of the thorax, rib cage, diaphragm, and abdomen. *Journal of Speech and Hearing Research, 19,* 297-356.

Honda, K. (1983). Relationship between pitch control and vowel articulation. *Haskins Laboratories Status Report on Speech Research, SR-73,* 269-282.

Hutchinson, J. (1974). Aerodynamic patterns of stuttered speech. In L.M. Webster & C. Furst (Eds.), *Vocal Tract Dynamics and Dysfluency.* New York: Speech and Hearing Institute of New York.

Isley, C. & Basmajian, J. (1973). Electromyography of the cheeks and lips. *Anatomical Record, 176,* 145-148.

Johnson, W., Darley, F. & Spriestersbach, D. (1963). *Diagnostic Methods in Speech Pathology.* New York: Harper and Row.

Kelso, J.A.S., Tuller, B. & Harris, K.S. (1984). A theoretical note on speech timing. *Haskins Laboratories Status Report on Speech Research, SR-79/80,* 161-166.

Kennedy, J.G. & Abbs, J.H. (1979). Anatomic studies of the perioral motor system: foundations for studies in speech physiology. In N. Lass (Ed.), *Speech and Language: Advances in Basic Research and Practice.* Vol. 1. New York, NY: Academic Press. 211-220.

Kent, R. (1972). Some considerations in the cinefluorographic analysis of tongue movement during speech. *Phonetica, 26,* 16-32.

Kiritani, S. (1977). Articulatory studies by the x-ray microbeam system. In M. Sawashima & F. Cooper (Eds.), *Dynamic Aspects of Speech Production.* Tokyo, Japan: University of Tokyo Press. 171-190.

Kitzing, P. (1982). Photo- and electroglottographical recording of the laryngeal vibratory pattern during different registers. *Folia Phoniatrica, 34,* 234-241.

Klatt, D. (1975). Voice onset time, frication and aspiration in wordinitial consonant clusters. *Journal of Speech and Hearing Research, 18,* 686-706.

Kuksht, M. (1975). *Electromyographic, aerodynamic and displacement characteristics of bilabial consonants.* Unpublished M.S. thesis, University of Washington, Seattle.

Leanderson, R. & Lindblom, B. (1972). Muscle activation for labial speech gestures. *Acta Otolaryngology, 73,* 362-363.

Lecluse, F.L.E. (1976). *Laboratory investigations in electroglottography.* XVIth International Congress of Logopedics. Basel, Switzerland: Karger, 294-296.

Lecluse, F.L.E., Brocaar, M. & Verschuure, J. (1975). The electroglottography and its relation to glottal activity. *Folia Phoniatrica, 27,* 215-224.

Lindblom, L. & Oeberg, K. (1974). An opto-electronic instrument for remote on-line movement monitoring. *Biotelemetry, 1,* 94-95.

Love, L. & Jeffress, L. (1971). Identification of brief pauses in the fluent speech of stutterers and non-stutterers. *Journal of Speech and Hearing Research, 14,* 229-240.

MacCurtain, F. & Fourcin, A. (1982). Application of the electroglottograph wave-form display. In V. Lawrence (Ed.), *Transcripts of the Tenth Symposium: Care of the Professional Voice.* New York, NY.: Voice Foundation.

McClean, M., Goldsmith, H. & Cerf, A. (1984). Lower-lip EMG and displacement during bilabial disfluencies in adult stutterers. *Journal of Speech and Hearing Research, 27,* 342-349.

Merits-Patterson, R. & Reed, C. (1981). Disfluencies in the speech of language-delayed children. *Journal of Speech and Hearing Research, 24,* 55-58.

Metz, D. Conture, E.G.& Caruso, A. (1979). Voice onset time, frication and aspiration during stutterers' fluent speech. *Journal of Speech and Hearing Research, 22,* 649-656.

Metz, D. Conture, E.G.& Colton, R. (1976). Temporal relationships among respiratory and laryngeal systems prior to fluent and stuttered utterances. *ASHA, 18,* 664. (Abstract)

Metz, D. & Folkins, J. (1985). Protection of human subjects in speech and hearing research. *ASHA, 27,* 25-29.

Metz, D., Samar, V. & Sacco, P. (1983). Acoustic analysis of stutterers' fluent speech before and after therapy. *Journal of Speech and Hearing Research, 26,* 531-536.

Metz, D., Whitehead, R. & Whitehead, B. (1984). Mechanics of vocal fold vibration and laryngeal articulatory gestures produced by hearing-impaired speakers. *Journal of Speech and Hearing Research, 27,* 62-69.

Minifie, F. Kelsey, C., Zagzebski, J. & King, T. (1971). Ultrasonic scans of the dorsal surface of the tongue. *Journal of the Acoustical Society of America, 49,* 1857-1860.

Morris, R., Blashfield, R. & Satz, P. (1981). Neuropsychology and cluster analysis: potentials and problems. *Journal of Clinical Neuropsychology, 3,* 79-99.

Muller, E. & Abbs, J.H. (1979). Strain gauge transduction of lip and jaw motion in the midsagital plane: Refinement of a prototype system. *Journal of the Acoustical Society of America, 65,* 481-486.

Ng, T. & Rothenberg, M.A. (1982). A matched delay approach to substantive linear phase high-pass filtering. *IEEE Transactions on Circuits and Systems, CAS-29,* 8, 584-587.

O'Dwyer, N, Quinn, P. Guitar, B., Andrews, G. & Neilson, P. (1981). Procedures for verification of electrode placement in EMG studies of orofacial and mandibular muscles. *Journal of Speech and Hearing Research, 24,* 273-288.

Perkins, W.H., Rudas, J., Johnson, L. & Bell, J. (1976). Stuttering: Discoordination of phonation with articulation and respiration. *Journal of Speech and Hearing Research, 19,* 509-522.

Preus, A. (1982). *Identifying subgroups of stutterers.* Oslo, Norway: Universitetsforlaget.

Prins, D. & Lohr, F. (1972). Behavioral dimensions of stuttered speech. *Journal of Speech and Hearing Research, 15,* 61-71.

Rentschler, G. (1984). Effects of subgrouping in stuttering research. *Journal of Fluency Disorders, 9,* 307-312.

Riley, G. (1972). A stuttering severity instrument for children and adults. *Journal of Speech and Hearing Disorders, 37,* 314-321.

Riley, G. (1980). *Stuttering Severity Instrument: For Children and Adults.* Tigand, OR: CC Publishing Inc.

Riley, G. & Riley, J. (1982). Evaluating stuttering problems in children. In H. Luper (Ed.), Intervention with the young stutterer. *Journal of Childhood Communication Disorders, VI,* No. 1.

Rothenberg, M.A. (1968). The breath-stream dynamics of simple-released-plosive production. *Biblioteca Phonetica,* No. 6.

Rothenberg, M.A. (1977). Measurement of airflow in speech. *Journal of Speech and Hearing Research, 20,* 155-176.

Rothenberg, M.A. (1981). Some relations between glottal air flow and vocal fold contact area. In C. Ludlow & M. Hart (Eds.), *Proceedings of the Conference on the Assessment of Vocal Pathology.* ASHA Reports 11, Danville, Ill.: Interstate Printers.

Sackner, M.A. (1979). Monitoring of ventilation without physical connection to the airway: A review. A paper presented at the Third International Symposium on Ambulatory Monitoring. Harrow, Middlesex, U.K.

Schwartz, H.D., Conture, E.G. & Gleason, J. (1982). Subgrouping young stutterers: preliminary observations. Paper presented to annual meeting of American Speech Language Hearing Association. Toronto, Ontario.

Schwartz, H.D. (1984). Subgrouping young stutterers: a behavioral/physiological perspective. Ph.D. dissertation. Syracuse University, Syracuse, New York.

Shapiro, A. (1980). An electromyographic analysis of the fluent and dysfluent utterances of several types of stutterers. *Journal of Fluency Disorders, 5,* 203-231.

St. Onge, A. (1963). The stuttering syndrome. *Journal of Speech and Hearing Research, 6,* 195-197.

Starkweather, C.W. (1982). Stuttering and laryngeal behavior: a review. *ASHA Monographs,* No. 21.

Stocker, B. (1976). *The Stocker Probe Technique Manual.* Tulsa, OK.: Modern Educational Corp.

Stromsta, C. & Fibiger, S. (1980). *Physiological correlates of the core behavior of stuttering.* Paper presented to XVIIIth IALP Congress, Washington, DC.

Sussman, H., MacNeilage, P.F. & Hanson, R. (1973). Labial and mandibular movement dynamics during the production of bilabial stop consonants. *Journal of Speech and Hearing Research, 16,* 379-420.

Tuller, B. & Kelso, J.A.S. (1984). The timing of articulatory gestures: evidence for relational invariants. *Haskins Laboratories Status Report on Speech Research, SR-79/80,* 49-64.

Van Riper, C. (1971). *Nature of Stuttering.* First Edition. Englewood Cliffs, NJ.: Prentice-Hall, Inc.

Van Riper, C. (1982). *Nature of Stuttering.* Second Edition. Englewood Cliffs, NJ.: Prentice-Hall, Inc.

Wall, M. & Myers, F. (1984). *Clinical Management of Childhood Stuttering.* Baltimore, Maryland: University Park Press.

Watkin, K., Minifie, F. & Kennedy, J.G. (1978). An ultrasonic-EMG transducer for biodynamic research. *Journal of Speech and Hearing Research, 21,* 174-182.

Watson, H. (1979). The technology of respiratory inductive plethysmograph. Paper presented to the Third International Symposium on Ambulatory Monitoring. Clinical Research Center, Harrow, Middlesex, U.K.

Watson, H. & Alfonso, P.J. (1982). A comparison of LRT and VOT values between stutterers and nonstutterers. *Journal of Fluency Disorders, 7,* 219-242.

Williams, D. (1978). Differential diagnosis of disorders of fluency. In F. Darley & D. Spriestersbach (Eds.), *Diagnostic Methods in Speech Pathology.* New York, NY.: Harper and Row. 284-321.

Zebrowski, P. Conture, E.G.& Colton, R. (1984). Temporal relations in young stutterers' fluent speech physiology. Paper presented to Annual Conference of American Speech-Hearing-Language Association. San Francisco, California.

Zebrowski, P. Conture, E.G.& Cudahy, E. (1985). Acoustic analysis of young stutterers' fluency: preliminary observations. *Journal of Fluency Disorders, 10,* 173-192.

Zimmermann, G. (1980a). Articulatory dynamics of fluent utterances of stutterers and nonstutterers. *Journal of Speech and Hearing Research, 23,* 95-107.

Zimmermann, G. (1980b). Articulatory behaviors associated with stuttering: a cinefluorographic analysis. *Journal of Speech and Hearing Research, 23,* 108-121.

Chapter **8**

Measuring Stutterers' Dynamical Vocal Tract Characteristics by X-ray Microbeam Pallet Tracking

Peter J. Alfonso, Ben C. Watson and Thomas Baer

Stuttering is generally considered to be a disorder of motor timing, yet neither the nature of the spatiotemporal interruptions of speech movements nor the physiological level(s) at which they occur is sufficiently understood. In particular, two critical questions that bear on the nature and treatment of stuttering, and by extension, the role of timing in various aspects of normal speech production remain unanswered. The first question concerns the anatomical locus of disordered motor timing. To what extent is the aberrant neuromuscular and kinematic activity that is associated with moments of stuttering specific to a single anatomical structure rather than spread throughout the speech production system? An aberrant state associated with a single structure, the larynx for example, might trigger abnormal activity in the respiratory and/or supralaryngeal systems. In this example, where laryngeal dysfunction precedes respiratory and supralaryngeal dysfunction, the activity of the latter systems might be viewed as compensatory rather than as an integral part of the stuttering breakdown. That is, the respiratory and supralaryngeal systems might be functioning to maintain appropriate temporal relationships with the abnormal laryngeal gestures. The alternative possibility to the stuttering locus question is that multiple components, for example the respiratory-laryngeal complex, or perhaps the complete speech production system, fail simultaneously. The second question is concerned with the temporal extent of the disruption. To what extent are the kinematic patterns in stutterers' perceptually fluent speech similar to those in the fluent speech of normal talkers? The answer to the second question will help determine whether the stutterers' speech motor system exhibits generalized spatiotemporal abnormalities regardless of the perceived fluency, or whether, alternatively, it behaves normally except during moments of observable stuttering.

One reason that the exact nature of the motor timing deficit is not better understood is related to the difficulties associated with obtaining sufficient amounts of physiological data, especially data pertaining to the activity patterns of the speech musculature and the movements of the speech structures. On the other hand, acoustic data are plentiful, owing to the fact that they are non-invasive and simple to collect. Indeed, the inferences about speech movements that we have made from acoustic signals have taught us much about various general characteristics of the disorder. Although the acoustic representation of speech reflects underlying articulatory events, the acoustic signal is related to speech movements in a complex way that does not permit the unambiguous recovery of the articulatory patterns responsible for its generation. For this reason, a major emphasis in the study of the physiological processes underlying stutterers' fluent and disfluent speech must be a direct examination of the articulatory kinematics involved in speech production, with analysis of simultaneous acoustic recordings.

The primary purpose of this chapter is to describe a powerful technique for gathering kinematic data on the supralaryngeal articulators, namely x-ray microbeam pellet-tracking. As an example of this technique, the methodologies employed in an x-ray microbeam experiment designed to address the two questions posed earlier will be presented. It should be noted that, in order to meet the primary purpose of the chapter, it is necessary to focus on supralaryngeal kinematics, even though the experiment monitored respiratory, laryngeal, and acoustic signals in parallel with x-ray microbeam pellet-tracking of the upper articulators. The benefits gained from analyzing kinematic data collected simultaneously from multiple components of the speech production system, particularly in the case of stutterers, have been presented elsewhere (Baer and Alfonso, 1984; Borden and Watson, 1986, this volume).

X-RAY MICROBEAM PELLET-TRACKING

Although less invasive techniques are available to capture the movements of the accessible articulators, for example tracking infrared light emitting diodes attached to the lips and jaw, cineradiography is the technique traditionally used to track movements of the most inaccessible articulators, namely the tongue and velum. A serious experimental drawback with conventional cineradiography is that, due to the radiation hazard to the subject, exposure times are limited to about three minutes. Clearly, this restricts the amount of data that can be obtained from a normal subject, but given the nature of stuttering, the restriction becomes increasingly severe. For example, the duration of a single disfluency can amount to a significant portion of the allowed exposure time. The subject safety hazard and the restrictive amount of data one can collect with cineradiography have spurred the development of other distinct-point measurement techniques to monitor movements of the inaccessible articulators. These include the alternating magnetic field system (Perkell & Cohen, 1985) and tongue pellet-tracking by ultrasound imaging (Shawker, Stone, and Sonies, 1985). Although these new techniques are potentially useful, technical improvements are needed before they can match the proven utility of x-ray microbeam pellet-tracking.

The x-ray microbeam pellet-tracking system prototype was developed at the Research Institute of Logopedics and Phoniatrics at the University of Tokyo, and has been operational since 1975. The system has been described in detail elsewhere (Fujimura, Kiritani, and Ishida, 1973; Kiritani, Itoh, and Fujimura, 1975). A second generation system, under development at the University of Wisconsin, will facilitate the collection of vocal-tract movement data along with simultaneous respiratory and laryngeal kinematic, EMG, and acoustic data. From a research point of view, the primary advantage of the microbeam system over traditional cineradiography is that allowable exposure times are significantly increased to about 45 to 60 minutes. With respect to subject safety, the x-ray microbeam system is advantageous in that the radiation level is significantly lower than cineradiography. These advantages are obtained because the microbeam system steers a narrow focused x-ray beam at relatively small regions of the head. The beam is directed by a computer-controlled system that predicts the two-dimensional position of each pellet based on its previous position, and then scans only the appropriate region. Thus, rather than radiate a large area of the subject's head as in traditional x-ray, the x-ray microbeam radiates only small areas around pellet locations, which usually include the lips, jaw, tongue, and velum. Exposure is further reduced because the pellet-locations are radiated for only a small portion of each measurement frame.

THE EXPERIMENT

This experiment examined the spatial and temporal coordination among the respiratory, laryngeal, and supralaryngeal systems during stutterers' fluent and disfluent speech in order to address the two questions stated above. To meet the primary purpose of this chapter, however, it is necessary to restrict the discussion to that portion of the experiment that compares the kinematics of the upper articulators in the perceptually fluent speech of one severe stutterer with that of a normal subject.

The experiment was carried out at the University of Tokyo using the x-ray microbeam pellet-tracking system to monitor the movements of the jaw, lips, tongue blade, and velum. Lead pellets, approximately 2.5 mm in diameter, were attached to each of these articulators. Because of their small size and mass, the pellets do not seem to impede normal articulation. Respitrace inductance plethysmography was used to monitor movements of the thorax and abdomen, and a Synchrovoice electroglottograph was used to infer movements of the vocal folds. For the portion of the experiment we report here, subjects were required to produce nonsense syllables, for example /etete/, in response to a pair of signals. Reaction-time is not the primary concern of the experiment. Rather, the paradigm represents a convenient way to measure relative displacement and appropriate peak velocity relationships derived from a quantifiable starting position.

The procedures used for this experiment were as follows. Subjects were instructed to begin inhalation when a computer-generated oscilloscope display indicated that the system had captured the locations of all the pellets. A programmable timer presented a sequence of two lights to the subject and a corresponding sequence of tones to the instrumentation recorder. The first light was presented at a random interval after inhalation onset. The subject was instructed to respond to this light by producing the vowel /e/ as quickly as possible and sustaining this vowel until the presentation of the second light. At that time, the subject was required to produce /pepe/, /tete/, /sese/, or /nene/ as quickly as possible. Primary stress was always on the first syllable. The interval between the first and second lights was either 500, 1000, or 2000 msec and the order of presentation was randomized. Subjects produced about 12 repetitions of each of the four nonsense syllables.

Figure 1 shows one sequence of events produced by the normal subject. The top record shows the 1 kHz pure tone. The onset of this tone corresponds to presentation of the first light, the offset to presentation of the second light. The next three records represent vertical displacement of the tongue blade, lower lip, and jaw respectively and were obtained by x-ray microbeam pellet-tracking. The jaw trajectory has been subtracted from the tongue and lip trajectories. The fifth record represents the electroglottograph

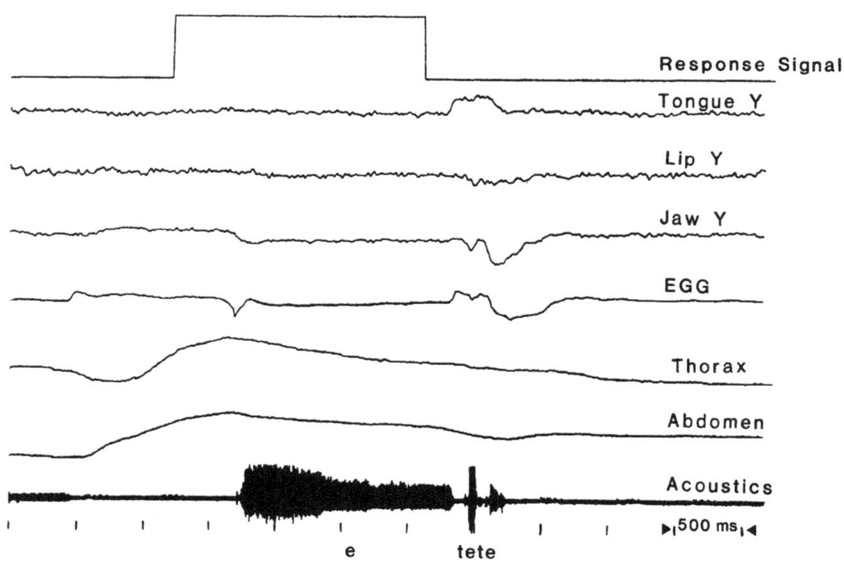

Figure 1. Normal subject's production of /etete/ in the nonsense syllable condition. A description of the data channels is given in the text.

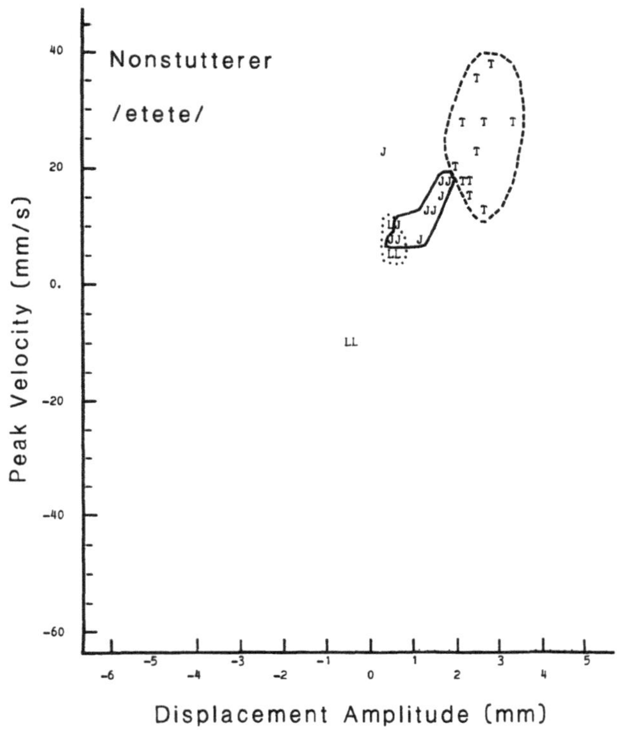

Figure 2. Displacement amplitude-peak velocity plot for the initial /t/ closing gesture in the nonstutterer's production of /etete/.

signal. Although this signal shows effects of high-pass filtering, the signal can be used to indicate the timing of vocal fold contact at adduction and separation of the vocal folds at abduction. Upward and downward displacement of this signal corresponds to decreasing and increasing vocal fold contact, respectively. The sixth and seventh records show thoracic and abdominal displacements. Expansion is upward, compression is downward. The bottom record shows the acoustic response.

Analyses of articulator movements following the first light extends the results of previous reaction-time experiments (Watson and Alfonso, 1982, 1983, 1987, this volume Chapter 13) in which respiratory and laryngeal prephonatory and phonatory movements were examined in parallel with the acoustic output in isolated vowel responses.

The data analyzed thus far seem to show that the severe stutterer used in the present experiment initiates respiratory compression before laryngeal adduction in producing the initial vowel as did the severe stutterers in previous work. Figure 1 demonstrates that respiratory-laryngeal-articulatory coordination in the present experiment can be analyzed similarly to respiratory-laryngeal coordination in isolated vowel responses.

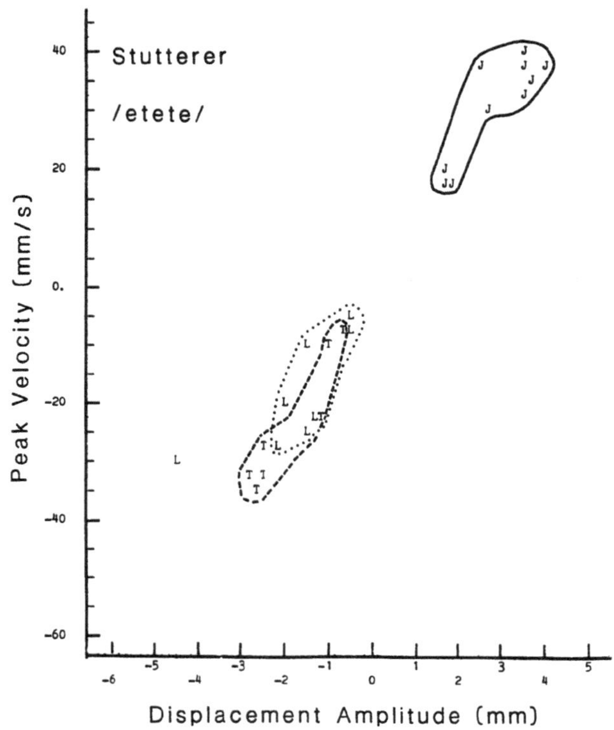

Figure 3. Displacement amplitude-peak velocity plot for the initial /t/ closing gesture in the stutterer's fluent productions of /etete/.

Articulation movements following the second light are shown in Figures 2 through 5. For all of the figures, the ordinate represents peak velocity in mm/sec and the abscissa represents displacement amplitude in mm. Figure 2 shows the relationship between these two parameters for closing gestures of the initial /t/ in /etete/ produced by the normal subject. The symbols L, T, and J represent individual token values for lower lip, tongue and jaw movements respectively. For example, the figure shows that five tokens of lip displacement and derived velocity, and 10 and 11 tokens of the same parameters for jaw and tongue movements, respectively, were measured. For the sake of clarity, the majority of data points for a single articulator have been enclosed within an ellipse. For the reasons given above, the discussion will concentrate primarily on jaw and tongue articulation. Note first that the same general relationship between displacement amplitude and peak velocity that has been reported for limb movements and lip and jaw movements (Kelso, Vatikiotis-Bateson, Saltzman, and Kay, 1985) holds for these data. That is, peak velocity increases as displacement amplitude increases. Note also that the range of displacement amplitudes and peak velocity for the tongue and jaw is distinct. Closure is achieved with elevation of both the tongue and jaw, where tongue elevation is always greater than jaw elevation.

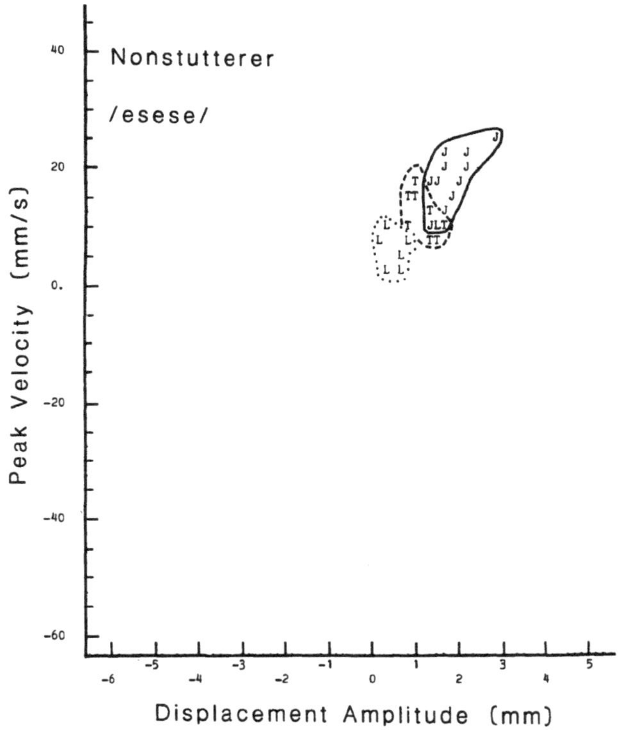

Figure 4. Displacement amplitude-peak velocity plot for the initial /s/ closing gesture in the nonstutterer's productions of /esese/.

Figure 3 shows displacement amplitude versus peak velocity for the stutterer's fluent productions of the same phonetic utterance shown in Figure 2. Note first that, in general, the linear relationship between displacement amplitude and peak velocity is present in the stutterer's data. In general, these and additional data indicate that the relationship between displacement amplitude and peak velocity does not distinguish stutterers from nonstutterers. However, a comparison of Figures 2 and 3 shows that the organization and precision of the closing gesture for /t/ is clearly different between the two subjects. Figure 2 shows that the nonstutterer achieves closure with complementary displacement of the jaw and tongue. Figure 3, on the other hand, shows that the stutterer achieves the same gesture with paradoxical jaw and tongue movements. That is, closure is achieved by jaw elevation and tongue blade lowering. More importantly, in view of the often reported idiosyncratic differences in tongue/jaw synergies, note that the stutterer produces the closing gesture with a wider range of displacement amplitude and peak velocity values than does the nonstutterer. Thus, the stutterer produces multiple repetitions of the same gesture with greater variability than the normal subject.

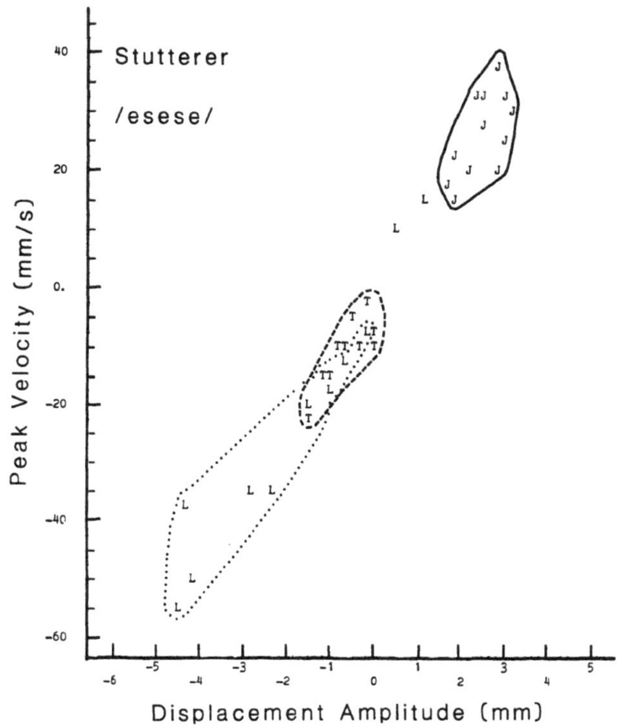

Figure 5. Displacement amplitude-peak velocity plot for the initial /s/ closing gesture in the stutterer's fluent productions of /esese/.

Figure 4 shows the same kinematic parameters for the nonstutterer's closing gesture for initial /s/ in /esese/. In general, the displacement-velocity relationship for /s/ appears similar to that shown for /t/ in Figure 2. Note, that as in Figure 2, the nonstutterer achieves closure with complementary displacement of the tongue and jaw, although the synergy is different for /s/ closure than for /t/ closure. For /s/, the normal subject uses greater jaw elevation than tongue elevation to achieve the target position. Recall that for /t/ closure, he uses greater tongue elevation than jaw elevation. This reversal appears to reflect the tongue's greater contribution to shape than to elevation for /s/ than for /t/, and the jaw's compensation for the decrease in tongue elevation for /s/. A comparison of Figures 2 and 4 also shows that articulator variability is somewhat reduced for /s/ closures as compared to /t/ closure. The data presented in Figure 4 are more representative of the variability associated with closure and release gestures for these and other phonetic environments produced by the normal subject. The data shown in Figure 2 represents the gesture that produced the greatest variability for this subject.

Figure 5 shows the stutterer's data for fluent productions of /esese/. As was the case for /t/ closure, the stutterer achieves /s/ closure primarily through jaw elevation with little or no vertical assist of the tongue. In general, the stutterer, unlike the normal subject, achieves /s/ and /t/ closure with paradoxical vertical movements of the tongue blade and jaw. Closure is achieved primarily through jaw elevation for both /s/ and /t/. With respect to the between subject comparison of the variability associated with articulator displacement amplitude and peak velocity, the differences noted in Figures 2 and 3 are also observed in Figures 4 and 5. That is, the ranges of displacement amplitude and peak velocity for each of the articulators in the stutterer's data are greater than those observed in the nonstutterer's data. In fact, the coefficient of variation (the ratio of the mean and standard deviation) for displacement amplitude for these and data not reported here is approximately two and a half times greater for the stutterer than for the nonstutterer.

SUMMARY

We must emphasize that the data presented here are preliminary in that they are based on few observations taken from two subjects. Additional stutterers and control subjects need to be studied. Nevertheless, the differences between the two subjects with respect to the variability associated with the organization of the tongue and jaw for repeated fluent productions of the same phonetic context are striking and most interesting. In fact, when one considers the constraints imposed by the experimental paradigm, and that the utterances are perceptually fluent, it is interesting that any differences were found at all.

Our understanding of the physiology of stutterers' disfluent and perceptually fluent speech should increase as our ability to monitor the movements of multiple articulators increases. For example, the recently available data on lip and jaw interaction, articulators that can be monitored with relative ease, have proven quite useful. Information about the tongue, and how it behaves in concert with other structures, should prove even more useful in that the tongue's contribution to overall vocal-tract shaping is greater than any other single articulator. Finally, x-ray microbeam pellet-tracking will not only increase the data base on the complete set of upper articulators, but it will also provide for the examination of the supralaryngeal system in reference to respiratory and laryngeal movements since signals from the three systems can be monitored simultaneously.

ACKNOWLEDGEMENTS

Research reported here was supported by NIH Grants NS-13617 and 1-T32-NS-07237 awarded to Haskins Laboratories and by a grant from the Stuttering Center, Baylor College of Medicine. We are indebted to the staff of the Research Institute of Logopedics and Phoniatrics, University of Tokyo, Japan for their assistance in subject selection and data collection.

REFERENCES

Baer, T. & Alfonso, P.J. (1984). On simultaneous neuromuscular, movement, and acoustic measures of speech articulation. In R.G. Daniloff (Ed.), *Articulation Assessment and Treatment Issues.* San Diego: College Hill Press. 195-214.

Borden, G. & Watson, B.C. (1987). Methodological aspects of simultaneous measurements: Limitations and possibilities. In H.F.M. Peters & W. Hulstijn (Eds.) *Speech motor dynamics in stuttering .* Wien: Springer Press.

Fujimura, O., Kiritani, S. & Ishida, H. (1973). Computer controlled radiography for observation of movement of articulatory and other human organs. *Comp. Biol. Med, 3,* 371-384.

Kelso, J.A.S., Vatikiotis-Bateson, E., Saltzman, E. & Kay, B. (1985). A qualitative analysis of reiterant speech production: Phase portraits, kinematics, and dynamic modeling. *Journal of the Acoustical Society of America, 77,* 1, 266-280.

Kiritani, S., Itoh, K. & Fujimura, O. (1975). Tongue-pellet tracking by a computer controlled microbeam system. *Journal of the Acoustical Society of America, 57.*

Perkell, J.S. & Cohen, M.H. (1985). Design and construction of an alternating magnetic field system for transducing articulatory movements in the midsagittal plane. *Journal of the Acoustical Society of America, 77,* S99.

Shawker, M.D., Stone, M. & Sonies, B.C. (1985). Tongue pellet tracking by ultrasound: Development of a reverberation pellet. *Journal of Phonetics,* in press.

Watson, B.C. & Alfonso, P.J. (1982). A comparison of LRT and VOT values between stutterers and nonstutterers. *Journal of Fluency Disorders, 7,* 219-241.

Watson, B.C. & Alfonso, P.J. (1983). Foreperiod and stuttering severity effects on acoustic laryngeal reaction time. *Journal of Fluency Disorders, 8,* 183-205.

Watson, B.C. & Alfonso, P.J. (1987). Coordination of prephonatory events in mild and severe stutterers. In H.F.M. Peters & W. Hulstijn (Eds.), *Speech motor dynamics in stuttering.* Wien: Springer Press.

Watson, B.C. & Alfonso, P.J. (In Press). Physiologcial bases of LRT in nonstutterers, mild stutterers, and severe stutterers. *Journal of Speech and Hearing Research.*

Chapter 9

Brain Electrical Activity Mapping: Applications to Vocal Motor Control Disorders

Kenneth Pool, Frances J. Freeman, Therese Finitzo

Brain Electrical Activity Mapping (BEAM) is a recently developed analytic tool for examining both electroencephalographic (EEG) and evoked potential (EP) data. Specifically BEAM overcomes several of the limitations which have hampered full use of these approaches, especially as applied to disorders of speech motor control. This chapter discusses rationale for development of BEAM, briefly describes the technology, and presents findings from initial studies of patients with two vocal motor control disorders - spasmodic dysphonia (SD) and stuttering (ST).

ELECTROENCEPHALOGRAPHY AND EVOKED POTENTIALS

In the past, EEG has been used to examine electrocortical activity in both spasmodic dysphonia and stuttering (Knott, Correll, and Shepherd, 1959; Robe, Brumlik, and Moore, 1960; Fritzell, Petersen, and Sellden, 1965; and Sayles, 1971). While reports have varied as to the frequency of abnormalities, certainly some changes were accurately observed in some patients. However, for the most part, findings have been non-specific and poorly localized and have not contributed significantly to our understanding of either disorder. For every positive report in the literature, there have been conflicting negative reports.

These ambiguous and non-specific findings are not surprising since the classical analysis of EEG is hampered by serious limitations. First, representation of electrical activity as an analog waveform makes interpretation highly dependent on gestalt pattern recognition. This is especially true since rigorously defined normal ranges cannot be easily applied to analog data. Second, the EEG contains a tremendous amount of information (between 500,000 to 24,000,000 pieces, depending on the items examined). With classical visual evaluation, this is more data than can be processed, so much is ignored. Third, in the analog recording all frequencies are intermixed so that the examiner must attempt to visually separate these for consideration. This problem is compounded since certain visual patterns (i.e. alpha rhythm in a normal recording speed) are more easily recognized than others. This visual sensitivity disparity leads to biased amplitude estimates of various frequencies. Finally, mechanical EEG output systems are limited in resolution, both in amplitude and time. Since amplitude and timing are critical factors in determining significance and localization, this is a crucial limit.

While these limitations have not prevented classical EEG from contributing greatly to our understanding and detection of certain disorders, they restrict and hamper recognition and definition of more subtle disruptions of electrocortical function.

In the last decade, our ability to examine CNS dysfunctions has been extended by the use of evoked potentials (EPs), which have revealed many new insights in neurologic diseases. The majority of these insights involve impulse transmission. Through this approach, white fiber tracts have come within our analytic range.

Generally, EPs are simultaneously recorded from a limited number of sites (typically 1 to 4). These sites are selected to maximize detection of specific waveforms. For peak latency measurements this approach has validity; however, it results in a very limited examination of the cortical surface area.

Further, examination of the EP waveform is generally limited to peak latencies. This information, for the most part, reveals white fiber tract transmission velocity rather than grey matter activity. In considering evoked potentials, it is important to remember that latencies are predominantly related to white fiber transmission time, whereas amplitudes are generally related to generator sites. Examination of amplitudes is seldom performed, except for occasional peak amplitude and amplitude ratios. More detailed examination of amplitude is limited by the amount of data and determination of baselines.

Recent studies of EPs in stutterers and spasmodic dysphonic subjects have suffered from these limitations, but have none-the-less generated intriguing findings. Auditory Brainstem Responses (ABR) have been most extensively examined. For stutterers (Pinsky and McAdam, 1980; Stager, Finitzo and Freeman, 1982; Decker, Healey and Howe, 1982) and patients with SD (Finitzo-Hieber et al., 1982; Schaefer et al., 1983) abnormalities in interpeak latency measurements have been noted. However, in SD, the most common abnormality has been found in Wave V latency prolongations when using high stimulus repetition rates to stress the auditory system.

BRAIN ELECTRICAL ACTIVITY MAPPING - BEAM TECHNIQUE AND METHODOLOGY

For this approach, EEG electrodes are placed at 25 sites over the scalp (including three extracerebral monitors and two earlobe references by the 10-20 International System (Figure 1). The data are amplified by standard EEG amplifiers. This amplified data are then digitized at a rate of 240 Hz (4 msec samples) into epochs of 10 second duration. The two second epochs are then visually inspected for artifacts and those epochs to be used in spectral analysis are selected. The selected epochs are subjected to fast fourier transformation (FFT) to produce amplitude-frequency curves from .5 Hz to 32 Hz in .5 Hz increments. This is performed on each two second epoch from each electrode. Generally, at least thirty, two second epochs are analyzed at each electrode. The epochs are the same for all electrodes. The FFT curves from each two second epoch are averaged for each electrode producing an average FFT for each electrode at the 20 sites over the scalp.

Similar EEG data collection has been carried out in the past on normal populations (separated by age decade in adults) and is contained in the resident data base of the system (Duffy, 1982). In addition to these normal average FFT curves, the standard deviation FFT curves have been determined. This data base allows calculation of the number of standard deviations a subject's data differs from the normal at each frequency step at each electrode.

Once this data has been collected and processed, it is displayed by color graphics. Data are used to generate images repre-

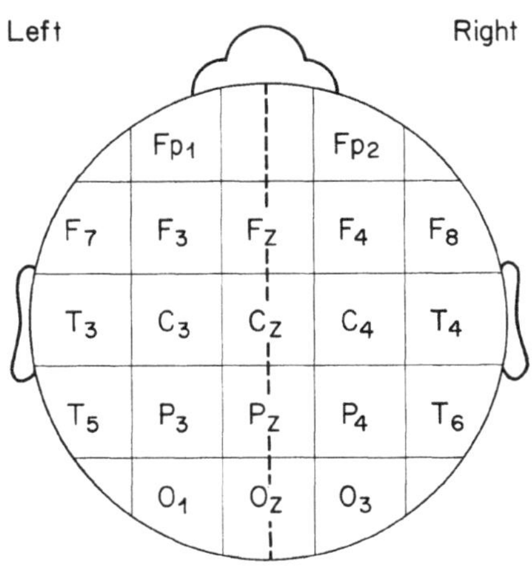

Figure 1. Schematic representation of recording sites.
A schematic, superior view of the head, identifying recording sites for BEAM studies. F identifies frontal; T is temporal; C is central; P is parietal; O is occipital; Odd numbers are sites on the Left; Even numbers are sites on the Right; z indicates midline sites. This schematic facilitates consideration of abnormalities identified in Tables 1-3. For example, "Left mid-Temporal" identifies abnormal electrocortical events at site T3.

senting amplitudes or standard deviations from normal. EEG data may be displayed over any selected frequency band. Typically, and in the present studies, bands used are Delta .5-3.5 Hz, Theta 4.0-7.5 Hz, Alpha 8.0-11.5 Hz, Beta1 12.0-15.5 Hz, Beta2 16.0-19.5 Hz, Beta3 20.0-23.5 Hz, and Total .5-32 Hz.

BEAM evoked potentials may be recorded with any stimulus technique. For the studies reported in this chapter, auditory and flash visual EPs are reported. EP waveforms are simultaneously recorded from each electrode used in the EEG analysis described above. The digitization rate remains 250 Hz. The stimuli are delivered pseudorandomly between 1.25 and 1.75 per stimulus. Activity is averaged for a 512 msec pre-stimulus period and a 512 msec post-stimulus period. Again, as with the EEG data, age-dependent normative collections have been made in the past, and these along with standard deviations of the amplitudes at each sample point are resident in the system. Similar color graphic displays are created representing amplitude, polarity or standard deviations for each 4 msec measurement. The 128 post stimulus images (mappings) are either viewed one at a time or displayed in rapid succession in a movie or cartoon format.

APPLICATION TO VOCAL MOTOR CONTROL DISORDERS

The BEAM studies described in the remainder of this chapter are part of an ongoing research effort at the Center for Vocal Motor Control of the University of Texas at Dallas. Our current line of research in stuttering and spasmodic dysphonia is based on three assumptions:

1) Both disorders have a common critical component - disordered vocal motor control.

2) At least substantial subgroups of patients with these disorders have CNS dysfunction(s) which underly disruption of normal vocal motor control.

3) Understanding of these two disorders, and of central nervous system mechanism(s) of vocal motor control, will be advanced more rapidly by comparison/contrast studies of these disorders than by the study of either in isolation.

Much of our approach is further based in the observation that neither disorder (in the majority of patients) involves gross or widespread CNS lesions - rather they represent relatively specific, focal, and/or subtle CNS dysfunction. Therefore we have focused on electrical measurements reflecting the dynamic character of the cortex. The VMC disorders represent disrupted *dynamics* in neurologic control, and electrical measurements are therefore highly likely to be productive.

The basis for grouping stuttering and spasmodic dysphonia together as disorders of vocal motor control can be traced to the Conference on Vocal Tract Dynamics and Dysfluency (Webster and Furst, 1975). Participants there attempted to draw together all existing evidence, direct or inferential, relating to the issue of hypothesized laryngeal involvement in stuttering. In this context McCall (1975) presented a paper which drew on his studies of SD (conducted in conjunction with Rabuzzi, 1972; Brewer, Colton and Skolnick, 1971). He compared critical features of spasmodic dysphonia with stuttering. In the discussion of his presentation, the term *vocal motor control disorders* was used, perhaps for the first time, with respect to these disorders.

McCall and the present authors, while recognizing the multiple clinical features which differentiate stuttering and SD, have chosen to concentrate on their common features, particularly the common dysfunction in fine control of volitional phonation. Support for such a view is drawn from EMG studies of vocal control in stuttering (Freeman, 1977; Freeman and Ushijima, 1978; Shapiro, 1980; Adams, Freeman, and Conture, 1984), from finding of ameliorative speaking conditions in SD (Freeman, Cannito, and Finitzo, 1984a, Freeman, Cannito and Finitzo, 1984b) and from studies demonstrating that SD is neither a psychogenic nor a peripheral neurogenic disorder (Feldman, Nixon, Finitzo, Freeman, 1984; Finitzo-Hieber, Freeman, Gerling et al., 1982; Schaefer, Freeman, Finitzo et al., 1985).

Hypotheses

The primary hypotheses of this study held that electrocortical activity in patients with VMC disorders would be abnormal in the fronto-temporal areas and in the paramedian frontal area. The motor control of the larynx in the fronto-temporal area was the basis for the first hypothesis and the supplementary speech area in the paramedian frontal area was the basis for the second. We predicted that other cortical areas would be normal in VMC subjects.

Subjects

A total of seventeen subjects are reported here. Thirteen of these have spasmodic dysphonia, three are stutterers and one has inspiratory laryngeal spasm. The patient with inspiratory adductor vocal fold spasms is included to allow differentiation of features which are specific to VMC from those which may represent less specific motor control disorders or contributions of respiratory abnormalities.

Results

Findings are presented in Tables 1-3 and summarized in Figure 2. In all cases, for an abnormality to be identified, the region must consistently be more than three standard deviations from the mean of the age-matched control group. Results in subjects with spasmodic dysphonia and preliminary findings in stutterers are remarkably similar in distribution. The principle difference between the groups, not clearly reflected in Figure 2, lies in the severity of their abnormalities.

Spasmodic dysphonic subjects generally demonstrated greater deviations from normal means than stutterers. The absence of EEG spectral changes, and generally less frequent and less abnormal EP amplitudes suggest more normal electrocortical function in stutterers. The number of stutterers examined to date is too few to allow definitive statements regarding disease specific comparisons, but

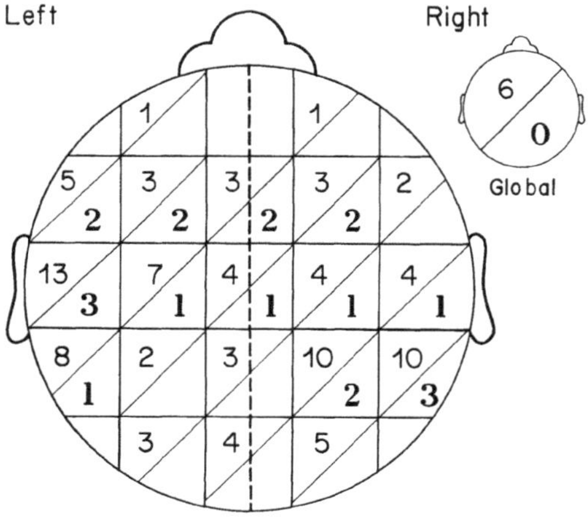

Figure 2. Total identified abnormalities: SD patients/stutterers.
A schematic, superior view of the head (parallel to Fig. 1) with total numbers of abnormalities noted in 13 SD patients for each site, indicated by light numbers on the upper/left, and total numbers of abnormalities noted in three Stuttering subjects for each site, indicated by dark numbers on the lower/right. The smaller figure in the upper right indicates the six global abnormalities identified in SD patients.

findings do suggest common regional dysfunction in these two disorders.

Abnormalities in the fronto-temporal regions in SD patients and stutterers are consistent with our first hypothesis. This represents the region of principle pyramidal control of the larynx. The anatomic resolution of the BEAM is not sufficient, as yet, to allow specific localization to the laryngeal motor cortex, but findings are consistent with such a localization.

Abnormalities in the paramedian frontal cortex are confirmatory of the second hypothesis. The expectation is that this represents electrical dysfunction in the supplementary speech area; but again insufficient anatomic resolution precludes precise localization.

Identification of these dysfunction areas is encouraging because of their relationship to classical concepts of speech generation. More detailed analyses of a larger number of subjects is clearly needed to elucidate relationship(s) of specific responses (i.e. generators) to clinical manifestations.

The absence of consistent abnormalities in the vocal control territories of the patient with inspiratory laryngeal spasms suggests that our findings are somewhat specific to vocal motor control. The number of non-VMC patients clearly must be extended to confirm this suspicion.

The occurrence of right parietal abnormalities in the VMC subjects was unexpected, but sufficiently consistent to necessitate consideration. The role of this area in motor processes in general and/or VMC processes in particular, is unclear. It is possible that this area is related to the underlying pathophysiology; or it is possible that this area is functioning in an abnormal manner as a result of the disordered motor control rather than as a mechanism in its generation.

Table 1. EEG analysis

Patient Number	Clinical Problem	Classical EEG Abnormalities	BEAM Spectral Analysis Abnormalities
1	SD	Global Beta Increase	Left Central Delta increase Global Beta 1 & 2 increase
2	SD	Left Temporal Slow	Left Temporal & Right Temporal Delta increase Left Temporal Theta increase
3	SD	Left Temporal & Right Frontal Slow (borderline)	Bilateral Occipital Posterior Temporal, Beta 1 increase Left Temporal increased Theta variability Right Temporal increased Alpha variability
4	SD	None	Global increased Delta (borderline)
5	SD	None	None
6	SD	None	Right Occipital Parietal Delta increased
7	SD	None	None
8	SD	None	Normal variant Mu Rhythm
9	SD	None	None
10	SD	None	Global Beta 3 increased
11	SD	(borderline)	None
12	SD	Diffuse Slow	Global increased Theta, greater Biparietally
13	ST	None	None
14	ST	None	Excessive Asymetry, Right Parietal Delta
15	ST	None	None
16	IS	None	None

SD - Spasmodic Dysphonia ST - Stutterer IS - Inspiratory Spasms

Table 1. (continued) AER analysis

Patient Number	Clinical Problem	Classical AER Abnormalities	BEAM AER Abnormalities
1	SD	Delayed with normal pattern	Paramedian Frontal
2	SD	None	Left Frontal Temporal Right Frontal Right Posterior Temporal Parietal
3	SD	None	Left Paramedian Frontal Bioccipitally (borderline)
4	SD	None	Left Temporal Right Temporal Parietal
5	SD	Delayed with normal patterns	Delayed: normal topology
6	SD	None	Left Frontal Temporal
7	SD	None	Paramedian Frontal Left Mid-temporal
8	SD	None	Left Temporal (borderline) Right Posterior Temporal Occipital
9	SD	None	Right Posterior Temporal Parietal
10	SD	None	Global changes (borderline)
11	SD	None	Left Temporal Central
12	SD	None	Left Temporal
13	ST	None	Right Temporal (mild)
14	ST	None	Bifrontal, greater Left Frontal Temporal
15	ST	None	Left Temporal Right Parietal
16	IS	None	None

SD - Spasmodic Dysphonia ST - Stutterer IS - Inspiratory Spasms

Table 1. (continued) VER analysis

Patient Number	Clinical Problem	Classical VER Abnormalities	BEAM VER Abnormalities
1	SD	None	None
2	SD	Waveform Morphology	Left Frontal Temporal Right Frontal Temporal Right Parietal
3	SD	None	Right Parietal Posterior Temporal Bilateral Central
4	SD	None	Paramedian Central Parietal
5	SD	None	None
6	SD	None	Left Frontal Temporal Right Central Temporal Parietal Occipital
7	SD	None	Left Frontal Temporal
8	SD	None	Right Temporal
9	SD	None	None
10	SD	None	Bioccipital (mild)
11	SD	None	Global, greater Central
12	SD	None	None
13	ST	None	Right Temporal (borderline)
14	ST	None	Bilateral Frontal Central Left Temporal
15	ST	None	Left Frontal Temporal Right Posterior Temporal Parietal
16	IS	None	None

SD - Spasmodic Dysphonia ST - Stutterer IS - Inspiratory Spasms

This study has provided us with dramatic and encouraging findings in subjects with VMC. The electrocortical measures need to be extended in terms of numbers of subjects, disorders examined, and scope of electrocortical measurements. Understanding the patterns and dynamics of electrocortical dysfunction in individuals with VMC will hopefully lead us to new insights in management.

ACKNOWLEDGEMENTS

This research has been supported by NINCDS Grant #NS18276. The contributions of Michael Cannito, Ph.D., are gratefully acknowledged. We further wish to thank Lisa Williams for her assistance in preparing this manuscript. We are also endebted to Don N. Shannon, M.D., for identification and referral of the patient with inspiratory spasms; and to all our patients, whose persevering cooperation make this work possible. We note that data on 10 of the SD subjects was originally reported by Cannito, M., Finitzo, T., Freeman, F. and Pool, K. at the Spring Meeting of the Acoustical Society of America, Austin, Texas, April, 1985 (ABS. Journal of the Acoustical Society of America, 1985: 77 Suppl 1: S87; 4: 37).

REFERENCES

Adams, M.R., Freeman, F. & Conture, E. (1984). Laryngeal Dynamics of Stutterers. In Curlee & Perkins (Eds.), *Nature and Treatment of Stuttering*. College Hill Press.

Decker, T., Hely, E. & Howe, S. (1982) Brainstem auditory electrical response characteristics of stutterers and nonstutterers: A preliminary report. *Journal of Fluency Disorders, 7,* 385-389.

Duffy, F. (1982). Topographical display of evoked potentials: clinical applications of Brain Electrical Activity Mapping (BEAM). *Annals NY Acad. Science, 388,* 183-196.

Feldman, M., Nixon, M., Finitzo-Hieber, T. & Freeman, F. (1984). Abnormal parasympathetic function in spasmodic dysphonia. *Annals of Internal Medicine, 100,* 491-495.

Finitzo-Hieber, T., Freeman, F., Gerling, I., Dobson, L. & Schaefer, S. (1982). Auditory brainstem response abnormalities in adductor spasmodic dysphonia. *American Journal of Otolaryngology, 3,* 26-30.

Fox, D.R. (1966). Electroencephalographic analysis during stuttering and nonstuttering. *Journal of Speech and Hearing Research, 9,* 488-497.

Freeman, F. (1977). *The Stuttering Larynx.* Doctoral Dissertation, City University of New York.

Freeman, F. & Ushijima, T. (1978). Laryngeal muscle activity during stuttering. *Journal of Speech and Hearing Research, 21,* 538-562.

Freeman, F., Cannito, M. & Finitzo, T. (1984a). Ameliorative speaking conditions in spasmodic dysphonia. 13th Juillard Conference on Care of the Professional Voice.

Freeman, F., Cannito, M. & Finitzo, T. (1984b). Getting to know spasmodic dysphonia patients. *Texas: Journal of the Texas Speech Hearing Association,* 12-19.

Fritzell, B., Petersen, I. & Sellden, U. (1965). An EEG study of stuttering and nonstuttering school children. *De Therapia Vocis et Loquelae, Vol. 1.* VIII Congr., Int. Soc. Logoped. Phoniat.

Knott, J.R., Correll, R.E. & Shepherd, J.N. (1959). Frequency analysis of electroencephalograms of stutterers and nonstutterers. *Journal of Speech and Hearing Research, 2,* 74-80.

McCall, G. (1975). Spasmodic Dysphonia and the Stuttering Block: Commonalities or Possible Connections. *Vocal Tract Dynamics and Dysfluency.* New York: Speech and Hearing Institute.

McCall, G.N., Skolnick, M.L. & Brewer, D. (1971). A preliminary report of some atypical movement patterns of the tongue, palate, hypopharynx and larynx of patients with spasmodic dysphonia. *Journal of Speech and Hearing Disorders, 36,* 466-470.

Pinsky, S.D. & McAdam, D.W. (1980). Electroencephalographic and dichotic indices of cerebral laterality in stutterers. *Brain and Language, 11,* 374-397.

Rabuzzi, D. & McCall, G. (1972). Spasmodic dysphonia: A clinical perspective. *Trans. Am. Acad. Opthalmol. Otolaryngol., 76,* 724-728.

Robe, E., Brumlik, J. & Moore, P. (1960). A study of spastic dysphonia, *Laryngoscope, 70,* 219-245.
Sayles, D.G. (1971). Cortical excitability, perseveration, and stuttering. *Journal of Speech and Hearing Research, 14,* 462-475.
Schaefer, S., Finitzo-Hieber, T., Gerling, I. & Freeman, F. (1983). Brainstem conduction abnormalities in spasmodic dysphonia. *Annals of Otology, Rhinology and Laryngology, 92,* 59-65.
Schaefer, S., Freeman, F., Finitzo, T., Close, L., Cannito, M., Ross, E., Reish, J. & Maravilla, K. (1985, in press). MRI findings in spasmodic dysphonia patients. *Annals of Otology Rhinology and Laryngology.*
Shapiro, A.I. (1980). An electromyographic analysis of the fluent and dysfluent utterances of several types of stutterers. *Journal of Fluency Disorders, 5,* 203-232.
Stager, S., Freeman, F. & Finitzo-Hieber, T. (1982). Patterns of auditory brain stem response in stutterers. American Speech-Language-Hearing Association, Toronto, Canada, November 1982.
Webster, M. & Furst, L. (Eds.) (1975). *Vocal Tract Dynamics and Dysfluency.* New York: Speech and Hearing Institute.

ADDITIONAL READINGS ON BEAM TECHNOLOGY

Burchfiel, J., Duffy, F., Bartels, P. & Needleman, H. (1980). The combined discriminating power of quantitative EEG and neuropsychologic measures in evaluating central nervous system effects of lead at low levels. In H.L. Needleman (Ed.), *Low Level Lead Exposure: The Clinical Implications of Current Research.* Raven Press.
Duffy, F. (1981). Brain electrical activity mapping (BEAM): Computerized access to complex brain function. *International Journal of Neuroscience, 13,* 55-65.
Duffy, F., Burchfiel, J. & Lombroso, C. (1979). Brain electrical activity mapping (BEAM): A method for extending the clinical utility of EEG and evoked potential data. *Annals of Neurology, 5,* 309-321.
Duffy, F., Denckla, M., Bartels, P., Sandini, G. & Kiessling (1980a). Dyslexia: Automated diagnosis by computerized classification of brain electrical activity. *Annals of Neurology, 7,* 421-426.
Duffy, F., Denckla, M., Bartels, P. & Sandini, G. (1980b). Dyslexia: Regional differences in brain electrical activity mapping. *Annals of Neurology, 7,* 412-420.
Morchesa, J., Duffy, F., Wyatt, R. (1983). Brain electrical activity mapping (BEAM) in schizophrenic patients. *Arch. Gen. Psychiatry, 40,* 719-728.

Chapter 10

Dynamic Characteristics of Vocal Frequency Tracking in Stutterers and Nonstutterers

Harvey B. Nudelman, K.E. Herbrich, B.D. Hoyt and D.B. Rosenfield

The production of speech requires delicate coordination between laryngeal, articulatory and respiratory systems. Neurophysiology suggests that this coordination is achieved through the use of negative feedback control systems. That is, the central nervous system monitors proprioceptive feedback from these systems while it also monitors speech output through the auditory system. Actual speech output is compared to desired output, and corrective adjustments are made. Systems that use feedback (closed looped systems), like the CNS, are capable of much finer control than those that do not (open loop systems) because of their ability to monitor performance and make adjustments in their output. The price paid for this increase in performance is the possibility of the system becoming unstable, i.e., the adjustments that are made tend to degrade the performance rather than improve it. It is proposed to model stuttering as such an instability in the speech motor system. By studying the causes of these instabilities, we can understand the conditions leading to the production of a stuttered disfluency.

To understand the causes of instability in the speech motor control system (SMCS), the dynamic relationships between its input and output must be determined. The complete description of these dynamic relationships requires a differential equation. This can be better understood using the following analogy:

Consider throwing a ball in the air ten times, each time the ball having a different trajectory. One can describe the dynamics of this experiment by using an algebraic expression to describe each trajectory as a function of time. This description of the dynamics requires separate expressions for each toss. However, a more efficient way of describing this experiment is to write the differential equation from Newton's Law that describes the position of the ball as a function of time. Here, the solution of the differential equation describes all the trajectories and each individual trajectory is determined by the application of the initial conditions, i.e., the position, speed and angle of the ball at release.

Systems Analysis provides an empirical method for determining the equivalent of the differential equation for a linear system. A system is linear if the following property holds:

```
I1 ----> SYSTEM ----> 01                Property
I2 ----> SYSTEM ----> 02                   1
(a x I1)+(b x I2) ----> SYSTEM ----> (a x 01)+(b x 02)
      where a and b are constants.
```

If a system is linear, a sine wave input (I1) into that system will result in a sine wave output (01) with a different amplitude and phase but the same frequency. Similarly, a different sine wave input (I2) will yield a sine wave output (02) having a different amplitude and phase but the same frequency:

$$A \sin(wt) \text{ ----> SYSTEM ----> } B \sin(wt + \phi)$$

where A and B are constants reflecting the amplitude of the sine waves.

Gain is defined as B/A, and phase is the angle ϕ. If we measure the gain and phase for various input frequencies, we then have the equivalent of the differential equation of the system. This is true because of Property 1 (above) and the fact that any arbitrary input function may be written as a weighted sum of sine waves. The dynamic relationship between the input and output of a complex nonlinear system may be approximated by a form of Taylor Series expansion, around an operating point, consisting of a linear term and a sum of nonlinear terms (Anand, 1974; Milsum, 1966).

We contend that during vocal tracking the complex nonlinear system of speech production (composed of the respiratory, laryngeal and articulatory motor systems) can be adequately described by the linear term, as described above. A vocal tracking paradigm was used in which the subject hummed and attempted to match the changing frequency of a computer generated tone (Leonard and Ringel, 1979). The dynamic relationships (gain and phase as defined above) between the subject's output and the computer generated input were measured. By calculating gain and phase for various input frequencies, an equivalent of the differential equation of the system was established. In other words, we have a testable mathematical approximation of the dynamics of the speech motor control system.

METHODS AND RESULTS

The input of our vocal frequency tracking paradigm is a computer generated pure tone which is frequency modulated, i.e. frequency varies as a function of time, around a center frequency (CF, an individually selected operating point chosen such that the modulations can be easily matched). The tone was modulated about this center frequency in the form of sine and square waves (.3 to 4 Hz modulation frequency), ramps, and random steps. These tones were presented to the subjects through a free field speaker at 80-90 dB SPL. The subjects were instructed to match, by humming, the frequency of these tones. They were allowed to listen once to each type of modulation. They were not allowed to practice the tracking task. This subject's voice, transduced by a throat mike, and the test signals were tape recorded. The recorded signals were A/D converted at 10 kHz and a cycle by cycle instantaneous frequency versus time was calculated using a slope and threshold criterion.

Three right-handed, adult male fluent speakers, ages 21-44, one of whom is a professional singer, were evaluated. These were compared to four right-handed, adult males, who were diagnosed as stutterers by at least two certified speech-language pathologists.

Figure 1 shows responses to ramps of several velocities.

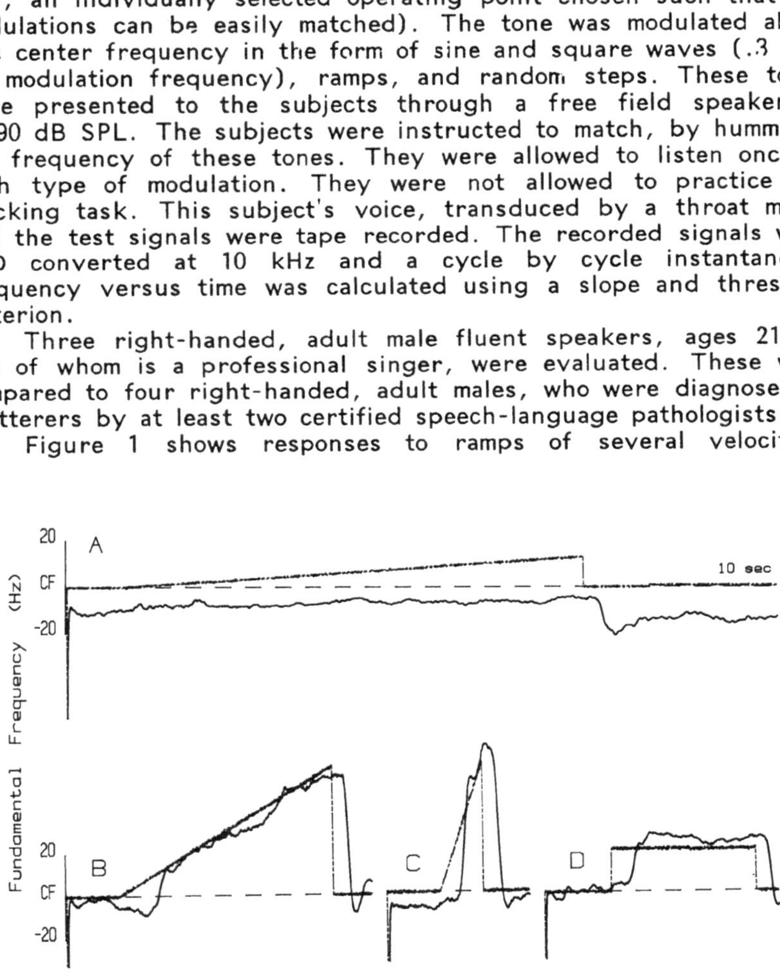

Figure 1. Plots of instantaneous fundamental frequency. The broken line represents the computer generated tone, the solid line represents the subject's voice.

(A) A male fluent speaker tracking a 2 Hz/sec ramp. Total amplitude of displacement=13 Hz, CF=135 Hz.

(B) A female fluent speaker tracking a 20 Hz/sec ramp. Total amplitude of displacement=60 Hz, CF=240 Hz.

(C) Same female tracking a 100 Hz/sec ramp. Total amplitude of displacement=60 Hz, CF=240 Hz.

(D) Same female tracking a step. Total amplitude of displacement=20Hz, CF=253 Hz.

Reaction time to the input ramp is inversely related to the ramp's velocity (i.e., faster ramps are associated with shorter reaction times). Note in Figure 1A that the subject responds only to the end of the ramp, indicating that he is responding to velocity as well as displacement of the tone.

Figure 2A and B are examples of the instantaneous frequencies of the tone the subject heard and the fundamental frequency that he produced to track it. *It is emphasized that these waveforms are not the sound waves but the time course of the fundamental frequency of the voice and tone sound waves.* The subject's response to the first modulated cycle exhibits a reaction time delay, but the responses to later cycles do not exhibit this delay. In this chapter, we shall analyze only these responses to periodic inputs, which are referred to as predictable responses (Stark, Vossius and Young, 1962).

The similarity of the response curve in Figure 2A to a sine wave suggests that the linear component of the response may predominate. This was tested by performing a FFT on each cycle of the longest segment of contiguous predictable data for each sinusoidal trial at ±20 Hz amplitude of modulation. The number of cycles analyzed varied from one at .3 Hz to 23 at 4.0 Hz modulation

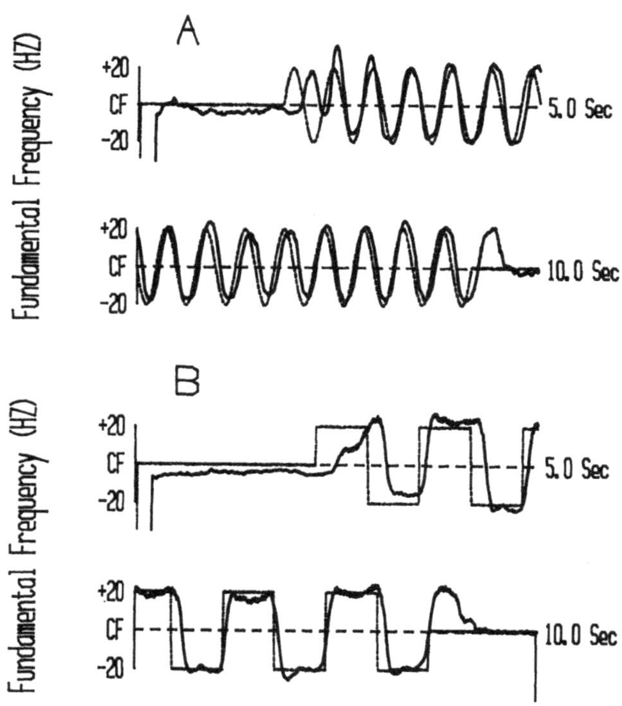

Figure 2. Plots of instantaneous fundamental frequency. The broken line represents the computer generated tone, the solid line represents the subject's voice. (A) A male fluent speaker tracking a 2.0 Hz sine wave at ±20 Hz amplitude of modulation. CF=122 Hz. (B) A male fluent speaker tracking a 0.78 Hz square wave, ±20 Hz amplitude of modulation. CF=131 Hz.

frequency. The FFT's show that the amplitude of the linear component (the one at the input frequency) averaged 5.5 ± 2.6 (range 1.7 to 13.1) times the largest nonlinear component (the ones not at the input frequency) across all modulation frequencies. These numbers suggest that the linear term may be a good approximation of the system. For the linear term, the gain and phase, with respect to the input sine wave, are the parameters of the system for this operating point. To arbitrarily decide whether or not a subject was "matching" the faster modulation frequencies (2, 3 & 4 Hz/second), the time it took for him to produce ten complete cycles was measured. If this time was within 5% of the time of ten tone cycles, then it was assumed that the subject was tracking the input modulation frequency.

Each subject's average gain and phase shift were calculated from the linear component, as determined from the FFT's, and plotted as a function of modulation frequency in Figure 3A. These individual curves are arranged in order of increasing performance, where ideal performance is defined as a gain of one for all modulation frequencies. Curves i-iv represent the stutterers and curve vii represents the professional singer. The average phase shifts for all stutterers and all fluent speakers are plotted in Figure 3B. Ideal performance corresponds to a phase shift of zero. Differences between individuals and groups are modulation frequency dependent. Stutterers are not a homogeneous group (Van Riper, 1971; Rosenfield, 1984), and our measures allow quantification of this heterogeneity. In our limited sample, all stutterers differ, within one standard deviation, from all nonstutterers at 2 and 3 Hz modulation frequency with respect to phase shift, and three are significantly different (at 2 Hz modulation frequency) with respect to gain.

If the linear term is a valid descriptor of the SMCS, conditions described by Property 1 should hold. This was easily tested because a square wave may be written as a weighted sum of sine waves of its odd harmonic frequencies (Anand, 1974). Each subject's response to square wave modulations was predicted by forming the sum of the square wave's components, adjusted for the subject's gains and phase shifts in the .3 Hz to 4 Hz range of this study. Figure 4 shows typical model predictions of responses to different input modulation frequencies and, for one subject(v), different amplitudes of modulation. Note that the model agrees in amplitude and phase for amplitudes of modulation larger (±30 Hz) and smaller (±10 Hz) than those from which the model parameters were derived (±20 Hz). This extends our description of SMCS dynamics to include the physiologic fundamental frequency range of English declarative sentences (Cooper & Sorenson, 1981).

Using Fourier analysis, SMCS adjustments during speech can be decomposed into sinusoids of different frequencies (i.e., their frequency content). For example, a 2 Hz modulation corresponds to a SMCS adjustment every 250 msec, close to the average syllable nucleus time in running speech (Shoup, Lass & Kuehn, 1982). It should be noted that fluent speakers' performance at a 2 Hz modulation frequency approaches ideal, whereas the stutterers deviate from ideal performance with respect to phase or gain or both.

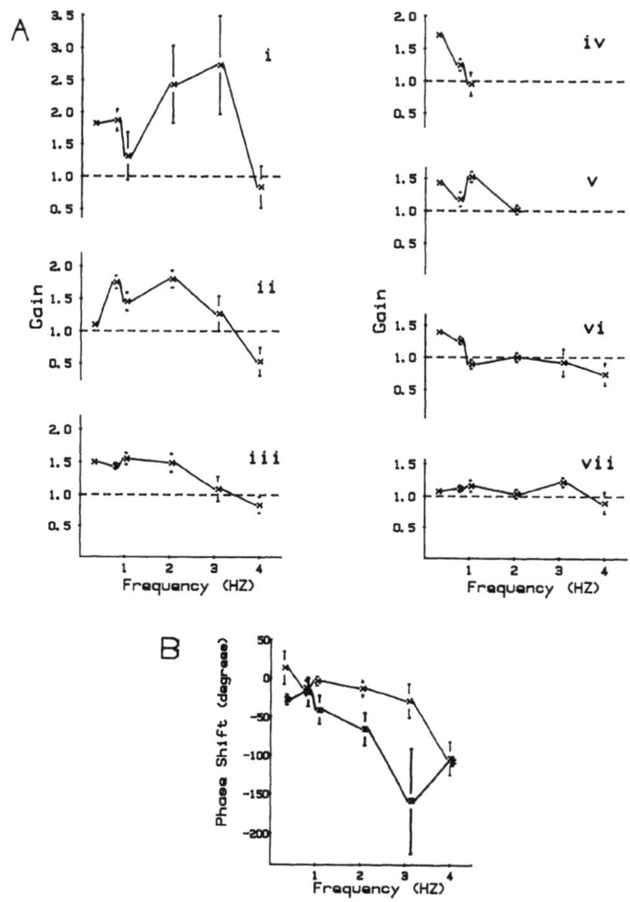

Figure 3. (A) Plots of gain vs modulation frequency for all seven subjects, arranged in order of increasing performance. i-iv represent the stutterers, v-vii the fluent speakers (see text). There are no error bars at 0.3 Hz because there was only one predictable cycle to measure at this modulation frequency. The missing data noted for subjects iv and v indicate that these subjects were not tracking at these modulation frequencies (see text). The number of cycles averaged varied from subject to subject and from one modulation frequency to another. The ranges of the number of cycles averaged for each modulation frequency are as follows:

0.3 Hz n=1	0.78 Hz n=3-4	1.0 Hz n=5-6
2.0 Hz n=5-12	3.0 Hz n=8-20	4.0 Hz n=6-23

(B) A plot of the mean of the average phase shifts of the two groups vs modulation frequency. At modulation frequencies of 1, 2 and 3 Hz, there is no overlap of the two groups within one standard deviation. The bold line represents the stutterers and the thin line represents the fluent speakers. The error bars show the standard deviation of the average of the individual means. Where there are no error bars the error is smaller than the size of the 'x'.

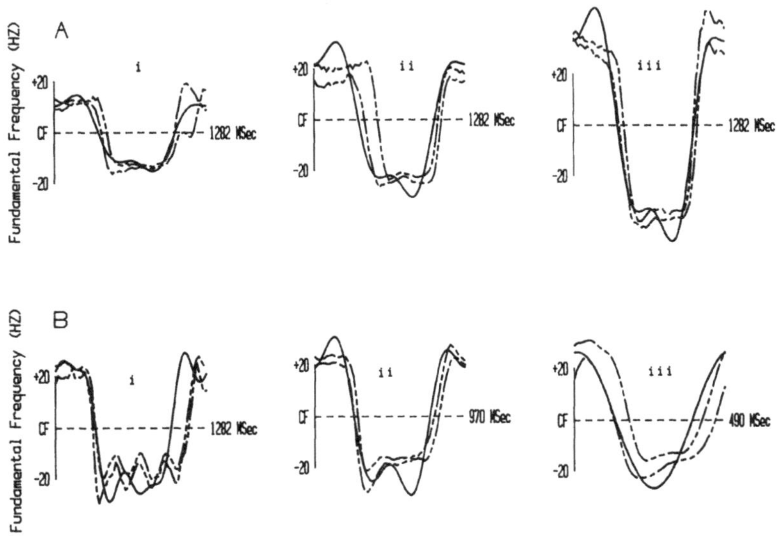

Figure 4. Model results. The solid line represents the predicted output. The broken line represents the average ± one standard deviation of the subject's actual response to square wave inputs. (A) The predicted responses of a fluent speaker to a square wave of 0.78 Hz, amplitude of modulation = (i) ±10 Hz, (ii) ±20 Hz, and (iii) ±30 Hz. CF=130 Hz. (B) The predicted responses of a different fluent speaker to square wave inputs of (i) 0.78 Hz, (ii) 1.0 Hz, and (iii) 2.0 Hz, amplitude of modulation= ±20 Hz. CF=170 Hz.

DISCUSSION

As noted earlier the use of feedback, although providing finer control, leads to the possibility of instabilities in a control system (i.e., disfluencies in speech). It can be better understood how these instabilities may occur by viewing speech as having two nested loops: 1) an inner phonatory control loop which produces sound, employing the respiratory, articulatory, and laryngeal motor systems, which is used by 2) an outer linguistic control loop which chooses and organizes the sounds that are produced. This experiment, measuring the dynamics of the inner phonatory control loop, demonstrates that stutterers have larger phase shifts around 2 - 3 Hz than do fluent speakers. How this relates to the stability of the total nested loop system of speech can be understood only after reviewing how a control system functions.

A negative feedback control system compares the desired output with the monitored actual output. This comparison requires subtraction of these two quantities. Instabilities arise when the monitored output has been phase shifted by 180 degrees (hence changing its sign) because the subtraction causes these two quantities to be added (i.e., the negative feedback has turned into positive feedback). If the system's gain is greater than one, the output will saturate (i.e., grow to the physical limits of the system).

At the highest frequency of modulation where a subject's gain is one, the term "phase margin" is defined as the amount of additional phase shift needed to make the systems' phase shift equal to 180 degrees (Anand, 1974). The data shows that stutterers have smaller phase margins than fluent speakers, meaning that the stutterer's SMCS is closer to instabilities. For example, at 2.5 Hz (see Figure 3B) fluent speakers are 160 degrees (approximately 177 msec) away from becoming unstable (i.e., 180 degrees out of phase), but the stutterers are only 70 degrees (approximately 77 msec) from this point. Recently Harrington (1987, this volume, Chapter 27) stated that an auditory delay time of 180 msec causes a fluent speaker to become disfluent. This is in good agreement with our calculations from the phase shift data that an additional delay of approximately 177 msec at 2.5 Hz should produce an instability in the SMCS of a fluent speaker. Approximately 77 msec is all that is necessary for the stutterer's SMCS to become unstable. Thus the stutterer has much less time for planning in the outer linguistic loop than does the fluent speaker.

We contend that speech disfluencies occur when sufficient delays (which act like phase shifts) in the outer linguistic loop are added into the SMCS, causing the system to become unstable. For example, anything prolonging time spent in the outer loop (stress?, anxiety?, affect-sensitivity?, etc.) can produce instability. Reducing the frequency content of speech by slowing the motor movements (slow prolonged speech (Howie & Andrews, 1984)) allows the stutterer to work in an area where his SMCS is unlikely to become unstable. Our model explains this as follows: (Recall: at 1 Hz 360 degrees = 1000 msec, at 3 Hz 360 degrees = 333 msec) at 1 Hz a stutterer has a phase shift of only 45 degrees, having an additional 135 degrees (approximately 375 msec at 1 Hz) for linguistic loop processing instead of the 77 he had at 2.5 Hz, where normal speech occurs. Any therapy causing the stutterers to spend excessive amounts of time concentrating/thinking about his speech production, for whatever reason, is unlikely to be as effective for speech produced at a normal rate, as it is for a slow prolonged rate. Successful therapies must automize speech so that less time is spent planning. Just because a stutterer can speak fluently at a slow rate, where he has more time for SMCS "planning", does not mean that he will speak fluently when his speech rate increases, when he has limited time for "planning". It is suggested that therapies must work on eliminating the phase delays in the speech systems of stutterers so that the speech becomes automatic. Only then will therapies provide long range effectiveness.

ACKNOWLEDGEMENTS

We thank the Ariel, Benjamin and Jeremiah Lowin Medical Foundation, the Kitty M. Perkins Foundation and the M.R. Bauer Foundation.

REFERENCES

Anand, D.K. (1974). *Introduction to Control Systems* Oxford: Pergamon.

Cooper, W.E. & Sorenson, J.M. (1981). *Fundamental Frequency in Sentence Production.* New York: Springer-Verlag.

Harrington, J. (1987). A model of stuttering and the production of speech under delayed auditory feedback conditions. In H.F.M. Peters & W. Hulstijn (Eds.), *Speech Motor Dynamics in Stuttering.* Wien: Springer Press.

Howie, P. & Andrews, G. (1984). Treatment of adult stutterers: Managing fluency. In R.F. Curlee & W.H. Perkins (Eds.), *Nature and Treatment of Stuttering - New Directions.* San Diego: College Hill.

Leonard, R.J. & Ringel, R.L. (1979). Vocal shadowing under conditions of normal and altered laryngeal sensation. *Journal of Speech and Hearing Research 22,* 794-817.

Milsum, J.H. (1966). *Biological Control Systems Analysis.* New York: McGraw Hill.

Rosenfield, D.B. (1984). Stuttering. *C.R.C. Critical Reviews in Clinical Neurobiology 1(2),* 117-139.

Shoup, J.E., Lass, N.J. & Kuehn, D.P. (1982). Acoustics of Speech. In N.J. Lass, L.V. McReynolds, J.L. Northern & D.E. Yoder (Eds.), *Speech, Language, and Hearing, Volume 1, Normal Processes.* Philadelphia: W.B. Saunders.

Stark, L. Vossius, G. & Young, L.R. (1962). Predictive control of eye tracking movements. *IRE Transactions on Human Factors in Electronics HFE-3,* 52-57.

Van Riper, C. (1971). *The Nature of Stuttering.* Englewood Cliffs, New Jersey: Prentice-Hall.

Part Four

Research on Coordination and Timing of Speech Motor Processes

Overview

Whereas studies in the past only involved the measurement of a single response, the theoretical developments (see Part one and Part two) as well as improvements in methods (see Part three) have led to an increase in the number of studies in which multiple responses are recorded simultaneously. In the present section (Part four) a number of these studies have been grouped together. They present a varied and representative picture of a field of study in which the coordination and timing of the various components of speech forms the main object. The question here is are stutterers characterized by a lack of or the faulty coordination of one or more speech mechanisms, and how can this be investigated? The chapters in this part of the book all approach the problem from a slightly different perspective. Some of them form the rudiments of years of research, while others describe purely pilot experiments. But each contributes another facet to the study of coordination and discoordination in stutterers' speech. This overview of the chapters in Part four contains a brief sketch and summary of all these approaches to the study of coordination.

The first three chapters of this part present reaction time studies. These studies, as well as the vast amount of literature that is referred to, make it quite clear that stutterers, at least in some conditions, show longer reaction times than normal subjects. What do these results really mean with regard to coordination or discoordination in stuttering? Coordination involves timing, yet it is too big a step to conclude from longer reaction times alone that some sort of timing mechanism is impaired. The imperfect operation of one single mechanism, such as laryngeal functioning, might just as easily be the cause. Previously learned strategies to slow speech down, cannot be ruled out in advance. Yet, the conjecture put forward most often is that stutterers encounter difficulties in the coordination of two or more subsystems that are required for the production of speech. It is only possible to decide between these alternatives if more than one response measure is monitored. In this way the delay in the stutterers' reaction time can be localized to one particular subset of all the possible mechanisms.

The first demonstration of the localization power of simultaneous measurements is given in a study by Bakker and Brutten (Chapter 11). In this study a large number of stutterers and nonstutterers had to rapidly initiate the utterances [pa] and [a], while their lip EMG activity and electroglottogram were being recorded. Stutterers differed from control subjects not so much in lip reaction time but in "voice onset time", i.e. the period between the onset of lip EMG activity and the first electroglottographic sign of vocal fold vibration.

A second study attempting to attribute the stutterers' delayed reaction time to a specific mechanism is described in Chapter 12. The authors Peters and Hulstijn, recorded the lip, larynx and masseter EMGs as well as the electrical activity of the vocal folds and the audio signal in a considerable number of stutterers and normal subjects. Stutterers were found to show longer "initiation" times - an interval which is comparable to Bakker and Brutten's "voice onset time" - but, in contrast to the results in their study, the initial part of the acoustic reaction time - the lip reaction times - varied. In addition to subdividing the acoustic reaction time into separate elements, the study was designed to test a motor programming hypothesis. It was thought that if stutterers have problems with the advance setting up of a motor program for an entire utterance then it would be reasonable to expect their reaction time to be delayed in the initial part of the reaction time and similarly, to encounter longer delays for more complex, utterances of greater length. Both these hypotheses were confirmed.

A third reaction time study is presented in Chapter 13, by Watson and Alfonso. Their study followed a simple reaction paradigm, requiring an isolated vowel response after a foreperiod (preparatory interval) that varied between 100 and 2000 msec. The acoustic signal, respiratory and laryngeal kinematic data were recorded in two nonstutterers and two mild and two severe stutterers. In line with their previously published results, they observed a difference in the acoustic reaction time between nonstutterers and severe stutterers. The mild stutterers' reaction time was equal to that of the severe group for short foreperiods and approaching the nonstutterers' reaction time for long foreperiods. In addition, the authors bring forward an interesting approach to the study of coordination, by presenting frequency distributions for the onset latencies of vocal fold closure and abdominal respiratory compression, for short and long foreperiods. In this way mild and severe stutterers could be differentiated on the basis of the coordination of prephonatory, respiratory and laryngeal events. The authors even conclude that these data suggest different anatomical loci for the stuttering in both groups.

The chapter by Borden and Armson (Chapter 14) presents a different method of studying coordination. Firstly, these authors present "voice onset times", an acoustic measure reflecting the interval between the stop release and the onset of voicing for the following vowel, which did not differ in the truly "fluent" utterances of four mild stutterers, four severe stutterers and ten control subjects. Clear examples of the simultaneous recording of lip/jaw displacement, slow and fast EGG and acoustic information in normal and stuttered speech are provided. Even in the example of stuttered speech, the multiple occurrance of supralaryngeal movement closely corresponded in time with specific laryngeal movement, thereby seemingly contradicting the hypothesis of a timing disorder in stutterers.

Schwarz (Chapter 15) studied the differences in coordination between several subgroups of young stutterers in a manner fairly similar to that described by Borden and Armson in the previous chapter. Simultaneous recordings of the respiratory activity, lip opening and closing and vocal fold contact were analysed in 15 young stutterers who each produced 10 stuttered speech utterances. Temporal onsets of these physiological activities were measured relative to the acoustic onset of the first fluently produced vowel or consonant which immediately preceded the stuttered word. No difference were found between the four behaviorally identified subgroups.

An entirely different way of investigating the coordination of subsystems is presented by Peters and Boves in Chapter 16. The most interesting aspect of their work is the extensive and careful recording of subglottal air pressure. This measure, in combination with electroglottography, in a sense reflects coordination in itself, since subglottal air pressure is the combined result of respiratory and laryngeal activity. Ten stutterers and seven nonstutterers took part in an experiment were a large number of short and long words had to be spoken in normal conditions and in two fluency enhancing conditions. Five categories of coordination - the authors refer to them more correctly as patterns of pressure build-up - could be distinguished and these are described. Four of them are rather unusual and occurred much more frequently in stutterers' speech.

In all the chapters introduced so far, coordination has simply been concluded from simultaneous measurements, but was never investigated by experimental means. The research described by Caruso, Gracco & Abbs in Chapter 17 is of great value because experimental techniques were employed, which have been borrowed from the study of coordination patterns in normally fluent speech. Unanticipated perturbations in the lower lip movement during oral closing for the utterance /p/ were evaluated. Upper and lower lip movements were recorded, as well as the EMG of five perioral muscles. Three stutterers and three nonstutterers took part in this study . The normal subjects, and the stutterers all manifested labial EMG and movement compensations to local perturbations, right from the first perturbation trial. However, in contrast to the nonstuttering subjects, both the upper and lower lip compensations were reduced in stutterers. In accordance with the ideas proposed by Gracco in Chapter 4, these findings suggest possible aberrations in the sensorimotor processes underlying the coordination and control of speech movements by stutterers.

The next chapter, Chapter 18, by Almé and McAllister, also presents data on upper and lower lip movement. In this pilot study labial coarticulation was studied without the lip activity itself being experimentally manipulated, by systematically varying the number of consonants that preceded a rounded vowel. Three normal speakers were compared with a mild and a severe stutterer. The stutterers exhibited a tendency towards having a longer interval between the start of the rounding of the lips and the acoustic onset of the rounded vowel sound. In addition, the temporal relation between the onset of the lip EMG and labial movement seemed to be more inconsistent.

Coordination is an important element in the final chapter, Chapter 19 by Stromsta. He reviews a number of his earlier studies that were directed at a special type of stuttering: intraphonemic disruptions. He considers these disruptions, occurring within phonemes, to be the core behavior of stuttering. Clear examples are given of the simultaneous recording of either a combination of a sound spectogram, labial EMG and EGG, or the combination of a speech, EGG and intra oral pressure, during these intraphonemic disruptions. The core behavior of stuttering is considered to be the result of faulty labial anticipatory coarticulation - a view which is in agreement with the results presented in the previous chapter. The second part of the chapter is devoted to a subject which was more prominent in the chapters at the beginning of Part four : reaction time. When a distinction is made between core stutterers - those with intraphonemic disruptions - and reacting stutterers - those with prolongations and tonic blocks, marked differences in the phonatory reaction time between both groups are observed. Only the reaction times of reacting stutterers were longer than those of the nonstutterers, a difference that disappeared, however, after a number of massed trials. These results once more raise the question of what one is actually measuring in reaction time studies: the direct effects of discoordination or learned strategies resulting in a speech delay?

Chapter 11

Labial and Laryngeal Reaction Times of Stutterers and Nonstutterers

Klaas Bakker and Gene J. Brutten

Simple reaction time experiments, in which speech-motor capacities of stutterers and nonstutterers were compared, most often have tested laryngeal functioning. In these studies subjects were required to phonate, as quickly as possible, when a cue-stimulus was presented. The results have tended to indicate that stutterers respond more slowly than do nonstutterers. This was true even though only fluent responses were analyzed to ensure that the results would not be contaminated by the presence of stuttering (Adams and Hayden, 1976; Cross and Luper, 1983; Prosek, 1978; Starkweather, Hirschman, and Tannenbaum, 1976; Watson and Alfonso, 1983).

The delay in the laryngeal reaction times of stutterers has given support to the hypothesis that they are likely to be neurologically less well equipped for speech than are nonstutterers (Adams and Hayden, 1976; Cross and Luper, 1978; Starkweather et al, 1976; Watson and Alfonso, 1983). It also has led some investigators to suggest that the observed between-group difference in reaction times was attributable to those aspects of the central nervous system that are specifically related to laryngeal functioning.

The conclusion that the stutterers' response time lag is limited to their laryngeal functioning may well have been precipitous. This is because the finding of delayed phonatory onsets among those who stutter is not sufficient to preclude the presence of other distinguishing response delays. It may merely reflect the fact that phonation was the function investigated. It remained possible, in other words, that reaction time lags also existed in other speech-related structures of stutterers or in their coordination during speech.

McFarlane and Prins (1979) appear to have been among the first to broaden the scope of the behaviors examined in speech-related reaction time studies. They investigated the lip reaction times of stutterers and nonstutterers who were cued by visual or auditory stimuli to say the syllables [pa] and [ba]. Specifically, they measured the time between the off-set of the cue-stimulus and the first appearance of EMG activity of the orbicularis oris muscle. As in similar studies, they avoided confounding by limiting the determination of reaction times to those utterances that were spoken fluently. Despite this precaution, the lip reaction time of the stutterers was slower than that of the nonstutterers when auditory stimuli cued the subjects' responses. This was not the case, however, when the cue-stimulus was visual.

McFarlane and Prins' results were noteworthy. In part, this was because they found that the response slowness observed among stutterers was not limited to laryngeal functioning. In part, too, it was because the reaction times did not differentiate stutterers from nonstutterers when the triggering stimulus was visual. Taken together, the data suggested that it would be worthwhile to determine if the delay in the reaction times of stutterers is predominantly accounted for by a limitation in motor programming and execution or is best understood in terms of the type of sensory modality.

In most of the reaction time experiments that were conducted with people who do or do not stutter, the response latency of only one aspect of motor performance was measured. And, as we have seen, when the cueing stimulus was auditory, the laryngeal or lip performance of those who stutter was slower than that of normal speakers. The findings did not, however, reflect on the coordination of these structures during speech. Thus, it is possible that the coordination between the larynx and the lips among those who stuttered was delayed also. This possibility has infrequently been addressed in reaction time experiments, even though there is some indirect evidence that a coordinational lag exists. For example, when Agnello (1975) analyzed the spectrographic recordings of his subjects' utterances of [pa] and [ba] he found that the time between the acoustic onset of the consonant and the onset of the following vowel was longer for the stutterers than for the nonstutterers. This group difference in consonant-vowel transition, or voice onset time, led him to conclude that stutterers have a reduced capacity to coordinate phonation with the activity of the articulators.

Agnello (1975) found a group difference in the voice onset times of stutterers and nonstutterers even though they were not required to respond quickly when a cue-stimulus was presented. It is possibile, therefore, that a still greater difference might have been obtained if their speech system had been pushed to the limit. This possibility was addressed by McFarlane and Shipley (1978), who required stutterers and nonstutterers to say [pa] and [ba] as quickly as possible when a visual or auditory cue-stimulus was presented. Measurement of the consonant to vowel transitions, defined as the time lapse between EMG onset at the lips and onset of phonation, made it evident that the stutterers' transitions were slower than those of the nonstutterers when auditory stimuli cued the subjects' responses. These results were consistent with those obtained by McFarlane and Prins (1979). Together they suggested that the motor performance of those who stutter is slower when auditory perception is involved in responding.

As we have seen, reaction time studies have tended to emphasize laryngeal functioning. Rarely have other speech-related responses been examined. When they have, as in the lip reaction and voice onset studies mentioned, stutterers showed evidence of a response lag when the cue-stimulus was auditory. Their reaction time did not differ from that of nonstutterers when the cue was visual, the only other stimulus modality that has so far been explored. These findings set the stage for the present investigation which was designed to determine if: (1) lip reaction times of people who stutter differ from those of nonstutterers, (2) voice initiation times of stutterers differ from those of nonstutterers, (3) voice onset times of stutterers and nonstutterers are different, and (4) if group differences in lip reaction times, voice initiation times, and voice onset times interact with stimulus modality.

METHOD

Subjects

Twenty-four stutterers and the same number of nonstutterers participated in the present reaction time experiment. Among the stutterers, whose ages ranged from 15 to 40 years, were 23 males and 1 female. Their mean age was 25 years. The nonstutterers ranged in age from 16 to 36 and their mean age was 24 years and 1 month. Included in this sample were 22 males and 2 females. In addition, all of the subjects of this study had normal hearing and vision. Individuals who reported neuro-physiological difficulties or used medication that might suppress reaction time were excluded from participation. So, too, were those who evidenced other speech and language problems. Most of the stutterers in this investigation had not had therapy. Of the few that had, none received therapy that was directed at prolonging their speech or altering their voice onset.

Procedure

All of the subjects were instructed to say [pa] or [a] as soon as a visual, auditory, or somato-sensory cue-stimulus was presented. Each of these stimuli were presented in blocks of 15 trials. The order of the stimulus blocks was counterbalanced across the subjects. So, too, were the response blocks; [pa] as the cued response preceded [a] half of the time.

The visual stimulus was a .1 sec flash of a quick responding light source. The auditory stimulus, a 1000 Hz tone at 70 dB presented to both ears through a Telefunken headphone (TH28, 2x400 Ohm), also lasted .1 sec. The somato-sensory stimulus was a discernable 50 microsecond shock presented to the surface of the right cheek, near the corner of the mouth, by a stimulator (Digital,

Type 3072). Each of the stimuli - the light, the tone, and the shock - were triggered by computer software that cued the subjects to respond at random intervals that ranged from 2 to 12 seconds.

The stimulus marks and the subjects' responses were stored on magnetic tape by an instrumentation recorder (Ampex, Fr 1300 A) which was run at a speed of 3.75 in/sec. The taped signals were subsequently printed out on a multi-channel ink writer (Schwarzer, RE412) at a paper speed of 5 cm/sec. The print-outs were used to obtain three response measures. Lip reaction time, one of the measures, was defined as the time lapse between stimulus onset and the first polygraphic evidence of EMG activity of the orbicularis oris inferior muscle when the subjects said [pa]. Another of the measures, voice initiation time, gauged the period between stimulus onset and the first electroglottographic sign of vocal fold vibration when the subjects said [a]. Voice onset time, the third measure employed in this study, was operationally defined as the temporal duration between the onset of EMG activity in the lips and the first appearance of vocal fold vibration in the electroglottographic signal when [pa] was uttered.

The lip reaction, voice initiation, and voice onset times were tested by means of a two-way analysis of variance that was repeated across the stimulus factor. Only two sources of variance were tested: the between-group main effect for each of the measured reaction times and the group by stimulus interaction.

RESULTS AND DISCUSSION

Table 1 shows the lip reaction times evidenced by the subject groups when they produced [pa]. Descriptively, the stutterers were somewhat slower than the nonstutterers in all of the stimulus conditions. However, these temporal differences were not statistically significant. There was neither a main effect for groups ($F(1,46) = .76$, $p < .05$) nor a group by stimulus interaction ($F(2,92) = .28$, $p < .05$). In other words, the lip reaction times for [pa] were not significantly different for the subject groups and the different cue-stimuli did not differentially affect the onset times of the stutterers and nonstutterers. There was no evidence, therefore, that lip reaction times of stutterers are slower or that stutterers are disadvantaged when they react to simple visual, auditory, or somato-sensory stimuli.

Table 1. Stutterers' and Nonstutterers Mean Lip Reaction Times for [pa] cued by a Visual, Auditory, or Somato-Sensory Stimulus.

	Visual Stimulus	Auditory Stimulus	Somato-Sensory Stimulus
Stutterers	247.2 ms	207.8 ms	260.6 ms
Nonstutterers	241.1 ms	190.4 ms	242.8 ms

The present data thus failed to confirm the McFarlane and Prins (1979) findings that the lip reaction times of stutterers are delayed when the cue-stimulus is auditory. There is reason, then, to question their position that an articulatory response lag results because of a disadvantage in auditory processing. In fact, the present results lead to the question of whether an articulatory delay exists, since the stutterers' and nonstutterers' lip reaction times were similar in all of the stimulus modalities.

As Table 2 indicates, the stutterers' Voice Initiation Times were descriptively longer than those of the nonstutterers. This was the case in all of the stimulus conditions. The between-group difference in voice initiation time across stimulus type was statistically significant ($F(1,46) = 6.57$, $p < .05$). In contrast, the interaction between subject and cue variables did not even approach significance ($F(2,92) = .20$, $p < .05$). This indicates that the difference in the voice initiation times of stutterers and nonstutterers was independent of the type of stimulus that was used to cue phonation.

Table 2. Stutterers' and Nonstutterers' Mean Voice Initiation Times for [a] cued by a Visual, Auditory, or Somato-Sensory Stimulus.

	Visual Stimulus	Auditory Stimulus	Somato-Sensory Stimulus
Stutterers	494.6 ms	446.8 ms	484.0 ms
Nonstutterers	402.4 ms	351.8 ms	402.2 ms

The finding of a significant main effect in voice initiation time is consistent with the results of the majority of reaction time studies involving phonatory onsets (Adams and Hayden, 1976; Starkweather et al, 1976). However, the absence of a group by stimulus interaction is not in keeping with the data from previous studies which indicated that stutterers and nonstutterers differ when an auditory but not a visual stimulus is employed to cue responding (McFarlane and Prins, 1979; McFarlane and Shipley, 1978). Stimulus modality was not found to differentially affect reaction time. The data of the present investigation did not, therefore, support the notion that the stutterers' lag in voice initiation time is due to a limitation in auditory processing. Indeed, the fact that stimulus type did not interact with the subject variable, suggests that sensory processing is not implicated in the response lag that we and others have observed.

Voice onset time for [pa], the time lapse between the onset of the consonant and the onset of the vowel in three different stimulus conditions, is displayed in Table 3. Apparent here is the fact that the average voice onset time of the stutterers was notably longer than that of the nonstutterers in each of the stimulus circumstances. Consistent with this finding is the fact that the between-group difference was statistically significant ($F(1,46) = 5.44$, $p <$

Table 3. Stutterers' and Nonstutterers' Mean Voice Onset Times of [pa] cued by a Visual, Auditory, or Somato-Sensory Stimulus.

	Visual Stimulus	Auditory Stimulus	Somato-Sensory Stimulus
Stutterers	238.8 ms	250.4 ms	257.8 ms
Nonstutterers	176.4 ms	173.4 ms	192.2 ms

.05). Cutting across stimulus type, the stutterers' voice onset times were slower than those of the nonstutterers to an extent that was not likely due to chance. The interaction between the two groups and three stimulus conditions was not significant, however ($F(2,92) = 2.20$, $p < .05$). In each of the stimulus conditions, the stutterers' onset times were slower than those of the nonstutterers to an extent that was essentially the same. Differences in the type of stimulus used to cue [pa] did not differentially influence the subjects' voice onset times. Once again, then, the data suggest that the stutterers' response lag is stimulus independent.

In summary, the reaction time lag of stutterers was limited to laryngeal functioning. While the lip reaction time of stutterers did not differ from that of nonstutterers, they were significantly slower in voice initiation and onset times. These between-group differences were stimulus independent. Still to be determined is whether similar results would be obtained if more complex cue-stimuli were employed and whether or not stutterers are generally slower than nonstutterers in perceiving and identifying sensory stimuli.

ACKNOWLEDGEMENTS

The help of the faculty and staff of the Department of Phoniatry (Medical School, University of Utrecht, The Netherlands) is gratefully acknowledged.

REFERENCES

Adams, M.R. & Hayden, P.A. (1976). The ability of stutterers and nonstutterers to initiate and terminate phonation during production of an isolated vowel. *Journal of Speech and Hearing Research, 19,* 290-296.

Agnello, J. G. (1975). Voice onset and voice termination features of stutterers. In Webster, L.M. & Furst, L.C. (Eds.), *Vocal Tract Dynamics and Dysfluency.* New York: Speech and Hearing Institute.

Cross, D.E. & Luper, H.L. (1978). Voice reaction time of stuttering and nonstuttering children and adults. *ASHA, 20,* 826.

Cross, D.E. & Luper, H.L. (1983). Relation between finger reaction times and voice reaction time in stuttering and nonstuttering children and adults. *Journal of Speech and Hearing Research, 26,* 356-361.

McFarlane, S.C. & Prins, D. (1979). Neural response time of stutterers and nonstutterers in selected oral reading tasks. *Journal of Speech and Hearing Research, 21,* 768-778.

McFarlane, S.C. & Shipley, K.G. (1978). Visual and auditory cueing effects on vocalization onset for stutterers and nonstutterers. *ASHA,* San Francisco.

Prosek, R.A. (1978). Acoustic and laryngeal reaction times of stutterers and nonstutterers. (abstract) *ASHA, 20,* San Francisco.

Starkweather, C.W., Hirschman, P. & Tannenbaum, R.S. (1976). Latency of vocalization onset: Stutterers versus nonstutterers. *Journal of Speech and Hearing Research, 19,* 481-492.

Watson, B.C. & Alfonso, P.J. (1983). Foreperiod and stuttering severity effects on acoustic laryngeal reaction time. *Journal of Fluency Disorders, 8,* 183-205.

Chapter 12

Programming and Initiation of Speech Utterances in Stuttering

Herman F.M. Peters and Wouter Hulstijn

INTRODUCTION

In the study of speech production it is a widely shared idea that fluent speech utterances are produced under the control of a "program" - a detailed representation of all or most of the utterance constructed in advance of the utterance itself. In such a view it is assumed that programming or in advance preparation of the utterance precedes the execution itself (Sternberg et al., 1978; Keele, 1981; Schmidt, 1982; Hulstijn & v. Galen, 1983). The programming process involves a limited number of successive processes. In the first stage an abstract representation, or program, of the type and sequence of movements is retrieved from long term memory. Next the setting of size, accuracy and timing parameters for actual execution are specified and finally the program is translated into actual muscle comments and initiated.

If stuttering is seen as a "disorder of movement" (Adams, 1975 Zimmermann, 1980; Andrews et al., 1983) then a possible disorder in advance preparation or the programming of speech motor activity in stuttering should be studied intensively, particularly since most disfluencies occur at the onset of words or phrases (St. Louis, 1979).

In laryngeal reaction time studies in stuttering significant slowness in initiating and terminating phonatory and articulatory movements is noted unequivocally (Adams, 1984). Assuming that letter and word recognition processes in reading are equally fast in stutterers and nonstutterers then an increase in reaction time may be the result of either an increased programming process or a longer initiation phase.

By simultaneous recording of responses in the laryngeal, articulatory and acoustic domain the time between the response signal and the onset of speech can be divided into two intervals: 1. the interval between the response signal and the first manifestation of physiologic activity (= latency time, LT) and 2. the interval between the start of the first physiologic activity and the onset of speech (= initiation time, IT). A lengthened latency time might reveal programming difficulties, if any, while a lengthened initiation time might give insight into initiation problems of either a special response system (f.i. in coordination among intrinsic laryngeal muscles or discoordination in oral movements) or problems in the coordination of the different subsystems involved (f.i. coordination of laryngeal movements with articulation and respiration). Figure 1 shows a schematic representation of the programming and initiation of physiological processes in speech utterances in reading.

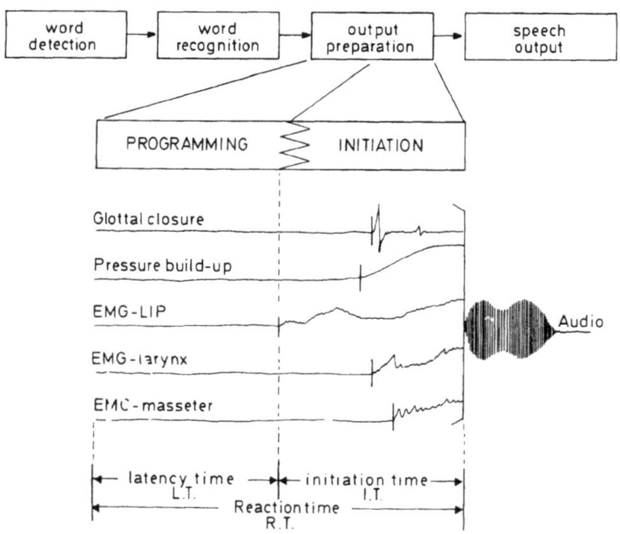

Figure 1. Schematic representation of programming and initiation of physiological processes in speech utterances in reading.

The aim of the overall experiment from which this study is a first report, is to examine the coordination of aerodynamic, laryngeal and supralaryngeal speech movements of stutterers from a motor programming perspective under different conditions.

The aim of the present study was to investigate whether a longer acoustic reaction time in fluent speech utterances of stutterers may be the result of a programming disorder or whether it is caused by a disturbance in motor initiation. It should be clear that premotor planning or programming is assumed to consume more time if utterances of increasing length have to be centrally organized. Therefore the length of speech utterances was systematically varied between one syllable words, polysyllabic words and short sentences. If stutterers encounter problems in the programming stage then it should be predicted that the difference between stutterers and nonstutterers in latency time should be larger in more lengthy or more complex utterances.

In a condition in which part or all the programming could be done before the response signal the hypothesized difference between both groups in latency time should decrease, contrary to a condition in which there is no time for preparatory programming of the utterance.

METHOD

Subjects

The subjects in this research were 11 male adult stutterers ranging in age between 19 and 28 years. They were selected from a larger group of 20 stutterers because they fulfilled the criterion of at least one fluent utterance in all subconditions of the experiment. Control subjects were 10 male nonstutterers matched for age.

None of the stutterers had been enrolled in any kind of therapy during the two years preceding the experiment. For this study only those utterances have been analysed which were judged to be spoken fluently. In order to be accepted as fluent an utterance had to satisfy two conditions. First, the word may not contain audible hesitations, prolongations or repetitions according to independent judgements of two trained raters, and further there may not be any visual sign of struggle in the face or body movements of the subject before or during the production of the utterance. Here the presence of visual signs of disfluency was established by the experimenter during the recording session.

Procedure

The experiment followed a reaction-time paradigm with two tasks conditions: an immediate and a delayed reading task.

In the immediate reading task first a 100 Hz tone of 200 msec was presented to the subject while at the same time a row of asterisks appeared on the TV-monitor. This auditory and visual warning signal indicated that the stimulusword should be presented on the monitor within a period of one to three seconds. The presentation of the stimulusword was attended with a 1000 Hz tone of 100 msec. The subject was instructed to read the word as soon as possible after the presentation of the response signal.

A three-second period during which the stimulusword was presented on the screen was followed by a variable intertrial interval of three to five seconds.

In the delayed reading task the procedure was quite the same with the only difference that the presentation of the stimulusword coincided with the warning signal. The subject was instructed to

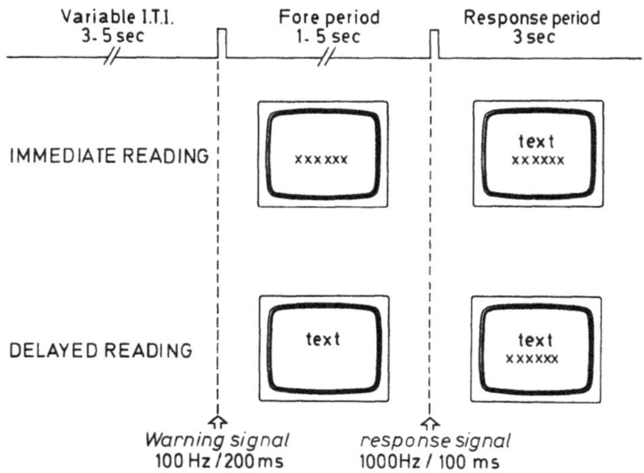

Figure 2. Procedure and stimulus presentation in the immediate and the delayed reading condition.

read the word or sentence as soon as possible after the simultaneous presentation of the auditory response signal (= 1000 Hz tone) and a visual response signal (= row of asterisks on the screen). In Figure 2 the stimulus presentation is showed schematically.

Stimulus presentation was drived by a Apple II + microcomputer. A randomisation program generated the variable foreperiod and the variable intertrial interval.

In each task 60 trials were presented, i.e. 20 one-syllable words, 20 three or four syllable words an 20 short sentences. In each category four initial sounds /a/, /o/, /p/ and /s/ were used with five trials for each. All subjects were given ten training sequences in both tasks before the start of the experiment. Moreover in each task five practice trials preceded the test stimuli. The subjects were instructed to make no speech movements before the onset of the response signal. The stimuli were presented in a balanced random order.

Conditions

The immediate and the delayed task condition were both presented in two speed conditions: a normal reaction time condition and a reaction time condition in which fast responding was additionally stressed. In the normal reaction time condition the subject was instructed to read the stimulusword as soon as possible after the response signal. In the time stress condition the subjects got feed back on their speech reaction times, measured by a voice key. Moreover the experimenter stressed the importance of extremely fast RTs several times during the first practice trials.

Instrumentation

Speech production was measured on different levels by simultaneous recordings in the laryngeal, articulatory and acoustic domain. A schematic diagram of the instrumentation set-up is presented in Figure 3. The signals recorded were:

1. Surface EMG-activity of the laryngeal area, the musculus orbicularis oris and the musculus masseter. The analog EMG-signals were amplified (Honeywell, Accudata 135), rectified and low-pass filtered.
2. Vocal fold activity was recorded by means of an electroglottograph, namely the device marketed Fourcin and Abberton under the name laryngograph.
3. The audiosignal, using an AKG type 451E condensor microphone, positioned approximately ten cm in front of the midline of the mouth.

All signals were recorded on a multichannel instrumentation tape recorder (Philips Analog 14) for subsequent processing. Computerized data processing and analysis followed for the two EMG recordings. Acoustic reaction time was measured from paper recordings made afterwards with a seven channel polygraph (Schönander-Elema), running at 50 mm/sec.

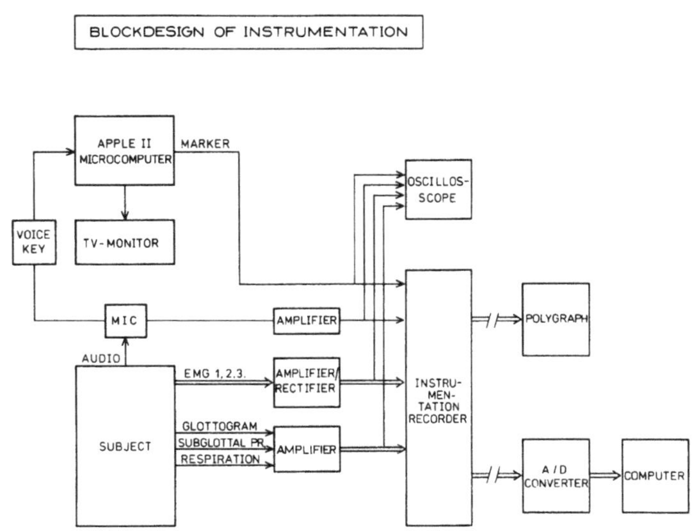

Figure 3. Schematic diagram of instrumentation set-up during the experiment.

RESULTS

Frequency of Disfluency

Utterance complexity seems to effect the frequency of disfluency very significantly. Figure 4 depicts the main results. In this figure the disfluencies (counted on all 20 subjects) are divided between initial disfluencies - occurring at the very first sound of the utterance - and "following" disfluencies, i.e. those that are produced in the rest of the utterance. Obviously the frequency of these latter disfluencies is a direct function of the number of syllables in the utterance. Therefore these "following" disfluencies are presented as a percentage of the total number of syllables in the utterance.

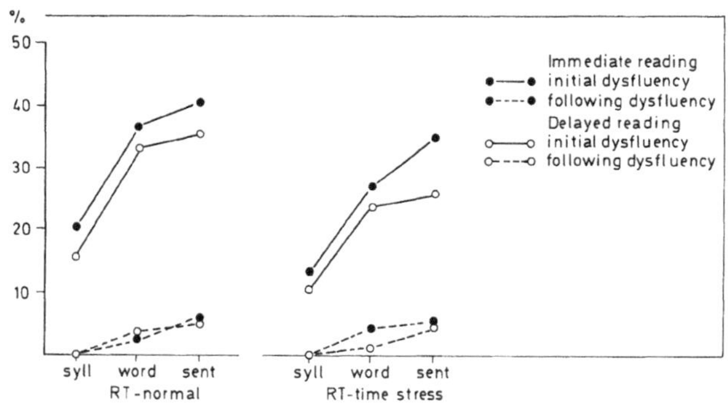

Figure 4. Stutterers dysfluency in condition RT-normal and condition RT-stress.

It is quite clear that the initial syllable elicits a much higher percentage of stuttering than the syllables that follow. A second effect, which is also quite marked is the effect of utterance length: in both speed-conditions and both task-conditions the percentage of initial disfluencies on polysyllabic words was about twice as high as on one-syllable words ($F(2,34) = 7.69$, $p < .002$).

The effects of task and speed conditions are smaller, but still significant ($F(2,17) = 8.13$, $p < .01$). In a delayed reading task in which the utterance can be programmed during the foreperiod, the percentage of initial disfluencies was about 5 percent lower. In addition quite unexpectedly in the time-stress RT condition the frequency of disfluency is lower (5-10%) than in the normal RT condition ($F(2,17) = 6.25$, $p < .02$). The last effect considered was the influence of the initial sound. Only the percentage of initial disfluencies on "p" was slightly higher, but this effect was far from significant. Therefore, in the rest of this chapter, the effect of the first sound will be left out of discussion.

Apart from the speed effect all other effects strongly point to stuttering as a defect in programming. The reduction in stuttering with time stress may be due to lessened accuracy demands in that condition. In the study of Peters and Boves was demonstrated that an instruction to care less about articulation reduces stuttering frequency. The well known speed-accuracy trade off has led subjects to produce less articulate utterances in the time-stress condition, which probably results in a lower percentage of disfluencies.

Latency Data

Part of the results of the latency data are presented in Figure 5. This figure depicts changes in four dependent variables: the acoustic RT and the latencies of the lip-, larynx- and masseter-EMG's. The data are given for stutterers (left side) and nonstutterers (right side of the figure) and are separated for both task-conditions. For reasons of clarity, only the time-stress condition is presented here. The latencies in the normal RT condition were much (and very significantly) higher, but in general produced the same picture as shown in this figure.

The four dependent variables all show the same effects to the same extent. In the analysis of variance on each of these four variables all main effects are highly significant. As might be expected the difference between immediate and delayed reading was quite large (Acoustic RT: $F(1,19) = 40.06$, $p < .001$; EMG LT lip: $F(1,19) = 137.63$, $p < .001$; EMG LT larynx: $F(1,19) = 207.35$, $p < .001$ and EMG LT Masseter: $F(1,19) = 119.03$, $p < .001$).

There was an increase of acoustic reaction time - at least from one syllable words to longer words - and, most important perhaps,

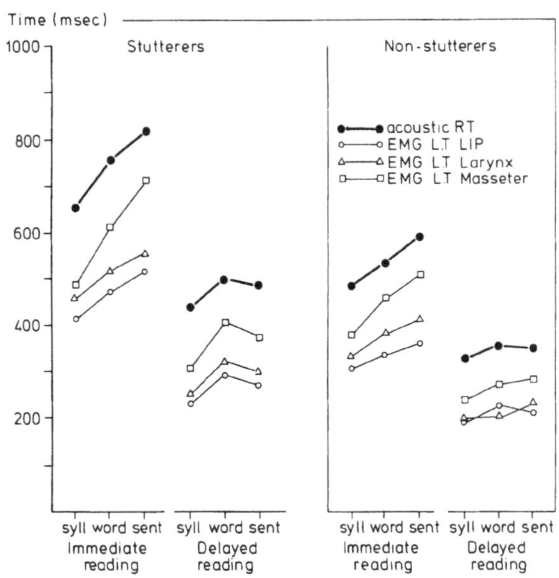

Figure 5. EMG-latency time and acoustic reaction time of stutterers and non-stutterers in RT condition-time stress.

the 11 stutterers initiated their fluent utterances much later than their nonstutterers controls. (Acoustic RT: ($F(1,19) = 29.24$, $p < .001$; EMG LT lip: $F(1,19) = 8.23$, $p < .01$; EMG LT larynx: $F(1.19) = 13.73$, $p < .001$ and EMG LT masseter: $F(1,19) = 14.88$, $p < .001$).

This last effect, replicates the findings of a number of other studies and in fact forms the starting point for the two main goals of this study, first, to investigate whether this increase in RT is larger in more complex utterances and secondly, whether this increase in RT is due to a longer latency time in the physiologic processes in speech or caused by an increase in voice initiation time. In Figure 6 the relevant details are presented.

As before only the data of the time-stress condition are given since the normal RT-condition produced about the same results. The acoustic RTs for both groups, in the immediate task as well as in the delayed reading task, are shown in the two curves on top.

Stutterers, as we have already seen in the preceding figure, have much larger RTs. In both groups there is an increase in RT with utterance length. In the delayed task condition however this effect is restricted to the increase from one syllable to polysyllabic words. Probably sentences are not programmed completely but only for the first two or three syllables. In the immediate reading task the increase in RT going from one syllable words to longer words is

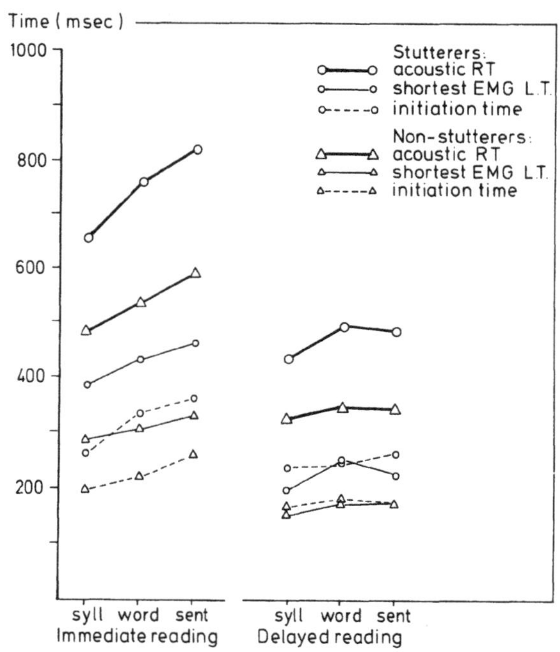

Figure 6. Latency time, initiation time and acoustic reaction time in RT condition-time stress.

larger than in the delayed reading task resulting in a significant interaction between length and task (Acoustic RT: ($F(2,38) = 14.19$, $p < .001$; EMG LT lip: $F(2,38) = 7.14$, $p < .01$; EMG LT larynx: $F(2.38) = 8.63$, $p < .001$ and EMG LT Masseter: $F(2,38) = 5.43$, $p < .01$). This is of course what might be expected since the RT in the immediate task condition is strongly influenced by letter and word recognition processes. These input-processes will understandably consume more time for longer utterances.

The interesting finding however, is that these increases in acoustic reaction time (from syllable to word) are larger in stutterers than in nonstutterers resulting in a significant interaction between groups and sequence length ($F(2.38) = 5.29$, $p < .01$).

In the lower part of this figure these acoustic RTs are subdivided into the latency time (thin lines) and the initiation time (dashed lines). It is quite clear that stutterers have longer latency times in laryngeal and articulatory activities that must be completed before the initiation of speech. However they also have longer initiation times in laryngeal and articulatory behavior.

To study the timing of articulatory movements the timing process was analysed separately for fluent utterances with initial /a/ and /o/. Figure 7 presents the relevant details. This figure summarizes the interval data between the response signal (R) at the left side of the figure and the onset of speech (S) at the right side of the figure. The interval between the response signal (R) and the first manifestation of laryngeal muscle activity (T) is as mentioned before very significantly longer in stutterers than in nonstutterers. There are the same differences between stutterers and nonstutterers in initial /a/ and initial /o/ for both tasks. So one may conclude that in general stutterers need much more time for programming their speech utterances.

In the interval between the first manifestation of laryngeal muscle activity (T) and the moment of closure vocal folds (G) there are no significant differences between stutterers and nonstutterers ($F(1.26) = .24$, n.s.). In the interval between vocal fold closure (G) and the onset of speech (S) stutterers are initiating phonation slower than nonstutterers. However this difference is not significant ($F(1,26) = 3.02$, $p = .09$). There seems to be no significant differences in the relative timing of laryngeal processes before the start of phonation. This indicates that stutterers seem to use the same motor programs in laryngeal manoeuvres before starting phonation. This seems to be not the case in the timing of phonatory and articulatory processes in the utterances beginning with an /o/. Nonstutterers start lip movement much the same time as the laryngeal muscle activity. Stutterers however seem to start lip movement much earlier than phonatory processes, resulting in a significant interaction between groups and sound ($F(1,26) = 5.34$, $p < .05$). The coordination or timing of laryngeal and articulatory processes is obviously not realised in the same way in stutterers as in nonstutterers.

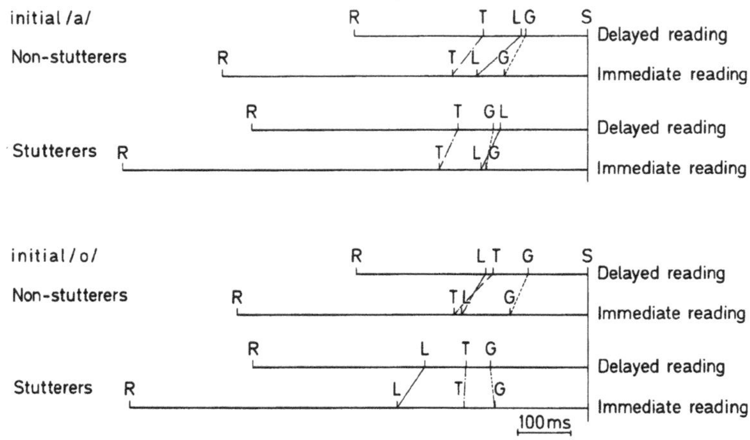

Figure 7. Timing of laryngeal and articulatory movements in fluent speech utterances with initial /a/ and /o/ in stutterers and non-stutterers (R = response signal; T = EMG latency time throat; L = EMG latency time lip; G = EGG latency time and S = onset of speech).

DISCUSSION

In summary our data on the frequency of disfluency replicate a well known finding that, by far, stuttering most frequently occurs at the start of an utterance. Because of time limits we did not give these data in detail. This finding however suggests that it is not the production of typical sounds that causes disturbance in stutterers but the programming or initiation of an utterance. By increasing the utterance length the extent of motor programming was assumed to be varied. This resulted in two effects: first the frequency of disfluencies increases markedly with utterance length and second, the increase in acoustic reaction time that was observed in longer utterances was greater in stutterers than in nonstutterers. These results suggest that, at least in part, stuttering is associated with a disturbance in motorprogramming.

Motorprogramming according to such authors as Sternberg, Keele and others, must be or will be, completed before the movement is initiated. Therefore, if the total acoustic reaction time is divided between a latency period in which no behavioral or physiologic manifestation is observed and a second initiation period we must expect the length of programming variables to have the most influence on the latency time. This was clearly the case. However in stutterers as well as in nonstutterers the effects of utterance length and task condition were equally evident in the initiation times. This suggests that motor programming may continue even after the first movement is made. This implies that programming and movement execution may occur more or less in parallel, a view that was exposed earlier by the second author to explain his reaction time results with handwriting as a motor task.

If parallel processing is adopted, then our findings are consistent with our earlier conclusion that stuttering is associated by ineffective motorprogramming, in as much as stutterers are slower in all our reaction time data and show larger effects of all independent variables on the latency and initiation times.

REFERENCES

Adams, M.R. (1975). A physiologic and aerodynamic interpretation of fluent and stutterers speech. *Journal of Fluency Disorders, 1*, 35-67.

Adams, M.R. (1984). Laryngeal onset and reaction time of stutterers. In R.F. Curlee & W.H. Perkins (Eds.), *Nature and treatment of stuttering: New directions.* San Diego: College-Hill Press.

Andrews, G., Craig, A., Feyer, A.M., Hoddinott, S., Howie, P. & Neilson, M. (1983). Stuttering: A review of research findings and theories circa 1982. *Journal of Speech and Hearing Disorders, 48*, 226-246.

Hulstijn, W. & Van Galen, G. (1983). Programming in handwriting: Reaction time and movement time as a function of sequence length. *Acta Psychologica, 54*, 23-49.

Keele, S.W. (1981). Behavior analysis in movement. In V. Brooks (Ed.), *Handbook of physiology, Vol. II: Motor control.* Baltimore: Williams & Wilkens.

Peters, H.F.M. & Hulstijn, W. (1984). *Programming of speech utterances in stuttering.* Paper presented at the annual convention of the American Speech and Hearing Association, San Francisco.

Schmidt, R.A. (1976). Control processes in motor skills. *Exercise and Sport Science, 4*, 229-261.

Sternberg, S., Monsell, S., Knoll, R.L. & Wright, C.E. (1978). The latency and duration of rapid movement sequences: Comparisons of speech and typewriting. In G.E. Stelmach (Ed.), *Information processing in motor control and learning.* New York: Academic Press.

St. Louis, K. (1979). Linguistic and motor aspects of stuttering. In N.J. Lass (Ed.), *Speech and language.* Vol I. New York: Academic Press.

Zimmermann, G. (1980). Stuttering: A disorder of movement. *Journal of Speech and Hearing Research, 23*, 122-136.

Chapter 13

Coordination of Prephonatory Events in Mild and Severe Stutterers

Ben C. Watson and Peter J. Alfonso

Many physiologically-based models of stuttering that associate laryngeal dysfunction with the disorder (Van Riper, 1971; Adams, 1978; Zimmermann, Smith & Hanley, 1981) share the hypothesis that stutterers have difficulty controlling the rapid initiation and termination of voicing. This hypothesis is supported by behavioral and physiological data drawn from samples of stutterers' connected speech. Behavioral data show that stutterers demonstrate greater frequency of disfluency and less adaptation when reading aloud passages containing both voiced and voiceless segments than passages containing only voiced segments (Adams and Reis, 1971, 1974; Adams, Riemenschnieder, Metz & Conture, 1975). Physiologic data, obtained from fiberoptic viewing of the vocal folds (Conture, McCall & Brewer, 1977) and the recording of electromyographic (EMG) signals from intrinsic laryngeal muscles (Freeman and Ushijima, 1978; Shapiro, 1980), reveal evidence of abnormal laryngeal activity during stutterers' disfluent utterances. However, it is not clear to what extent data reported in these studies reflect the potentially disruptive effects of stutterers' attempts to coordinate the timing of vocal fold adduction and abduction with the rapid changes in respiratory and articulatory activities inherent in the production of connected speech or deficits confined to the independent control of the larynx.

Investigation of laryngeal activity during voice onset and offset is facilitated by the use of the reaction time paradigm. The dependent variable in this paradigm is the onset latency of the acoustic signal corresponding to vocal fold vibration relative to an external reaction signal (for example, a tone or a light). We refer to this latency as acoustic laryngeal reaction time, or LRT. Certain studies report acoustic LRT values for the production of isolated, voiced vowels (Adams and Hayden, 1976; Cross and Luper, 1979; Cross, Shadden, and Luper, 1979; Reich, Till & Goldsmith, 1981; Watson and Alfonso, 1982, 1983). Since activity of the articulatory system may be minimized for the vocalic response, LRT values obtained in these studies more likely reflect respiratory and laryngeal activity than articulatory activity. Consequently, significant between group acoustic LRT differences reported in most of these studies suggest that stutterers have greater difficulty than nonstutterers in coordinating respiratory and laryngeal activity necessary for rapid voice onset and/or offset.

In a previous reaction time study (Watson and Alfonso, 1983), we observed a composite stuttering severity and foreperiod effect on stutterers' acoustic LRT values. That is, mild, but not severe, stutterers' LRT values approached nonstutterers' values as foreperiod increased from 100 to 3000 msec. Foreperiod is the interval between presentation of a warning cue and a phonate cue. Sufficiently long foreperiods (i.e., beyond one second) can provide subjects time to prepare for the known response. Therefore, improvement in only mild stutterers' LRT values with increasing foreperiod suggests that mild and severe stutterers may be distinguished by their ability to execute prephonatory movements during and after the foreperiod. This distinction is described by the differential deficit hypothesis (Watson and Alfonso, 1983). Briefly, this hypothesis suggests that mild stutterers' delayed phonation onsets are related to their inability to execute respiratory and laryngeal movements during short foreperiods while severe stutterers' delayed phonation onsets are related to their inability to execute these movements both during and after the foreperiod, regardless of foreperiod duration. Alternatively, both groups may have similar deficits, but the magnitude of the deficit is determined by the severity of the disorder. The study reported here continues our investigation of the differential deficit hypothesis by recording prephonatory respiratory and laryngeal movements in parallel with the acoustic signal.

METHOD

Respiratory and laryngeal kinematic data were recorded by use of Respitrace (Cohn, Watson, Weisshaut, Stott & Sackner, 1977) and transillumination (Lisker, Abramson, Cooper & Schvey, 1969) instrumentation, respectively. Kinematic data were analyzed in terms of subjects' success in attaining functional physiological targets during and after the foreperiod (Watson, 1983). The functional target during the foreperiod is inflation of the respiratory system. The functional target after the foreperiod is the initiation of phonation.

Data are presented for two nonstutterers and for two mild and two severe stutterers. Classification by stuttering severity was based on agreement between one subjective and two objective (Riley, 1972; Ryan, 1974) measures of the frequency and type of disfluency observed during samples of reading and conversational

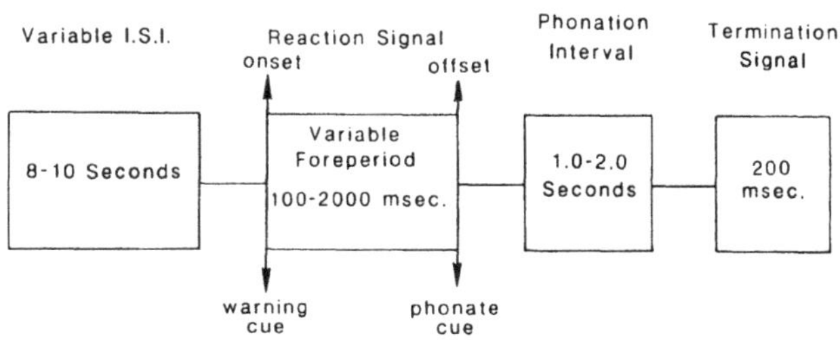

Figure 1. Schematic of the stimulus sequence. Subjects were instructed to prepare for the isolated vowel response following presentation of the warning cue and to initiate phonation after presentation of the phonate cue.

speech. Responses were included in the final data corpus only if they were perceptually fluent and there was no evidence of inaudible disfluencies in the acoustic signal; for example, isolated pitch pulses before the onset of continuous phonation. All subjects used the soft mode of vocal attack.

Figure 1 displays an example of one sequence of stimuli that allows us to test the effect of a variable foreperiod on LRT values. Each sequence is separated by a variable inter-stimulus interval (ISI) of 8 to 10 seconds. The reaction signal is the synthetic vowel /i/ varying in duration from 100 to 2000 msec in 11 steps. Onset of the reaction signal serves as the warning cue and offset serves as the phonate cue. Subjects are instructed to phonate the vowel /i/ immediately at the offset of the reaction signal. After a variable phonation interval, a terminate phonation signal is presented. The terminate signal consists of the synthetic vowel /a/. Each of the 11 sequences was replicated 8 times, randomized, and output on audiotape using the Haskins Laboratories PCM system.

Figure 2 displays an example of simultaneous acoustic and movement data for one response. The top record shows the reaction signal. The second record shows the transillumination signal. Upward displacement of this signal represents vocal fold opening and downward displacement represents vocal fold closing. For example, the arrow labelled A indicates the moment of vocal fold closure. The third and fourth records show Respitrace signals for the thoracic and abdominal walls, respectively. Upward displacement of these signals represents cavity expansion and downward displacement represents cavity compression. For example, the arrow labelled B indicates the onset of abdominal compression. Finally, the fifth record displays the acoustic signal.

The coordination of prephonatory laryngeal and respiratory movements executed to attain functional targets was evaluated in terms of their timing and organization. For this reaction time paradigm, the timing of prephonatory movements is reflected in their absolute onset latencies relative to presentation of either the warning cue or phonate cue. The organization of these movements is reflected in their relative onset latencies. Significant between group differences were observed in both measurement domains for movements leading to respiratory inflation and phonation initiation. For

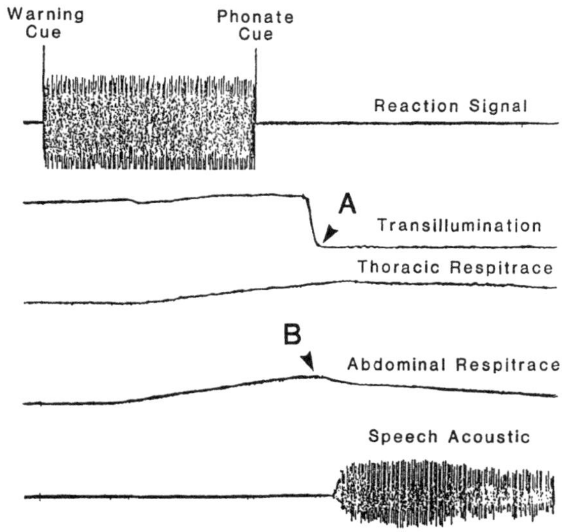

Figure 2. Example of simultaneous acoustic and movement data channels for one response.

example, during all foreperiods, nonstutterers and mild stutterers demonstrated well organized sequences characterized by the onset of vocal fold opening before the onset of inspiratory gestures. Conversely, severe stutterers demonstrated poorly organized sequences characterized by the onset of inspiratory gestures before the onset of vocal fold opening. However, this report is limited to a discussion of between group differences in the absolute and relative onset latencies of movements associated with initiation activities occurring after the foreperiod; that is, laryngeal and respiratory movements leading to phonation onset.

RESULTS

Figure 3 displays group mean acoustic LRT values as a function of foreperiod. The top function shows severe stutterers' values, the middle function shows mild stutterers' values, and the bottom function shows nonstutterers' values. Two aspects of these data are important. First, these data replicate our original observation of a composite stuttering severity and foreperiod effect on LRT values (Watson and Alfonso, 1983). Second, closer examination of this figure reveals that the range of foreperiods can be divided into two regions. Specifically, mild and severe stutterers' LRT values are similar at foreperiods between 100 and 700 msec, while mild stutterers' and nonstutterers' LRT values are similar at foreperiods beyond 700 msec. In order to identify characteristics of respiratory and laryngeal movements underlying the similarity between mild and

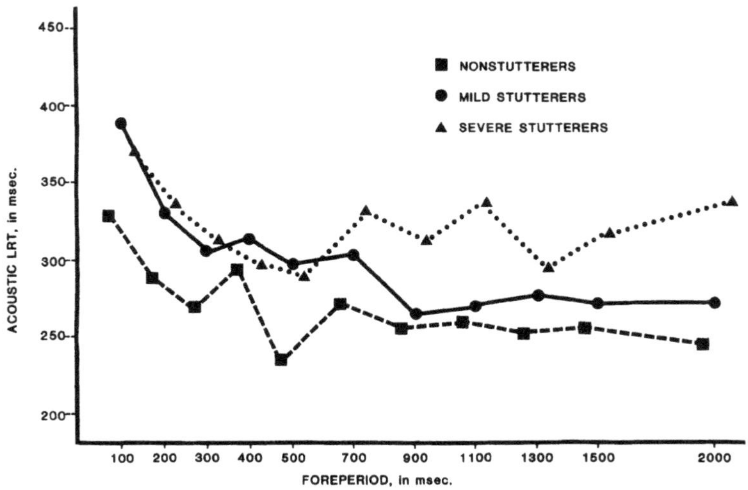

Figure 3. Mean acoustic LRT values as a function of foreperiod for two nonstutterers, two mild stutterers, and two severe stutterers. All subjects received the same foreperiod conditions. Mean LRT values at each foreperiod are offset for clarity.

severe stutterers' LRT values at short foreperiods and between mild stutterers' and nonstutterers' LRT values at long foreperiods, between group comparisons were made for movements occurring after short foreperiods (between 100 and 700 msec) and after long foreperiods (beyond 700 msec). To summarize, our aim is to identify between group differences in the timing and organization of prephonatory respiratory and laryngeal movements occurring after the foreperiod that can account for the observed between group differences in acoustic LRT values.

Figure 4 displays frequency distributions for the absolute onset latencies of vocal fold closure and abdominal compression for all groups after short foreperiods. The abdominal compression gesture was selected for analysis of respiratory movements because most subjects began thoracic compression after phonation onset. Values along the abscissa represent 20 msec intervals after presentation of the phonate cue. Note that the time scales differ for each group. Values along the ordinate represent frequency of occurrence expressed as the percent of valid responses. Thus, each data point represents the percent of valid responses for which a particular event was initiated during a specific 20 msec interval. Pair-wise Chi-square comparisons of onset latency distributions for vocal fold closure after short foreperiods reveal significant differences between nonstutterers and mild stutterers ($x^2 = 26.3$, $p < .05$) and between nonstutterers and severe stutterers ($x^2 = 34.2$, $p < .01$). The difference between mild and severe stutterers is not significant. Pair-wise comparisons of onset latency distributions for abdominal compression reveal significant differences between nonstutterers and mild stutterers ($x^2 = 32.8$, $p < .05$) and between

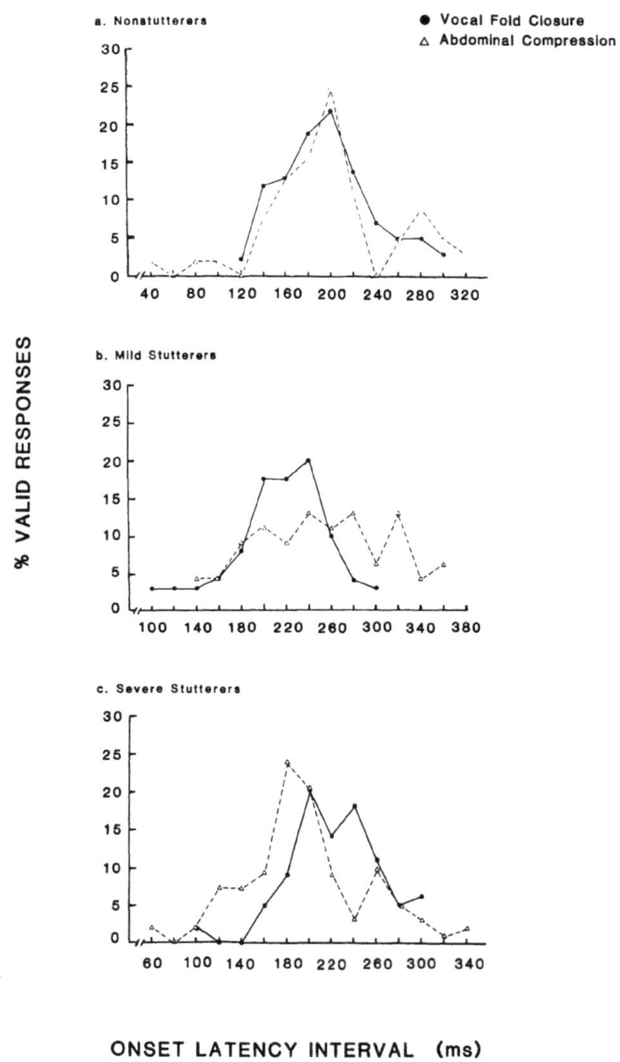

Figure 4. Frequency distributions of the onset latencies of abdominal compression and vocal fold closure after short foreperiods. Frequency values represent the percent of valid responses in which a movement began during a 20 ms interval following presentation of the warning cue.

mild and severe stutterers (x^2 = 39.5, $p < .01$). The difference between nonstutterers and severe stutterers is not significant. Thus, after short foreperiods, mild and severe stutterers are significantly slower than nonstutterers in attaining vocal fold closure, while mild stutterers are significantly slower than both nonstutterers and severe stutterers in initiating abdominal compression.

We turn now to a comparison of the relative timing relationship between vocal fold closure and the onset of abdominal compression for each group after short foreperiods. Here we compare the loci of the peaks in the frequency distributions for vocal fold closure and for abdominal compression. For the nonstutterers and mild stutterers, peaks in the distribution for vocal fold closure occur simultaneously with, or immediately before, peaks in the distribution for abdominal compression. That is, nonstutterers and mild stutterers generally attain vocal fold closure simultaneously with, or immediately before, the onset of abdominal compression. Thus, the organization of prephonatory laryngeal and respiratory movements for these subjects is appropriate for the soft mode of attack. However, severe stutterers demonstrate a peak in the distribution for abdominal compression before the peak for vocal fold closure. That is, severe stutterers' organization of prephonatory laryngeal and respiratory movements is inappropriate for the soft mode of attack. To summarize, after short foreperiods, mild stutterers demonstrate delayed onset of well organized laryngeal and respiratory movements, while severe stutterers demonstrate delayed onset of vocal fold closure and poorly organized prephonatory movements.

Figure 5 displays frequency distributions for the absolute onset latencies of vocal fold closure and abdominal compression after long foreperiods. Once again, values along the abscissa represent 20 msec intervals after presentation of the phonate cue and values along the ordinate represent frequency of occurrence as the percent of valid responses. Pair-wise comparisons of the frequency distributions for vocal fold closure reveal significant differences between nonstutterers and severe stutterers ($x^2 = 74.2$, $p < .01$) and between mild and severe stutterers ($x^2 = 23.9$, $p < .01$). However, the difference between nonstutterers and mild stutterers is not significant. Pair-wise comparisons of the distributions for abdominal compression reveal significant differences between nonstutterers and mild stutterers ($x^2 = 31.8$, $p < .01$) and between mild and severe stutterers ($x^2 = 23.9$, $p < .05$). The difference between nonstutterers and severe stutterers is not significant. Thus, only severe stutterers are significantly slower than nonstutterers in attaining vocal fold closure, while mild stutterers continue to be significantly slower in initiating abdominal compression. However, note that the mild stutterers' onset latency frequency distribution for abdominal compression is bimodal. We will discuss the implications of this observation below.

We turn now to an analysis of the relative timing relationship between vocal fold closure and the onset of abdominal compression for each group after long foreperiods. As was the case at short foreperiods, comparisons of the loci of the peaks in the frequency distributions reveal that both nonstutterers and mild stutterers demonstrate appropriate organization of laryngeal and respiratory movements for the soft mode of attack. With respect to the mild stutterers, the bimodal distribution for abdominal compression reflects the fact that one mild stutterer initiated this gesture simultaneously with the moment of vocal fold closure, while the other mild stutterer began abdominal compression after, but never before, vocal fold closure. For this latter subject, the acoustic signal indicates that overall respiratory pressure was sufficient to

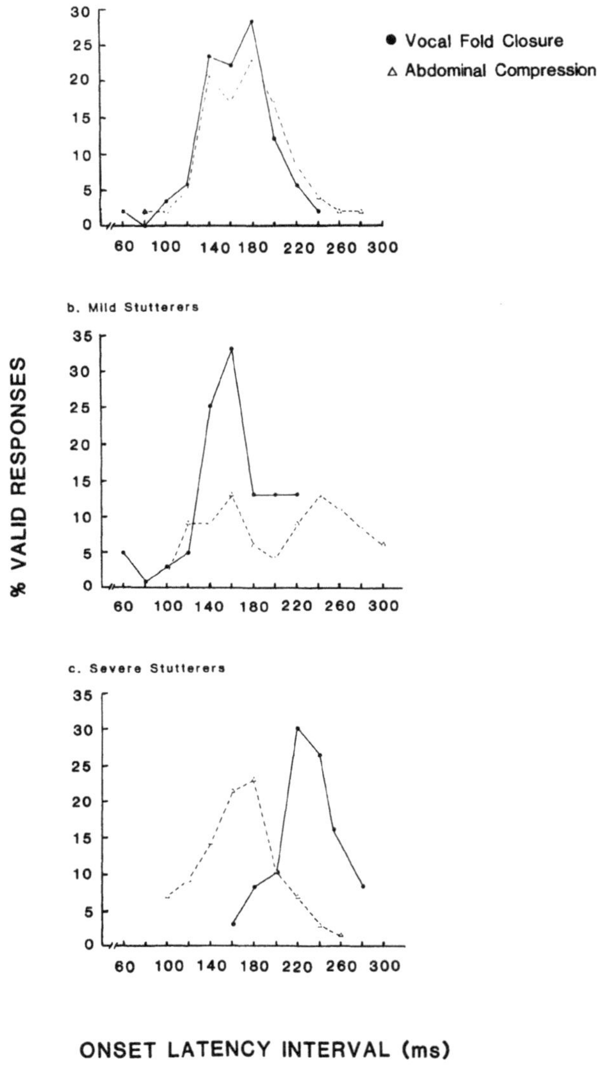

Figure 5. Frequency distributions of the onset latencys of abdominal compression and vocal fold closure after long foreperiods. Frequency values represent the percent of valid responses in which a movement began during a 20 ms interval following presentation of the phonate cue.

initiate vocal fold vibration even though abdominal compression occurred later. Conversely, severe stutterers' organization of laryngeal and respiratory movements remains inappropriate. Specifically, abdominal compression begins well before the moment of vocal fold closure. In summary, after long foreperiods, mild stutterers demonstrate delayed onset of abdominal compression and well organized prephonatory movements, while severe stutterers demonstrate delayed onset of vocal fold closure and poorly organized prephonatory movements.

DISCUSSION

Due to the relatively invasive nature of fiberoptic endoscopy, it is difficult to perform this procedure on a large number of naive subjects. However, we successfully recorded Respitrace and transillumination signals from nine stutterers. The data from five of these subjects were not reported in this study because they did not meet the fluency criteria, did not represent the soft mode of vocal attack, or did not unambiguously distinguish the subject as either a mild or severe stutterer. However, acoustic LRT values for the four stutterers reported here are nearly identical to the values for the ten stutterers reported in a previous study (Watson and Alfonso, 1983). Therefore, we assume that the two mild and two severe stutterers described in this experiment are representative of larger groups of similar severity ratings. As is often the case in physiologically-based studies, we are forced to draw what conclusions we can from a relatively small sample of the population.

The present analysis of the timing and organization of prephonatory respiratory and laryngeal movements reveals differential deficits in the stuttering subjects. These deficits can account for differences between mild and severe stutterers' acoustic LRT values as a function of increasing foreperiod duration. For example, severe stutterers demonstrate significant delays in attaining vocal fold closure as well as consistently poor organization of prephonatory respiratory and laryngeal movements after both short and long foreperiods. Taken together, these factors likely contribute to severe stutterers' prolonged acoustic LRT values at both short and long foreperiods. Conversely, mild stutterers demonstrate delays in attaining vocal fold closure only after short foreperiods. Presumably, they use the increased preparatory time afforded by longer foreperiods to achieve vocal fold closure before presentation of the phonate cue. Mild stutterers also demonstrate well organized prephonatory respiratory and laryngeal movements after all foreperiods. These factors likely contribute to the observed improvement in mild stutterers' acoustic LRT values at long versus short foreperiods.

These results are significant in two respects. First, these data support the differential deficit hypothesis for a subject classification protocol based on stuttering severity. That is, mild and severe stutterers attain, or fail to attain, functional prephonatory targets in quantitatively and qualitatively different ways. This difference may be an important factor underlying the heterogeneity of the stuttering population. Of course, other factors such as the prominent type (i.e., repetitions vs prolongations) (Stromsta, 1984) or locus (i.e., lingual vs. labial) (Shapiro, 1980) of disfluency have also been suggested as reliable grouping characteristics. However, since our subjects did not meet grouping criteria other than severity, it is unlikely that the between group differences observed in this study can be attributed to either the "type" or "locus" of disfluency. Second, observation of simultaneous respiratory and laryngeal movements implies that, at least for severe stutterers in this study, the physiological deficits underlying slower acoustic LRT values may occur in both the respiratory and laryngeal systems. In conclusion, these results support the notion that physiological differences characterize mild and severe stutterers and support multiple anatomical loci models of stuttering.

ACKNOWLEDGEMENTS

This research was supported by NIH Grants NS-13870 and 1-T32-NS-07237 awarded to Haskins Laboratories.

REFERENCES

Adams, M.R. & Reis, R. (1971). The influence of the onset of phonation on the frequency of stuttering. *Journal of Speech and Hearing Research, 14,* 639-644.

Adams, M.R. & Reis, R. (1974). Influence of the onset of phonation on the frequency of stuttering: A replication and re-evaluation. *Journal of Speech and Hearing Research, 17,* 752-754.

Adams, M.R., Riemenschnieder, S., Metz, D. & Conture, E. (1975). Voice onset and articulatory constriction requirements in a speech segment and their relation to the amount of stuttering adaptation. *Journal of Fluency Disorders, 1,* 24-31.

Adams, M.R. & Hayden, P. (1976). The ability of stutterers and nonstutterers to initiate and terminate phonation during production of an isolated vowel. *Journal of Speech and Hearing Research, 19,* 290-296.

Adams, M.R. (1978). Stuttering theory, research, and therapy: The present and future. *Journal of Fluency Disorders, 3,* 139-147.

Cohn, D.E., Watson, H., Weisshaut, R., Stott, F. & Sackner, M. (1977). *A transducer for non-invasive monitoring of respiration.* Paper presented at the 2nd International Symposium on Ambulatory Monitoring, Harrow, Middlesex, U.K.

Conture, E.G., McCall, G.N. & Brewer, D.W. (1977). Laryngeal behavior during stuttering. *Journal of Speech and Hearing Research, 20,* 661-668.

Cross, D.E. & Luper, H.L. (1979). Voice reaction time of stuttering and non-stuttering children and adults. *Journal of Fluency Disorders, 4,* 59-77.

Cross, D.E., Shadden, B.B. & Luper, H.L. (1979). Effects of stimulus ear presentation on the voice reaction time of adult stutterers and non-stutterers. *Journal of Fluency Disorders, 4,* 45-58.

Freeman, F.J. & Ushijima, T. (1978). Laryngeal muscle activity during stuttering. *Journal of Speech and Hearing Research, 21,* 538-562.

Lisker, L., Abramson, A., Cooper, F.S. & Schvey, M. (1969). "Transillumination of the larynx in running speech." *Journal of the Acoustical Society of America, 45,* 1544-1546.

Reich, A., Till, J. & Goldsmith, H. (1981). Laryngeal and manual reaction times of stuttering and nonstuttering adults. *Journal of Speech and Hearing Research, 24,* 192-196.

Riley, G. (1972). A stuttering severity instrument for children and adults. *Journal of Speech and Hearing Research, 37,* 314-322.

Ryan, B. (1974). *Programmed Therapy for Stuttering Children and Adults.* Springfield, IL: Charles C. Thomas.

Shapiro, A. (1980). An electromyographic analysis of the fluent and disfluent utterances of several types of stutterers. *Journal of Fluency Disorders, 5,* 203-231.

Stromsta, C. (1983). Phonatory reaction time of stutterers as a function of masking and therapeutic intervention. In M. Edwards (Ed.), *Proceedings of the XIX Congress of the International Association of Logopaedics and Phoniatrics,* Vol. 2, Edinburgh, Scotland.

Van Riper, C. (1971). *The nature of stuttering.* Englewood Cliffs, New Jersey: Prentice-Hall.

Watson, B.C. & Alfonso, P.J. (1982). A comparison of LRT and VOT values between stutterers and nonstutterers. *Journal of Fluency Disorders, 7,* 219-241.

Watson, B.C. & Alfonso, P.J. (1983). Foreperiod and stuttering severity effects on acoustic laryngeal reaction time. *Journal of Fluency Disorders, 8,* 183-205.

Watson, B.C. (1983). *Simultaneous fiberoptic, transillumination, Respitrace, and acoustic analysis of laryngeal reaction time in stutterers and nonstutterers.* Unpublished Ph.D. Dissertation, University of Connecticut.

Zimmermann, G.N., Smith, A. & Hanley, J.M. (1981). Stuttering: In need of a unifying conceptual framework. *Journal of Speech and Hearing Research, 24,* 25-31.

Chapter 14

Coordination of Laryngeal and Supralaryngeal Behavior in Stutterers

Gloria J. Borden and Joy Armson

In 1971 Van Riper suggested that the temporal disruptions in speech which constitute stuttering result from the speaker possessing a deficient timing mechanism for speech. Recently Kent (1984) has reiterated this idea by postulating that the essence of stuttering is a reduced ability to generate temporal programs. A related explanation of stuttering is expressed in the discoordination hypothesis advanced by Perkins and colleagues (1976). According to the discoordination hypothesis, stuttering results from a speaker's difficulty in coordinating phonation with articulation and respiration. This hypothesis expresses in weakened form, the view that the larynx has a central role in precipitating moments of stuttering, a notion which prompted much research in the 1970s. In general, these studies have left the question of laryngeal focus unresolved, although they have revealed evidence of a strong laryngeal component in stuttering (Conture, McCall & Brewer, 1977; Freeman & Ushijima, 1978). In order both to better understand the nature of speech timing in stutterers and to resolve the laryngeal focus question, it is appropriate to study how the three major speech systems interact or coordinate when stutterers are speaking. In this chapter, we will be dealing with the topic of laryngeal/supralaryngeal coordination. We will begin by outlining information about the interaction of these systems in normal speakers, then present some relevant data regarding stutterers, and end with a description of a study which proposes to more completely investigate this interaction.

One aspect of laryngeal/supralaryngeal cooperation during speech that has been well researched in normal speakers is that which underlies production of the voicing contrast. For example, we know from the work of Lisker and Abramson (1964) that speakers of different languages coordinate laryngeal and supralaryngeal activity for this contrast according to the relative timing constraints imposed by particular languages. Voice onset time (VOT), the measure defined by Lisker and Abramson, is obtained from the acoustic record, and shows that the supralaryngeal release of a stop consonant is coordinated with onset of voicing for a following vowel differently for voiced than for voiceless stops, that the difference lies in relative timing, and is lawful as well as language specific. In contrast to the many acoustic studies of the voicing contrast which followed Lisker and Abramsons' seminal study, Löfqvist's (1980) work provides the only analysis of which we are aware that attempts to provide a physiological description of the coordination of supralaryngeal and laryngeal articulations during stop consonant production. Using transillumination and aerodynamic measures, Löfqvist found timing of laryngeal-supralaryngeal interactions to be the critical factor used to control degree of aspiration in a voiceless stop consonant. His work showed that peak glottal opening occurred at approximately the same time as the release of the aspirated stop. It is worth noting that there are no published studies that probe the kinematics of both systems as they operate in parallel. From the information which is available, however, it is apparent that coarticulation of laryngeal and supralaryngeal systems for production of the voicing contrast involves relatively precise temporal coordination, and as such, provides an appropriate context for studying motor control in a population which has difficulty generating temporal patterns.

Most of what we know about the interaction of laryngeal and supralaryngeal behavior in the speech of stutterers also comes from studies of the acoustic measure of voice onset time. Results are equivocal. Some studies report VOT to be longer than normal in the perceptually fluent utterances of stutterers (Agnello & Wendall, 1972; Hillman & Gilbert, 1977), while other studies contradict or qualify the longer VOT results (Metz, Conture & Caruso, 1979; Watson & Alfonso, 1983). The lack of agreement in these studies may be the result of differences in the number of covert blocks in the speech samples accepted as 'fluent'. Evidence that perceptual fluency is not synonymous with physiological fluency is illustrated by the findings of the EMG studies conducted by Freeman and Ushijima (1978) and Shapiro (1980). Both found instances of abnormal muscle activity and disruptions in normal coordination characteristic of stuttering during some of the perceptually fluent utterances of stutterers. In a study by Borden, Baer, and Kenney (1985), an attempt was made to eliminate as many covert blocks as possible. To begin with, utterances were elicited using the adaptation procedure; i.e., subjects repeated each utterance until fluency was achieved. Next, prior to analysis, movement data gathered concomitantly with the acoustic data were inspected for abnormal fluctuations. Any perceptually fluent utterances for which there was evidence of abnormal movement were eliminated from the sample.

VOTs for the 16 subjects in this study are shown in Figure 1. Each bar of the histogram represents the mean VOT for one subject. Means are based on 10, or in cases where utterances were disqualified, somewhat fewer productions of the word "two".

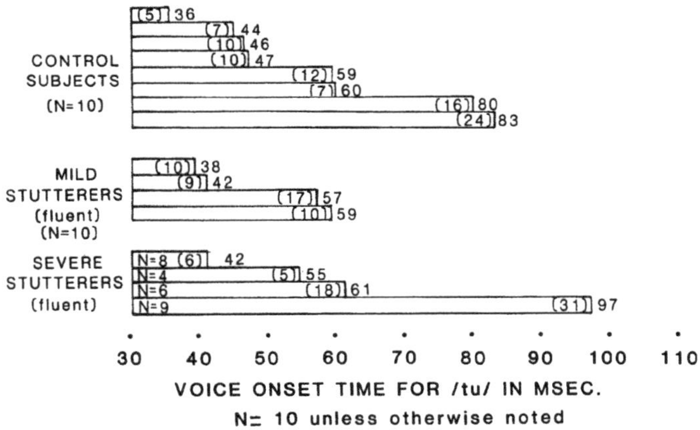

Figure 1. Voice onset time (VOT) as measured from sound spectrograms of the fluent utterances [tu] of the stutterers during the adaptation task and those of the control subjects. Each of the 8 control subjects and the 4 mild stutterers yielded 10 samples of [tu]. Fewer than 10 fluent samples were obtained from the four severe stutterers.

Voice onset time measured from the utterances of nonstuttering control subjects ranged from an average of 36 msec to 83 msec. Mild stutterers were well within normal limits of VOT when they were perceptually and physiologically fluent as were most of the severe stutterers. One of the severe stutterers was somewhat slower in VOT than the other subjects but group differences were not significant. These data suggest that when stutterers are "physiologically" as well as perceptually fluent, they demonstrate normal relative timing between laryngeal and supralaryngeal systems for at least this CV combination.

Since we are interested in relative timing, recording and measuring the articulatory movements provide us with information that supplements the acoustic record: onsets of movements, durations of movements, and phasing of interarticulator movements. This information enables us to better describe the coordination and discoordination that produce the acoustic effects found. We are currently analyzing data of this type from stutterers and nonstutterers.

In Figure 2 movement records taken simultaneously with the acoustic record show coordination of the laryngeal and supralaryngeal systems for a normal speaker. Shown here from top to bottom are: first, lip/jaw movement, where upward deflection of the tracing represents lip/jaw closure and downward deflection shows the opening gesture; second, slow EGG where again peaks represent closure and valleys represent opening; third, fast EGG, and on the bottom, the record of the acoustic signal. The speaker is saying "3425" here. For production of the words "four" and "five" these tracings show initiation of lip opening for /f/ to be closely timed with the peak of glottal opening. The temporal coordination shown here for an English voiceless fricative is similar to Löfqvist's findings for a Swedish aspirated stop.

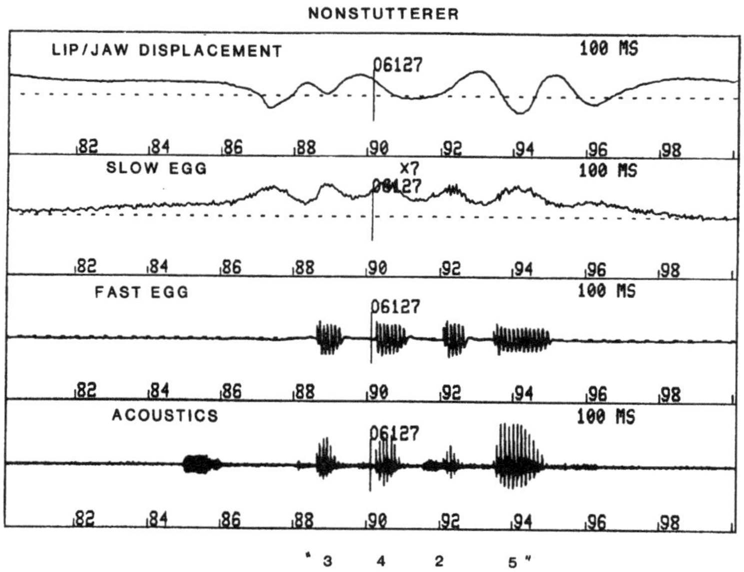

Figure 2. Laryngeal and supralaryngeal movements for the utterance '3425' spoken by a nonstutterer. In the acoustic trace the first burst was produced by the response signal. The timing of lip/jaw release from the fricative [f] constriction for '4' and '5' (indicated by downward arrows) closely corresponds with peak vocal fold abduction for the [f] (indicated by upward arrows). Vertical lines through each trace served as line up points.

Figure 3 shows records obtained during an instance of stuttering. The stutterer is attempting to say the word 'four'. Voice onset for 'four' was delayed in this instance for approximately 2800 msec after the preliminary lip/jaw lowering and vocal adductory movements, yet the two systems retained their phase relationship across the four trials shown here. For each trial, peak vocal fold opening (indicated by the up arrows on the slow EGG tracing) is coordinated with the initiation of lip/jaw lowering (indicated by the down arrows on the lip/jaw displacement tracing). This corresponds to the laryngeal-supralaryngeal pre-voice posturing that was evident in the figure for the nonstutterer. So, although speech is discoordinated during stuttering, here is an instance in which the pre-voicing movements remain coordinated.

One might ask what it is that prevents voicing from being initiated in this case. A clue to this lies in the lip and fast EGG waveforms - the first and third shown in the figure. Here we can see evidence of a physiological tremor of about 7 Hz in both systems. Abnormal muscle activity of this type must necessarily affect system dynamics, conceivably in such a way as would impede the forward flow of speech. As to what is responsible for this abnormal muscle activity pattern there are no clues in these data. However, in this instance, we are at least able to rule out a mistiming of initial lip and laryngeal adjustments as a possible precipitating condition. In view of the laryngeal focus question, we might

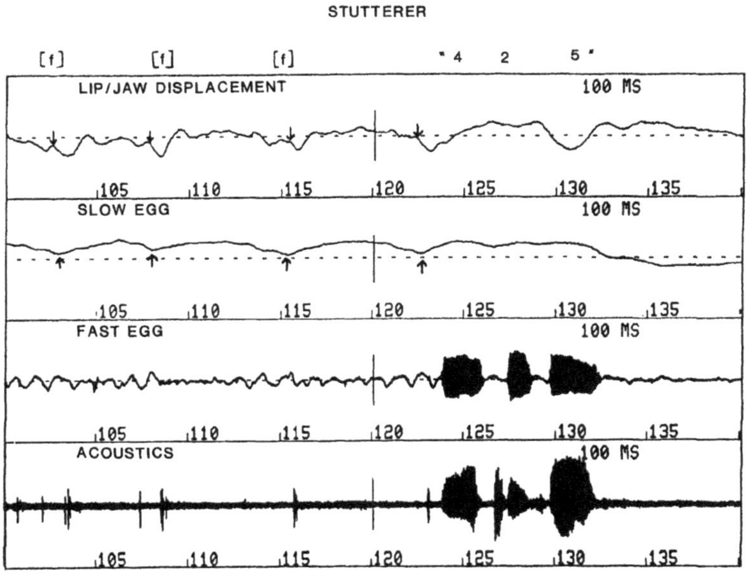

Figure 3. Laryngeal and supralaryngeal movements for the last three digits of the utterance '3425' spoken by a stutterer who repeated the voiceless fricative [f]. Although there are simultaneous tremors in the lip/jaw displacement and the vocal fold displacement (fast EEG) traces, the lower frequency repetitive [f] trials reveal the proximity of lip/jaw release of the [f] constriction and peak vocal fold abduction (as indicated in the slow EGG signal) that was evident in the traces of the nonstutterer.

also be interested to know whether the tremor began in one system and radiated to another or whether the tremors were set up simultaneously, as a result of a higher level problem in motor commands common to both systems. At this level of investigation it is impossible to determine this. Electromyographic data, however, could presumably provide access to this type of information.

Clearly research into interarticulator coordination of stutterers is in an early stage. Although valuable information may be contributed to this topic by analysis based on acoustic and kinematic records, interpretation of such findings is likely to be greatly facilitated if accompanied by EMG data as was suggested in the foregoing discussion. For this reason we have designed a study which requires simultaneous measures of movement (as indicated by lip/jaw optical tracking records and EGG records) and muscle activity (from recordings of the orbicularis oris muscle and selected laryngeal muscles). Laryngeal/supralaryngeal coordination for production of labial stop consonants will be analyzed under three conditions: stuttered speech, the fluent speech of stutterers, and the speech of nonstutterers. By relating speech movement indices to records of muscle activity levels we should obtain an in depth physiological description of the labial/laryngeal interaction for production of the voicing contrast. From such a physiological description it is hoped that inferences can be drawn about the nature of speech timing in stutterers as well as the role of the larynx as either a trigger or merely a participant in the breakdown of fluency.

REFERENCES

Agnello, J., Wingate, M. & Wendall, M. (1974). *Voice onset and voice termination times of children and adult stutterers.* Paper presented at the Acoustical Society of America, St. Louis, MO.

Borden, G.J., Baer, T.B. & Kenney, M.K. (1985). Onset of voicing in stuttered and fluent utterances. *Journal of Speech and Hearing Research, 28,* 363-372.

Conture, E.G., McCall, G.N. & Brewer, D.W. (1977). Laryngeal behavior during stuttering. *Journal of Speech and Hearing Research, 20,* 661-668.

Freeman, F.J. & Ushijima, T. (1978). Laryngeal muscle activity during stuttering. *Journal of Speech and Hearing Research, 21,* 538-562.

Hillman, R.E. & Gilbert, H. (1977). Voice onset time for voiceless stop consonants in the fluent reading of stutterers and nonstutterers. *Journal of the Acoustical Society of America, 61,* 610-611.

Kent, R.D. (1984). Stuttering as a temporal programming disorder. In R.F. Curlee & W.H. Perkins (Eds.), *Nature and treatment of stuttering: New directions* (pp. 283-301). San Diego, CA: College-Hill Press.

Lisker, L. & Abramson, A. (1964). A cross-language study of voicing in initial stops: Acoustical measurements. *Word, 20,* 384-422.

Löfqvist, A. (1980). Interarticulator programming in stop production. *Journal of Phonetics, 8,* 475-490.

Metz, D.E., Conture, E.G. & Caruso, A. (1979). Voice onset time, frication, and aspiration during stutterers' fluent speech. *Journal of Speech and Hearing Research, 22,* 649-656.

Perkins, W.H., Rudas, J., Johnson, L. & Bell, J. (1976). Stuttering: Discoordination of phonation with articulation and respiration. *Journal of Speech and Hearing Research, 19,* 509-522.

Shapiro, A. (1980). An electromyographic analysis of the fluent and dysfluent utterances of several types of stutterers. *Journal of Fluency Disorders, 5,* 203-231.

Van Riper, C. (1971). *The nature of stuttering.* Englewood Cliffs, NJ: Prentice Hall.

Watson, B.C. & Alfonso, P.J. (1983). Foreperiod and stuttering severity effects on acoustic laryngeal reaction time. *Journal of Fluency Disorders, 8,* 183-206.

Chapter 15

Subgrouping Young Stutterers: A Physiological Perspective

Howard D. Schwartz

Identification and description of subgroups of stutterers has been related to both the etiology and treatment of stuttering (Preus, 1981). Andrews and Harris (1964) proposed an etiological classification where they attempted to group young stutterers by using a large number of psycho-social variables, for example, birth order, child rearing practices and intelligence. Treatment subgroups were examined by Douglass and Quarrington (1952) who suggested that diagnostic procedures would reveal different types of stutterers who may require different types of therapeutic management. In a somewhat different manner, Prins and Lohr (1972), examined the characteristics of the stuttered speech and described the different speech and nonspeech behaviors associated with the production of stuttered words. These investigators suggested that quantification of behaviors associated with stuttering may have implications for the manner in which we consider "etiologies and therapies" for stuttering.

Using a method similar to Prins and Lohr (1972), Schwartz and Conture (1986) suggested that identification of subgroups should focus on the speech and nonspeech behaviors associated with stuttering so that the differences that appear to differentiate normally fluent speaker from stutterers may also help to differentiate among the stutterers themselves. As a result, Schwartz and Conture (1986) suggested that by quantifying the most frequently occurring disfluency type (sound/syllable repetitions and sound prolongations) and examining the number and variety of behaviors associated with stuttering, young stutterers could be divided into five subgroups.

While differences have been noted among stutterers in speech disfluency type and associated behaviors, it has been suggested that stutterers may also exhibit a disordered timing mechanism relative to their speech production. Recently, Kent (1984) has speculated that "... a primary difference between stutterers and nonstutterers lies in their capacity to generate temporal programs, or time structures of action". Perkins, Rudas, Johnson, and Bell (1976) examined the relationship between the articulatory and phonatory systems and suggested that stuttering results from a discoordination between these two systems. The question then arises as to whether observable characteristics associated with stuttering (speech disfluency type; number and variety of associated behaviors) reflect the suggested differences in the temporal characteristics of speech physiology associated with young stutterers' stuttering.

Therefore, as the second part of the experiment reported by Schwartz and Conture (1986), the purpose of the present investigation was to examine the temporal onsets of speech physiology associated with stuttering to determine if the temporal aspects of speech physiology further differentiates among behavioral subgroups.

METHOD

Subjects

Fifteen young stutterers took part in this investigation. These 15 young stutterers were a subsample (N = 15) of a larger corpus of 43 subjects whose stuttering and associated speech and nonspeech behaviors were also investigated (see Schwartz & Conture, 1986). It should be noted that although it was believed that 15 subjects would provide a representative sample of children from all behavioral clusters, none of the 15 children examined were placed in Cluster 5 and thus no physiological data was available for analysis. The 15 young stutterers (8 females and 7 males) had a mean age of 5 years, 7 months with range from 3 years, 10 months to 7 years, 5 months. All 15 stutterers exhibited sound/syllable repetitions and sound prolongations with a mean stuttering frequency of 12 stutterings per 100 words of conversational speech (range = 3 to 42 within-word disfluencies per 100 words of conversational speech).

Speech Stimuli and Conditions

In order to obtain stutterings and their associated temporal physiological characteristics, stutterings were obtained during conversational speech and structured speaking activities. The conversational samples ranged from 81 words to 300 words for these 15 children.

Data Collection

Recording. The recording of the physiological signals occurred in a single session during conversations between the examiner and the client. This session was also audio/video recorded to obtain speech and nonspeech behaviors associated with stuttering (see Schwartz and Conture, 1986). The collection of physiological signals from the respiratory, supralaryngeal, and laryngeal systems occurred in a specially designed clinical room that was electrically connected to a laboratory containing recording devices (e.g. multi-channel FM recorder Honeywell, Model 101).

Respiratory System. Respiratory activity was sensed using a non-invasive inductive plethysmograph or Respitrace (Sackner, 1979; Watson, 1979; Bless, Hunker & Weismer, 1981) which provided displacement measures of rib and abdominal activity. The two respiratory signals were recorded on separate channels of the FM recorder.

Supralaryngeal Articulatory System. Supralaryngeal articulatory activity focused on electrical interference patterns associated with lip muscle opening and closing during the production of stutterings. Surface electromyographic (EMG) electrodes were used to obtain recordings from electrode sites anatomically associated with lip muscle activity involved with lip opening (Depressor Labi Inferior, DLI) and lip closing (Orbicularis Oris Inferior, OOI). EMG electrode placements were based upon earlier work with young children completed at Syracuse University as well as recommendations in a number of published reports (Isley and Basmajian, 1973; Kennedy and Abbs, 1975; O'Dwyer, Quinn, Guitar, Andrews, and Neilson, 1981).

Laryngeal System. Onset of vocal fold contact associated with the initiation of phonation was sensed using an electroglottograph (EGG) (Abberton, 1971; Conture, Rothenberg & Molitor, 1986; Fourcin, 1974, 1981; MacCurtain and Fourcin, 1981; Gilbert, Potter & Hoodin, 1984; Michel, Pfister, and Luchsinger, 1970; Rothenberg, 1981). To reduce low frequency distortion, the EGG signal was high pass filtered (Ng and Rothenberg, 1982) and subsequently recorded on one channel of the FM recorder.

Data Measurement

Processing for Subsequent Analysis. Ten stutterings were selected from the conversational samples of each subject and analyzed during the behavioral portion of this investigation (see Schwartz and Conture, 1986). These same ten stutterings were selected for physiological analysis and were derived from FM tape recordings for the 15 subjects under investigation (150 stutterings in total).

The five physiological signals and the acoustic signals were output from the FM recorder to a multi-channel storage oscilloscope whose face was video recorded (Sony, BVU 200A) (60 videofields per second) on 3/4" videotape for subsequent data measurement. Proper segmentation of each instance of stuttering was controlled by replaying the FM recorder and videotape while it moved across the face of the oscilloscope.

Criteria. The measurement of the temporal aspects of speech physiology associated with stuttering was made relative to the onset (time zero) of acoustic energy (voicing) associated with the first fluently produced vowel or consonant which immediately followed the stuttered sound, syllable, or monosyllabic whole-word. The identification of the time zero point and onsets of speech physiology were accomplished using a computer-assisted measurement program.

This measurement program involved the movement of a visible dot or cursor across the face of the television monitor. For every stuttered word, the time zero point was located and stored in the computer. This time zero point became the reference point for all subsequent temporal measurements (in milliseconds) with those occurring prior to time zero being labeled with a negative (-) value.

The onset of respiratory behavior was determined to be the highest voltage associated with the stuttered word prior to time zero. Onset of supralaryngeal articulatory activity (OOI and DLI) was measured at 10% of the peak amplitude (highest voltage) *prior* to time zero. Onset of laryngeal activity was measured when the positive excursion of the EGG waveform first exceeded 25% of the peak positive value during the first occurrence of the vowel in the disfluent word.

Data Analysis

The analysis of the physiological characteristics of stuttered speech involved the measurement of temporal onsets and relative sequences of temporal onsets for the five signals examined (Rib deflation, Abdomen Deflation, Lip muscle activity associated with lip muscle closing, Lip muscle activity associated with lip muscle opening, and Vocal Fold contact. Descriptive statistics (e.g. mean, standard deviations, and rank ordering) were used with for all of these measurements.

Reliability of Physiological Measures

One within-word disfluency (representing the distribution of speech disfluency type, and place and manner of articulatory productions in the total corpus of 150 stutterings) was selected from each of the 15 subjects whose speech physiology was measured (N-15 10% of total stutterings), in order to determine intra and interjudge reliability of physiological measurements. The number of sound prolongations (N = 9) and sound/syllable repetitions (N = 6) as well as place (bilabial/labial = 7 and dental/alveolar = 8) and manner (stops = 6, continuants = 5, fricatives = 4) of articulatory productions of 15 stutterings selected for remeasurement closely approximated the distribution of these variables within the entire corpus of 150 stutterings. Using a computer-assisted measurement program, two independent judges remeasured the physiological onsets (in milliseconds) of five signals associated with the stuttered sound, syllable or monosyllabic whole-word. Onset values were calculated for all five physiological signals where all the signals were present during the initial and rejudgement tasks (total number of measurements = 69). All measurements were made relative to the onset of the fluent consonant or vowel following the stuttering (time zero). Mean difference values for interjudge reliability were 45.06 msec (mean error = 69.32 msec) and mean differences for intrajudge reliability were 55.68 msec (mean error = 69.45 msec).

RESULTS

The speech physiology data to be reported will represent mean temporal onsets and sequences of physiological onsets among the speech physiology signals associated with 150 stutterings exhibited by 15 young stutterers in four of five behavioral subgroups. Although every attempt was made to include at least one subject from each of the five behavioral clusters, speech physiology data was not collected for any member of cluster 5.

Temporal aspects of speech physiology to be reported include the *onset* of: rib cage deflation, abdomen deflation, OOI activity associated with lip closing, DLI activity associated with lip opening, and vocal fold contact all associated with the production of a stuttering.

Sequence of Physiological Onsets for Behavioral Subgroups

Table 1 shows mean onset of speech physiology signals associated with stuttering for Clusters 1 through 4. It should be noted that the two most populated behavioral clusters (Clusters 1 and 3) are the clusters most represented in the physiological analysis. Examination of the relative sequence of the physiological onsets among the speech physiology signals for all clusters suggested that for all clusters investigated, respiratory deflation onsets first, followed by supralaryngeal lip muscle activity and finally laryngeal activity. Table 1 shows that the exact order of onset is not identical across the four groups; however, this appears to be a function of the manner of articulatory production of the stutterings observed (e.g. plosives versus fricatives) rather than actual physiological differences among the four subgroups. It should be pointed out that the diversity of stuttered words in regard to both manner and place of articulatory production occurred as a result of the investigators attempt to obtain stuttered words from conversational samples rather than limiting the clients to predetermined phonetically restricted phrases.

Sequence of Physiological Onsets for Stuttered Words Containing all Five Physiological Signals

Further examination of Table 1 indicated that the four clusters differed in terms of the number of tokens in which all five physiological signals were included. In attempts to achieve more adequate comparisons of the sequence of physiological onsets between clusters, only those stuttered words (N = 84) which contained all five physiological signals were examined (Table 2). It should be noted however, that two of the fifteen subjects could not be included in this portion of the investigation because they were missing at least one physiological signal for each of their ten disfluencies examined.

Table 1. Mean and standard deviation (intra- and inter-subject variability) of mean physiological onsets (in msec.) and rank ordered sequence of physiological onsets (first [1] to last [5]) associated with stuttering for 15 young stutterers' respiratory deflation (ABDOMEN and RIB), supralaryngeal lip muscle onset (OOI, DLI) and laryngeal onset (LX) associated with 150 within-word speech disfluencies for Clusters One through Four determined by hierarchical cluster analysis procedures (Schwartz and Conture 1986).

	RANK ORDERED ONSET SEQUENCE	VARIABLE	NUMBER TOKENS	MEAN (in msec)	STANDARD DEVIATION
CLUSTER 1 (subjects=5)	1	ABD	50	-1108	499
	2	RIB	50	- 955	484
	3	DLI	32	- 911	500
	4	OOI	35	- 818	508
	5	LX	50	- 592	504
CLUSTER 2 (subjects=2)	1	ABD	20	-2001	980
	2	RIB	20	-1817	960
	3	OOI	19	-1730	970
	4	DLI	19	-1678	1036
	5	LX	20	-1353	1149
CLUSTER 3 (subjects=7)	1	ABD	69	-1499	873
	2	RIB	70	-1352	817
	3	DLI	43	-1350	863
	4	OOI	48	-1310	848
	5	LX	60	- 859	823
CLUSTER 4 (subjects=1)	1	ABD	10	-1743	380*
	2	DLI	7	-1575	690
	3	RIB	10	-1387	405
	4	OOI	3	-1051	556
	5	LX	10	- 876	571

* Intra-subject variability only

Table 2 shows that the sequence of physiological onsets for Clusters 1 through 4 continued to exhibit the same sequence of respiratory, supralaryngeal, and laryngeal onsets. In an attempt to further examine the onset data containing all five physiological signals, the stutterings were categorized according to place of articulatory production with Table 3 showing the sequence of onsets for stuttered words (N = 34) beginning with labial and bilabial sounds, the place of production with the largest number of stutterings.

Results of this restricted comparisons show the same sequence of physiological onset: respiratory, supralaryngeal and laryngeal onset.

Mean Temporal Onsets for Clusters One through Four

The comparison of mean temporal onsets will focus on those stuttered words (N = 84) characterized by all five physiological

Table 2. Mean and standard deviation (intra- and inter-subject variability) of mean physiological onsets (in msec.) and rank ordered sequence of physiological onsets (first [1] to last [5]) associated with stuttering for 13 young stutterers' respiratory deflation (ABDOMEN and RIB), supralaryngeal lip muscle onset (OOI, DLI) and laryngeal onset (LX) associated with all stutterings (N=84) that exhibited all five physiological signals for Clusters One through Four (Schwartz and Conture, 1985). Two subjects were not included because at least one signal was missing for every stuttering.

	RANK ORDERED ONSET SEQUENCE	VARIABLE	NUMBER TOKENS	MEAN (in msec)	STANDARD DEVIATION
CLUSTER 1					
(subjects=5)	1	ABD	26	-1241	523
	2	RIB	26	-1061	524
	3	DLI	26	- 932	521
	4	OOI	26	- 902	510
	5	LX	26	- 674	601
CLUSTER 2					
(subjects=2)	1	ABD	19	-1960	989
	2	RIB	19	-1760	951
	3	OOI	19	-1730	970
	4	DLI	19	-1678	1036
	5	LX	19	-1419	1142
CLUSTER 3					
(subjects=5)	1	ABD	36	-1616	930
	2	RIB	36	-1485	861
	3	OOI	36	-1333	888
	4	DLI	36	-1315	887
	5	LX	36	- 972	917
CLUSTER 4					
(subjects=1)	1	ABD	3	-1581	374*
	2	RIB	3	-1546	310
	3	LX	3	-1148	243
	4	DLI	3	-1051	453
	5	OOI	3	-1051	556

* Intra-subjects variability only

signals exhibited by 13 of the 15 young stutterers in four subgroups (see Table 1). It should be noted that discussion of mean temporal onset essentially involves describing the *duration* from the initiation of the physiological signal associated with the stuttered segment to the onset (time zero) of the fluent sound, syllable or word.

Initial examination of Cluster 1 suggested that the mean signal onsets for all signals occurred closer (shorter duration) to time zero than the other three clusters examined. Cluster 2 on the other hand exhibited signals that were further from time zero (longest duration) when compared to the other clusters. Cluster 2's relatively early signal onsets (long durations) are especially evident for the onset of laryngeal activity which occurs on the average, 1.4 seconds before the onset of the fluent word. Clusters 3 and 4 exhibited mean onsets of physiological behavior that appeared to fall within the range of physiological onsets reported for Clusters 1 or

Table 3. Mean and standard deviation (intra- and inter-subject variability) of mean physiological onsets (in msec.) and rank ordered sequence of physiological onsets (first [1] to last [5]) associated with stuttering for 13 young stutterers' respiratory deflation (ABDOMEN and RIB), supralaryngeal lip muscle onset (OOI, DLI) and laryngeal onset (LX) associated with all stutterings (N=34) beginning with BILABIAL and LABIAL sounds that exhibit all five physiological signals. CLuster 4 did not exhibit any stuttered words beginning with labial of bilabial sounds and two subjects did not exhibit at least one signal for each stuttering.

	RANK ORDERED ONSET SEQUENCE	VARIABLE	NUMBER TOKENS	MEAN (in msec)	STANDARD DEVIATION
CLUSTER 1					
	1	ABD	10	-1026	338
	2	RIB	10	- 888	460
	3	OOI	10	- 598	242
	4	DLI	10	- 659	375
	5	LX	10	- 557	356
CLUSTER 2					
	1	ABD	13	-1761	660
	2	OOI	13	-1601	659
	3	RIB	13	-1581	687
	4	DLI	13	-1417	734
	5	LX	13	-1173	784
CLUSTER 3					
	1	ABD	11	-1551	584
	2	OOI	11	-1442	837
	3	RIB	11	-1400	610
	4	DLI	11	-1227	908
	5	LX	11	- 943	791

2. Generally, for Clusters 3 and 4, the mean onset of physiological activity began about 1.6 seconds prior to time zero (abdomen onset) while the mean onset of the last physiological signal (laryngeal onset) began at 950 msec for both clusters. In terms of signal onsets, these two clusters appear to fall between extreme range of scores for Clusters 1 and 2.

DISCUSSION

In recent years, several researchers have stressed the importance of time and temporally related phenomenon to the onset and development of stuttering. (Adams, Freeman & Conture 1984; Cooper and Allen, 1977; Conture, 1982; Kent, 1984; Perkins et al., 1976; Perkins, Bell, Johnson & Stocks 1979; Van Riper, 1971, 1982;) In seminal research investigating the timing aspects of stuttering, Perkins et al., (1976, 1979) reported that stuttering involves a temporal discoordination of the phonatory and respiratory systems which results in a breakdown in the mechanisms responsible for fluent speech production. In view of the reported concerns regarding a temporal breakdown in stuttering, the discussion of the results will take place.

Previously, it was suggested that the characteristics of stuttering (e.g. speech disfluency type, number and variety of associated behaviors) differentiated among stutterers (Schwartz and Conture, 1986). Given this information and the speculation that stuttering involves "disordered timing" and "discoordination", among the various components (respiratory, supralaryngeal, and laryngeal) of the speech production mechanism, the temporal onsets and sequence of temporal onsets of speech physiology associated with stuttering were investigated.

Discussion of the present physiological findings needs to be prefaced by the fact that the collection of physiological onsets associated with stuttering was completed during conversational tasks. This procedure attempted to provide a relatively natural setting conducive to conversation in order to obtain stutterings that characterized the child's speech outside of experimental setting. However, the nature and number of disfluent words produced by each subject was beyond the examiner's control and often resulted in the production of stuttered words that are difficult or impossible to analyze as they did not include all five physiological signals (e.g. lip muscle activity associated with a stuttered vowel in the initial position of a word). As a result, direct, subject to subject, or cluster to cluster comparisons of mean physiological onsets was extremely difficult in this investigation.

Results in the present investigation indicated that the onsets of speech physiology associated with stuttering did not differentiate among the behavioral subgroups. This lack of differentiation can be examined from various perspectives. First, the similarity of sequence of onsets supports the idea that young stutterers' ability to sequence the respiratory, supralaryngeal, and laryngeal systems is generally intact and comparable to results discussed for normally fluent speakers (Kuksht, 1975; Baken, McManus, & Cavallo 1983; Caruso, 1983). This finding contradicts the Perkins et al. (1976, 1979) "discoordination hypothesis" at least on one level of comparison. Perkins et al. hypothesized that because the frequency of stuttering decreased in their experiment from a voicing condition to whispering to silent articulation then "some condition existed during this experiment powerful enough to exert almost complete control of stuttering". The authors suggested that stuttering occurred due to a breakdown in the coordination between phonatory and respiratory coordination. Intuitively and clinically this hypothesis has some appeal as clients often appear to exhibit some inability to coordinate the various physiological systems necessary for fluent speech. However, examination of this hypothesis in view of the results in the present investigation suggested that in general during stuttering, the relative sequence of physiological onsets was similar across subjects in the behavioral clusters. Although the present results contradict a generalized or molar discoordination among the respiratory, supralaryngeal, and laryngeal systems, it may be that a more finely tuned or molecular analysis of young stutterers "timing systems" needs to explored.

Cooper and Allen (1977) have suggested that "stuttering is a manifestation of poorer basic timing ability", which they believe to be related to an internal "neural clock" that helps to regulate speech and nonspeech motor activities. The fact that stutterings were shown to occur for as long as two seconds in the present investigation suggests that timing at some level is disrupted in stutterers. In the present investigation it was shown that the young children were able to produce most stutterings according to the same generally consistent, predictable, and seemingly appropriate sequence of physiological onsets; however, it may be that a timing problem exists in moving from one system to another. For example, for most subjects the respiratory system onsets first and this was followed by supralaryngeal lip muscle activity. Although the general sequence of onset was consistent, the durations between respiratory onset and supralaryngeal onset varied across the clusters. Even in the most restricted case of labial and bilabials (see Table 3), Cluster 1 showed a 400 msec difference between respiratory and supralaryngeal onset while Clusters 2 and 3 exhibited a 100 msec duration between onset of the systems. It may be possible that the timing relationship between any two of the three systems is as important as the relative sequence of physiological onsets among all three physiological systems. Investigation of these relationships using a more restricted speech sample should provide further information.

A second concept worth considering relates to the discussion of adaptation/adaptive strategies that characterize each child. It was evident that although the general sequence of physiological onsets was similar for each subgroup, there was a degree of variation among individual subjects. If we view these variations in speech physiology as being related to each child's ability to produce speech and his/her adaptation strategy for "coping with" communicative and environmental stress, it is possible that as the stuttering problem continues to develop, the sequence of temporal onsets of speech physiology *may* also be affected to some degree. Conture (1982) speculated that changes in the speech disfluency type are typically associated with changes or increases in "...physiological disruptions in fluent-disfluent speech". Further, adult stutterers have been shown to exhibit disturbances in laryngeal functioning associated with stuttering (e.g. Freeman and Ushijima, 1978) and disturbances in articulatory functioning associated with fluent speech (e.g. Zimmermann, 1980). Perhaps we can speculate that for young children, their initial adaptation strategy or method of reacting to their problem results in changes in speech disfluency type and the number and nature of associated behaviors. If we speculate that Clusters 3, 4, and 5 exhibit a well defined stuttering problem, it may be possible that the stutterer begins to react to his communication problem by also disrupting the temporal sequence of physiological onsets associated with the stuttering. Perhaps a similar examination of adult stutterers would shed further light on the adaptation strategies of older stutterers and the impact of these strategies on temporal onsets of speech physiology.

ACKNOWLEDGEMENTS

Research supported in part by a contract from NINCDS to Syracuse University (NDI-NS-0-8 and conference attendance), supported in part by a new faculty development award from the NYS/UUP Professional and Quality of Working Life Committee.

REFERENCES

Abberton, E. (1971). First application of a new laryngograph. *Medical and Biological Illustrations, 21,* 172-183.

Adams, M.R., Freeman, F. & Conture, E. (1984). Laryngeal dynamics in stuttering. In R. Curlee & W. Perkins (Eds.), *Nature and Treatment of Stuttering: New Directions.* San Diego, CA: College Hill Press, 89-130.

Andrews, G. & Harris, M. (1964). *The Syndrome of Stuttering.* London: Spastics Society Medical Education and Information Unit in Association with Wm. Heinemann Medical Books ltd.

Baken, R.J., McManus, D.A. & Cavallo, S.A. (1983). Prephonatory chest wall posturing in stutterers. *Journal of Speech and Hearing Research, 26,* 444-450.

Bless, D.M., Hunker, C.J. & Weismer, G. (1981). Comparison of noninvasive methods to obtain chest-wall displacement and aerodynamic measures during speech. *Ninth Symposium: Care of the Professional Voice.* New York: Voice Foundation, Inc.

Caruso, A.J. (1983). *Speech Physiology During Young Stutterers' Stuttering.* Unpublished Ph.D dissertation, Syracuse University.

Conture, E.G. (1982). *Stuttering.* Englewood Cliffs, NJ.: Prentice-Hall, Inc.

Conture, E.G., Rothenberg, M.R. & Molitor, R. (1986 In press). Electroglottographic observations of young stutterers' fluency. Paper submitted to *Journal of Speech and Hearing Research.*

Cooper, M.H. & Allen, G.D. (1977). Time control accuracy in normal speakers and stutterers. *Journal of Speech and Hearing Research, 20,* 55-71.

Douglass, E. & Quarrington, B. (1952). The differentiation of interiorized and exteriorized secondary stuttering. *Journal of Speech and Hearing Research, 17,* 377-385.

Fourcin, A.J. (1974). Laryngographic examination of vocal fold vibration. In B. Wyke (Ed.), *Ventilatory and Phonatory Control Systems.* London, England: Oxford University Press.

Fourcin, A.J. (1981). Laryngographic assessment of phonatory function. In C. Ludlow & M. Hart (Eds.), *Proceedings of the Conference on the Assessment of Vocal Pathology.* Rockville, Maryland: ASHA reports 11.

Freeman, F. & Ushijima, T. (1978). Laryngeal muscle activity during stuttering. *Journal of Speech and Hearing Research, 21,* 538-562.

Gilbert, H.R., Potter, C.R. & Hoodin, R. (1984). Laryngograph as a measure of vocal fold contact area. *Journal of Speech and Hearing Research, 27,* 178-182.

Isley, C.L. & Basmajian, J. (1973). Electromyography of the cheeks and lips. *Anatomical Record, 176,* 145-148.

Kennedy, J.G. & Abbs, J.H. (1979). Anatomic studies of the perioral motor system: foundations for studies in speech physiology. In N. Lass (Ed.), *Speech and Language: Advances in Basic Research and Practice.* Vol. 1. New York: Academic Press. 211-270.

Kent, R.D. (1984). Stuttering as a temporal programming disorder. In R.F. Curlee & W.H. Perkins (Eds.), *Nature and treatment of stuttering: New directions.* San Diego, CA: College-Hill Press. 283-301.

Kuksht, M.J. (1975). *Electromyographic, aerodynamic and displacement characteristics of bilabial consonants.* Unpublished M.S. thesis, University of Washington.

MacCurtain, F. & Fourcin, A. (1981). Application of the electroglottograph wave-form display. In V. Lawrence (Ed.), *Transcripts of the Tenth Symposium: Care of the Professional Voice.* New York, NY.: Voice Foundation, Inc.

Michel, C., Pfister, K. & Luchsinger, R. (1970). Electro-glottographie et cinematographie laryngee ultra-rapide. *Folia Phoniatrica, 22,* 81-91.

Ng, T. & Rothenberg, M. (1982). A matched delay approach to substantive linear phase high-pass filtering. *IEEE Transactions on Circuits and Systems, 8.*

O'Dwyer, N.J., Quinn, P. Guitar, B., Andrews, G. & Neilson, P. (1981). Procedures for verification of electrode placement in EMG studies of orofacial and mandibular muscles. *Journal of Speech and Hearing Research, 24,* 273-288.

Perkins, W.H., Rudas, J. Johnson, L. & Bell, J. (1976). Stuttering: Discoordination of phonation with articulation and respiration. *Journal of Speech and Hearing Research, 19,* 509-522.

Perkins, W.H., Bell, J., Johnson, L. & Stocks, J. (1979). Phone rate and effective planning time hypothesis of stuttering. *Journal of Speech and Hearing Research, 22,* 747-755.

Preus, A. (1981). *Identifying Subgroups of Stutterers.* Oslo, Norway: Universitetsforlaget.

Prins, D. & Lohr, F. (1972). Behavioral dimensions of stuttered speech. *Journal of Speech and Hearing Research, 15,* 61-71.

Rothenberg, M.R. (1981). Some relations between glottal air flow and vocal fold contact area. In C. Ludlow & M. Hart (Eds.), *Proceedings of the Conference on the Assessment of Vocal Pathology.* ASHA Reports 11. Rockville, Maryland: Interstate Printers.

Sackner, M.A. (1979). *Monitoring of ventilation without physical connection to the airway: A review.* A paper presented at the Third International Symposium on Ambulatory Monitoring. Harrow, Middlesex, U.K.

Schwartz, H.D. & Conture, E.G. (1986). Subgrouping Young Stutterers: A Behavioral Perspective. Manuscript submitted to *Journal of Speech and Hearing Research.*

Van Riper, C. (1982). *The Nature of Stuttering.* Englewood Cliffs, New Jersey: Prentice-Hall, Inc.

Watson, H. (1979). *The technology of respiratory inductive plethysmography.* Paper presented to the Third International Symposium on Ambulatory Monitoring. Clinical Research Center, Harrow, Middlesex, U.K.

Zimmermann, G. (1980). Articulatory dynamics of fluent utterances of stutterers and nonstutterers. *Journal of Speech and Hearing Research, 23,* 95-107.

Chapter 16

Aerodynamic Functions in Fluent Speech Utterances of Stutterers and Nonstutterers in Different Speech Conditions

Herman F.M. Peters and Louis Boves

INTRODUCTION

The production of fluent speech requires a precise coordination of respiratory, phonatory and articulatory manoeuvres. A number of authors (Van Riper, 1982; Adams, 1974; Wingate, 1976; Agnello, 1975), have suggested that the failure to coordinate expiratory actions and global adjustment of the laryngeal musculature in preparation for phonation is a major cause of disfluencies in stuttering. This suggestion seems to be substantiated by recent experimental work of Conture (1977), Freeman (1979), Shapiro (1980) and Yoshioka and Löfqvist (1981), who reported substantial differences in laryngeal activity between nonstutterers and stutterers when producing auditorily fluent utterances. Although there is general agreement on the fact that subglottal pressure must be increased to a certain level before phonation can start, very little is known about the details of the way in which the pressure is controlled. This applies equally to normal speech production and speech production of stutterers. Obviously, there may be interactions between laryngeal behavior preceding phonation and the control of subglottal pressure. In this contribution we will deal with both aspects, but the attention will be focussed on the control of subglottal pressure.

To learn to understand the complex process of phonation, multiple physiological processes on several levels should be measured simultaneously. Using the electroglottogram one can obtain information on the behavior of the vocal folds, because the glottogram reflects the time variations of the area of contact between the vocal folds. In the present investigation the EGG was recorded as a means for obtaining crude information on the behavior and state of the larynx. For instance, glottal closure necessary to increase subglottal pressure in utterances that begin with a vowel can be detected as an isolated sharp peak in the EGG. Also, the start of phonation can be seen very clearly in the EGG.

Over the years a number of techniques have been developed for measuring subglottal air pressure (Van den Berg, 1960). However, because of the invasive character, the restricted bandwidth of measurements as well as interference with phonation these methods are not very suitable for investigations in continuous speech. Since the introduction of miniature pressure transducers mounted at the distal end of a very thin catheter, subglottal pressure registrations can cover a wider frequency range (Koike, 1981; Boves, 1984). Also, the catheter, if properly positioned, does not interfere with normal phonation and articulation.

If speech is a complex multi-level process, problems in speech production may originate from almost everywhere. Thus it is only natural that different stuttering therapies address different aspects of speech production, according to which parts of the process are considered as responsible for the disfluencies. In fluency shaping programs a large number of different strategies directed towards breathing "Airflow Technique", Schwartz (1976); "Breath Stream Management", Perkins (1973); " Regulated Breathing Approach", Azrin and Nunn (1974), phonation ("easy voice onset"), Ryan (1974) and Agnello (1975); " effortless phonation", Adams (1975); "gentle voice onset", Webster (1978) and articulation ("prolonged speech"), Ryan (1974); Shames and Florance (1980); " easy relaxed speech", Gregory and Hill (1980) are used to change these behaviors. It is not clear whether all these aspects must be treated independently or whether one may hope that the results obtained from training at one level automatically will carry over to other levels. In this study we have tried to investigate this carry-over effect by making measurements in three different speech conditions, viz. one which can be considered as normal speech, another in which the subjects employed a very gentle voice onset, and a third that can be characterized as consciously reduced articulatory effort.

The purpose of the present chapter is first to describe the way in which the build-up of subglottal pressure proceeds. Next we try to answer the question whether the patterns of pressure build-up found in perceptually fluent utterances of stutterers are different from the patterns found in the speech of nonstutterers. Thirdly, we would like to know if conscious changes in voice onset affect the patterns of pressure build-up, and if so, whether the effects are different from the results of a conscious reduction of articulatory effort.

METHOD

Subjects

Fifteen adult male stutterers aged between 19 and 28 years and fifteen nonstuttering males, matched for age, served as the subjects in this experiment. With 5 stutterers and 8 control subjects it appeared to be impossible to insert the catheter for measuring subglottal pressure in a proper way due to a number of practical problems. These problems mostly concern anatomical obstructions in the nasal and nasopharyngeal pathway or hypersensibility of the mucous membranes. Also, because of its stiffness the catheter sometimes drops besides the vocal folds in the sinus piriformis or in the anterior commissure instead of the posterior commissure. This leaves us with 10 stutterers and 7 control speakers from whom speech material is available for analysis. All subjects had a normal hearing acuity and normal language and voice quality.

None of the stutterers had been enrolled in any kind of therapy during the two years preceding the experiment. Because the measurements are invasive and a somewhat unpleasant experience for the subject, it was decided not to try and make the control group equally large as the group of stutterers. Although this decision may complicate the statistical analysis of the data it can still be warranted. Straightforward analysis will not be possible anyhow since the controls do not stutter. The smaller number of controls produce a larger number of fluent stutterers.

Stutterers were classified as mild, moderate or severe stutterers. This classification was based on a combination of scale-ratings of stuttering severity in conversational speech and text reading.

Speech Conditions

Each subject was tested under three different conditions. The first condition is referred to as the normal speech condition. In this condition subjects were simply asked to produce the words as soon as possible after the response signal. In the remaining two conditions the subjects were asked to produce the words either with an extremely gentle voice onset or with deliberately reduced articulatory effort. The obligation to respond as soon as possible after the warning signal was repeated in the instruction for the two manipulated conditions. The training was given by a very experienced speech therapist. Although the training never took much more than about 30 minutes, care was taken to ensure that all subjects had reached approximately the same level of proficiency before the start of the experiment. The criterion was - by necessity - the auditory and visual judgement of the speech therapist. Proficiency in performing a gentle voice onset was considered adequate if the subjects were able to consistently produce vowels with a gradual increase in loudness from hardly audible to normal. In the condition with deliberately reduced articulatory effort subjects must be

Speech Material

The speech material used in this experiment consisted of 80 words in each speech condition. Half of the words were one-syllable words of the VC and CVC type. The other half contained three or four syllables. All polysyllabic words had the main stress on the first syllable. In half of the words the initial sounds were two contrasted vowels /a/ and /o/ and in the remaining half two contrasted consonants /p/ and /s/. All word-initial phonemes occurred with the same frequency in both the monosyllables and in the polysyllabic words. In order to obtain this balance, some of the monosyllables had to be nonsense words. The polysyllabic words do exist in the Dutch language, although a few of them are not used very frequently. The choice of the word-initial phonemes was primarily motivated by the requirements of a more comprehensive study of speech motor behavior in stuttering. For the present experiment we will not distinguish between /a/ and /o/ as word-initial vowels. There will, however, be made a distinction between words beginning with a vowel and words beginning with a (voiceless) consonant. In the latter category a further distinction between plosives and fricatives must be made. From the 80 stimulus words three complete lists were constructed by putting the words in different balanced random orders. The lists were intended for use in the three conditions that made up the experiment.

Speech Task

The procedure in the speech task basically followed a reaction time paradigm. In the experimental setting subjects were seated in front of a TV-monitor. Subjects were asked to read out the stimuli that were presented visually on the TV-screen. Stimulus presentation was controlled by an Apple II+-microcomputer. A randomization program generated a variable fore-period of 1-3 seconds after an auditory (100 Hz tone during 100 msec) and a visual warning signal (a row of asterisks displayed on the screen). Subjects were instructed to produce the stimulus words as soon as possible after an auditory response signal (a 1 kHz tone lasting 100 msec). After each stimulus word a variable inter trial interval of 3-5 seconds followed before the next warning signal.

Fluency Criteria

For this study only those speech utterances have been analyzed which were judged to be spoken fluently. In order to be accepted as fluent a word had to satisfy three conditions. Firstly, there must be a complete absence of any visual sign of struggle in the facial or body movements of the subject before or during the production of the word. The presence of visual signs of disfluency was established by the experimenter during the experiment. Secondly, the utterance may not contain audible hesitations, prolongations or repetitions. To establish the presence of audible disfluencies after the experiment an audio-recording of subjects speech was independently judged by two trained raters. Thirdly, the word must be produced within a reasonable time span following the response signal.

The percentage of fluent utterances ranged from 16.3 to 100 in the group of stutterers, while in the group of nonstutterers subjects had a fluency percentage of 98.7-100.

Instrumentation

A schematic diagram of the instrumentation set-up during the experiment is presented in Figure 1. As mentioned before the experiment was completely controlled by an Apple II+ microcomputer. All signals were recorded on a FM recorder (Philips Analog 14) running at a tape speed of 15 inch per second for subsequent processing. Vocal fold activity was recorded by means of an electroglottograph; use was made of the device marketed by Fourcin and Abberton under the name Laryngograph (Fourcin, 1981). Subglottal air pressure was measured by means of a Millar PC-350 micro tip catheter, inserted into the trachea via the nasal pathway and the glottis. The speech signal was recorded using an AKG type C451E condensor microphone.

Thanks to the high tape speed employed the frequency response of all recordings was flat up to at least 5 kHz. The recordings were displayed by playing the FM tapes at a reduced speed into a polygraph. All measurements were taken from these paper recordings made with a paper speed of 5 cm/sec.

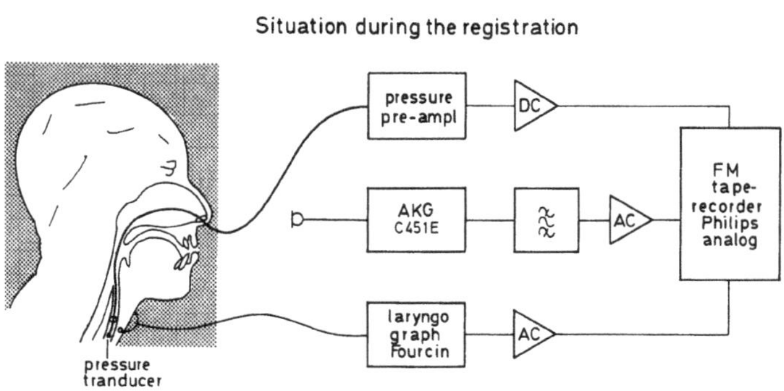

Figure 1. Schematic representation of the experimental set-up during the experiment.

Data Analysis and Results

The experimental data consisted of 10 × 80 = 800 words produced by the stutterers and 7 × 80 = 560 words produced by control subjects. Of the 800 items of the stutterers 27 words could not be used in the analysis either because of the subjects' coughing in the interval between the warning and response signal, or because of failures of the instrumentation. Of the 773 analyzed words 573 were considered as produced in a completely fluent way. These 573 words form the data base for the stutterers. Of the 560 words produced by the control subjects seven words were not amenable to analysis due to coughs or failures of the instrumentation and one word could not be considered as fluent, so 553 words rested for further analysis.

Pressure Build-Up

Given the present state of knowledge about subglottal pressure signals it is virtually impossible to subject these signals to a meaningful automated analysis. Therefore, the analysis was restricted to a detailed visual inspection of the signals from the moment of its first rise to the onset of phonation. The latter moment can easily be established on the basis of the appearance of pitch frequency oscillations superimposed on the low frequency traces.

In the attempt to devise a scheme for classifying the pressure envelopes seven different types of pressure build-up were found sufficient to cover the relevant characteristics of the traces. Using our knowledge of the physiology of phonation and the subglottal pressure traces of the nonstutterers as a reference, we concluded that of the seven types of pressure build-up three can be considered as normal, whereas the remaining four must be considered as deviant. The eventual classification of the traces was based on a consensus between the two authors. With very few exceptions the classifications made by the authors when working individually were identical. Where the initial classifications differed, it proved to be easy to reach a consensus after very short discussions. The normal types of pressure build-up (Type 1a, b and c) are shown in Figure 2, the deviant types (Type 2, 3, 4 and 5) in Figure 3. Here we will give a concise description and explanation of each type.

Normal Types of Pressure Build-Up

Type 1a. This type is the most frequent pattern for words which start on a vowel. The pressure rise as a function of time is monotone and smooth; its overall shape is much like an integral symbol. Phonation starts shortly before the pressure has reached its maximum level. This type of pressure build-up is seen both in VC... and CVC... words. The start of phonation can be determined from the point in time where a high frequency ripple on the pressure curve becomes visible. Similar indications of the onset of phonation are present in the audio signal and in the EGG. This type of pressure build-up corresponds with normal non-abrupt voice onset. Phonation starts from a closed glottis condition. The initial closure of the glottis in preparation for phonation can be seen as a single large amplitude peak in the EGG. Note that this excursion coincides with the moment were the subglottal pressure first starts to rise.

Type 1b. The pressure builds up monotonely with an integral symbol shaped pattern. Phonation only starts at the moment where the pressure reaches its maximum level (both in VC... and CVC... words) or, alternately, some time after the maximum has been reached (only in CVC... words). In the last case phonation seems to be initiated from an open glottis condition, which is quite normal in words beginning with a consonant.

Type 1c. Pressure builds up monotonely, with an integral symbol-like pattern from an open glottis and complete closure of the vocal

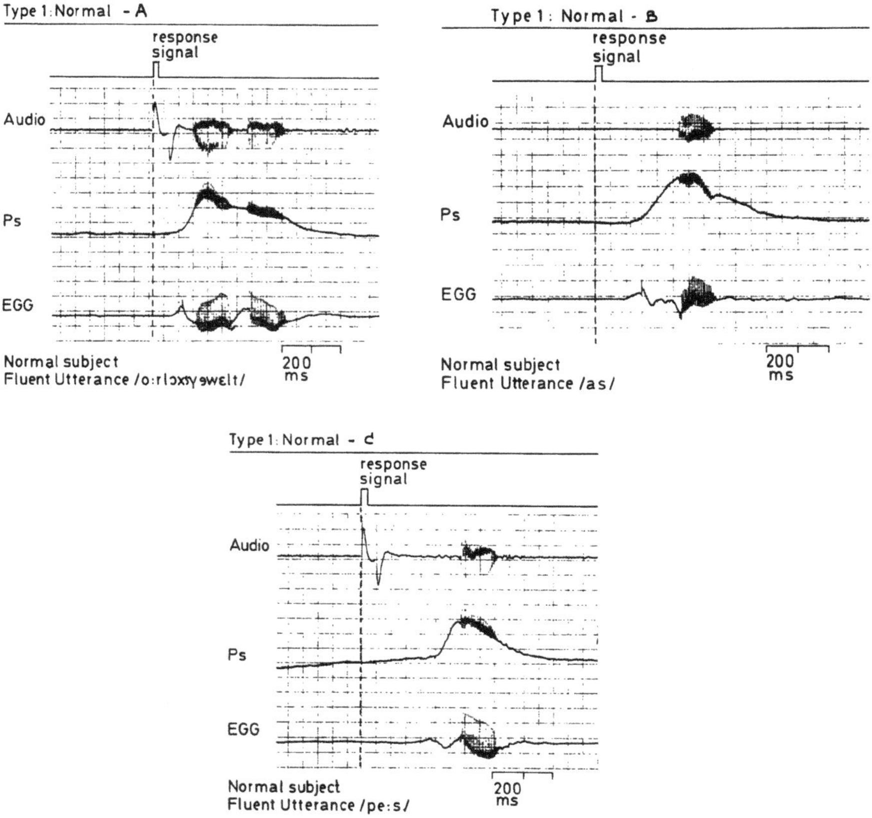

Figure 2. Recordings of normal types of subglottal pressure build-up (type 1A, 1B, 1C). Recorded signals: Audio = speech signal; Ps = subglottal pressure and EGG = electroglottogram.

tract associated with stop articulation. However, a small drop of pressure is observed preceding the start of phonation. Phonation starts during pressure recovery or immediately after the moment where the pressure reaches its eventual maximum. In our material this type is restricted to words beginning with /p/. The pressure drop is most certainly associated with aspiration of the consonant, which is not a frequent but neither an abnormal phenomenon in Dutch.

Deviant Types of Pressure Build-Up

Type 2. The pressure increases monotonely in a smooth way but phonation starts at least 100 milliseconds after pressure has reached its eventual maximum. This type, which has been restricted to words beginning with a vowel, should be considered as an indication that the speaker is having problems in the coordination of the respiratory and phonatory (and/or perhaps also articulatory)

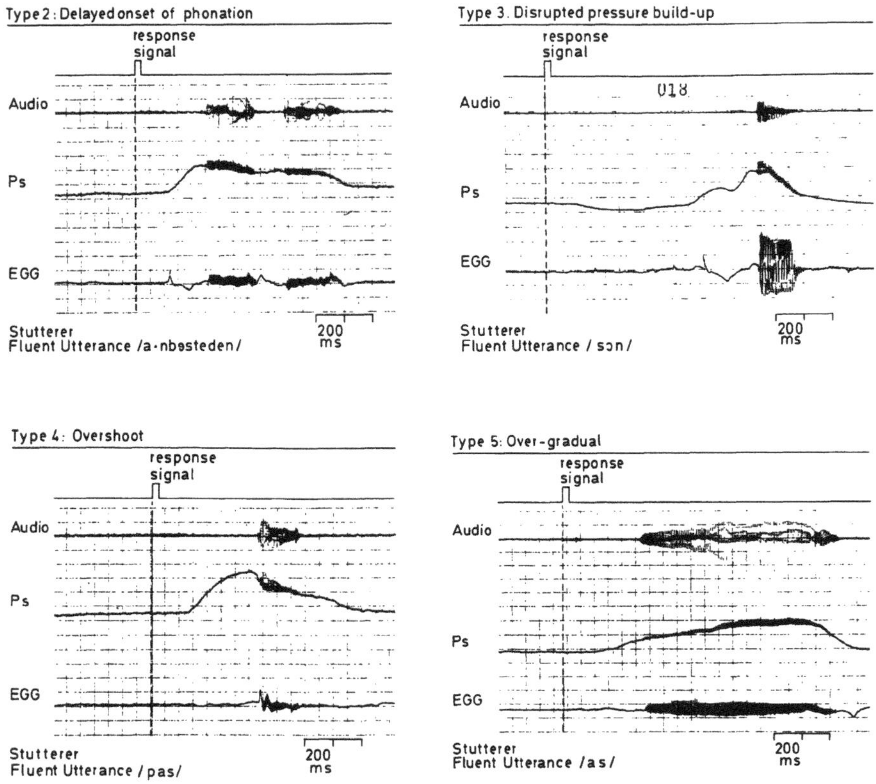

Figure 3. Recordings of deviant types of subglottal pressure build up (type 2, 3, 4, and 5). Recorded signals: Audio = speech signal; Ps = subglottal pressure and EGG = electroglottogram.

systems. It may perhaps be considered as a very short covert blockade.

Type 3. In this type of pressure build-up the smooth and continuous increase in pressure found in the previous types is disrupted and, therefore, can be described as a non-monotone behavior of the pressure trace before the start of phonation. We consider this type of pressure build-up as a result of problems in the control of the respiratory system or a failure to coordinate expiratory manoeuvres and the concomitant adjustments of the phonatory and/or articulatory systems.

Type 4. In this type the pressure builds up smoothly, usually to a level that is too high for comfortable phonation. After having reached its maximum, the pressure drops considerably before phonation starts eventually. This type can be considered as evidence of an overshoot in the functioning of the respiratory system which is responsible for controlling the subglottal pressure. This type is seen more frequently on words beginning with /p/ than on words beginning with /s/ or /a, o/. Thus it can be considered as evidence of an insufficient coordination of respiratory and articulatory gestures.

Type 5. In this type pressure build-up is exceedingly slow. Phonation starts at a very low pressure level, long before subglottal pressure attains its eventual level. It is closely associated with deliberate and extremely gentle voice onset. Most probably the vocal folds are adducted very gently, perhaps even without touching each other. Therefore, we may not expect to find an indication of glottal closure in the EGG. Consequently, it is not possible to say whether phonation starts from an open or from a closed glottis condition.

Differences between Groups and Subjects

After having identified the different types of pressure build-up, their frequency of occurrence as a function of the group of subjects and as a function of the speech condition was investigated. The group effects will be discussed first and after that the subject effect. In order to minimize the risk that we are studying artefacts caused by the manipulations of the manner of speech production the analysis was restricted to the normal speech condition.

Group Effect. In order to be able to compare the group of stutterers with the control group the absolute numbers of occurrence of the pressure build-up types were first converted to proportions of the number of fluent utterances for each subject. The results for both groups are shown graphically in Figure 4. The numerical data for the individual subjects and both groups are given in Table 1. From the right hand part of Figure 4 it can be seen that the pressure build-up types 2, 3 and 4 occur roughly with the same frequency. The over-gradual build-up (type 5) is clearly under-represented in the normal speech condition. These remarks apply equally to both groups.

The groups differ significantly, however, with respect to the

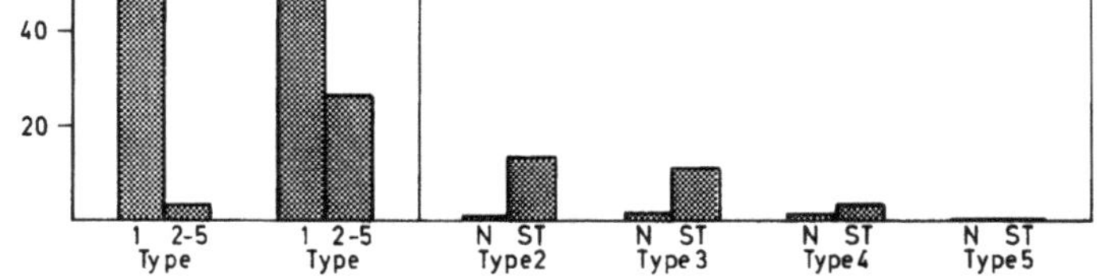

Figure 4. Relative frequency of normal types of pressure build-up (type 1A+1B+1C), the total number of deviant type of pressure build-up (type 2+3+4+5) and individual types of deviant pressure build-up in stutterers (ST) and non-stutterers (N).

Table 1. Summary of the pressure build-up data in the normal speech condition. Subjects are ordered on the basis of the proportion of fluent utterances in the experiment. The column "Stuttering classification" gives the clinical judgement of stuttering severity (I: mild; II: moderate; III: severe).

Subjects	Stuttering classification	Number of fluent utterances	% fluent	Type 1	Type 2	Type 3	Type 4	Type 5
Non-stutterers								
N4	--	78	98.7	93.6	--	2.6	3.8	--
N1	--	80	100	98.7	--	1.3	--	--
N2	--	80	100	100	--	--	--	--
N3	--	78	100	94.9	--	5.1	--	--
N5	--	79	100	98.7	1.3	--	--	--
N6	--	77	100	96.1	--	--	3.9	--
N7	--	80	100	96.3	2.5	1.3	--	--
Stutterers								
ST1	III	13	16.3	--	61.5	46.2	7.6	--
ST6	III	21	26.3	90.6	4.6	4.6	--	--
ST2	III	56	76.7	87.5	5.4	5.4	1.8	--
ST4	I	61	79.2	67.2	24.6	--	8.2	--
ST7	II	63	79.7	63.5	--	31.7	9.5	--
ST8	III	60	84.5	75.0	20.0	5.0	--	--
ST5	III	66	84.6	93.9	--	4.5	1.5	--
ST3	II	76	97.4	82.9	15.8	1.1	--	--
ST9	II	80	100	88.8	2.5	1.3	7.5	--
ST10	II	77	100	88.4	--	14.3	1.3	--
Mean non-stutterers			99.8	96.9	0.5	1.5	1.1	--
Mean stutterers			74.6	73.4	13.4	11.4	3.7	--

proportion of normal pressure build-up types ($t = -2.675$, $df = 9$, $p < .05$, assuming unequal variances in the two populations), and also with respect to the proportion of deviant pressure build-up types ($t = 2.477$, $df = 9$, $p < .05$, again assuming unequal variances).

Thus we are forced to conclude that even in perceptually fluent utterances of stutterers the way in which respiratory and phonatory processes are coordinated seems to differ from that in the speech of nonstutterers. This finding confirms previous results of research into glottal activity (Conture et al., 1977; Freeman, 1979; Yoshioka & Löfqvist, 1981).

Subject Effect. Table 1 also shows a breakdown of the results for the individual subjects. From this table it appears that there is no relation between the severity of stuttering and the number of occurrence of other pressure build-up patterns than type 1 (Kendall's *tau* = -.279, $z = -1.127$, $p = .13$). This becomes especially clear if one compares subjects 1, 3 and 6 in the group of stutterers. Both 1 and 6 are severe stutterers, but whereas number 1 produces a type 1 pattern in none of his fluent utterances, number

6 does so in 90.6%. The mild stutterer 3, on the other hand, produces a type 1 pattern in no more than 82.9% of his fluent utterances.

Condition Effect

In both manipulated conditions the percentage of disfluencies decreases significantly compared to the normal condition ($F(2.18)$ = 3.845, $p < .05$). In the normal speech condition the mean disfluency percentage is 26.4; however, in the gentle voice onset condition it is only 6.3; and in the reduced articulatory effort condition not more than 9.8% of the utterances are not fluent. Thus, it is quite clear that a conscious change of the normal speech motor behavior leads to a significant decrease in the proportion of disfluencies. A post-hoc contrast test shows that the two manipulated conditions do not differ between each other as far as the proportion of stutters is concerned (t = .607, $p < .5$). So for the time being it seems that any reduction in phonatory or articulatory effort affects the stuttering frequency. Or, alternatively, it is the fact that attention is focussed on the speech behavior that causes the effect.

Frequency of Subglottal Pressure Types. The effect of the manipulated conditions on the frequency of occurrence of the different types of pressure build-up was very significant as can be seen in Figure 5. In Table 2 the numerical data are given for the individual subjects in both groups for the gentle voice onset condition, in Table 3 for the reduced articulatory effort condition. Both in stutterers and nonstutterers the frequency of over-gradual pressure build-up (type 5) increases dramatically in the gentle voice onset condition. For both groups the effect is significant in a one-way analysis of variance with repeated measures ($F(2.18)$ = 13.68, $p < .001$ for the group of the stutterers and $F(2.12)$ = 16.445, $p < .001$ for the control subjects). Thus there appear to be

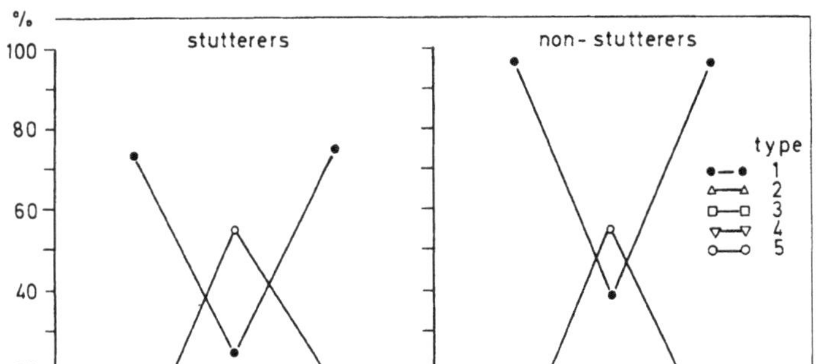

Figure 5. Relative frequency of occurrance of pressure build-up patterns in normal speech, speaking with a gentle voice onset and speaking with reduced articulatory effort.

Table 2. Relative frequency of types of pressure build-up for individual subjects in gentle voice onset condition. (cf. Table 1)

Subjects	Stutte-ring classi-cation	Number of fluent utterances	% fluent	Type 1	Type 2	Type 3	Type 4	Type 5
Non-stutterers								
N4		79	98.7	7.6	--	1.2	--	91.1
N1		76	98.7	82.8	--	3.9	1.3	11.8
N2		80	100	77.5	--	--	7.5	15.0
N3		79	100	18.9	10.1	10.1	2.5	60.7
N5		79	100	5.1	--	3.8	--	91.1
N6		77	97.5	64.9	--	--	2.6	32.5
N7		79	100	15.2	--	--	--	84.8
Stutterers								
ST1	III	64	84.2	12.5	28.1	6.2	20.3	48.4
ST6	III	77	97.5	81.8	--	2.6	10.4	5.2
ST2	III	71	89.9	26.8	9.8	14.8	--	49.3
ST4	I	76	100	--	--	--	--	100
ST7	II	70	88.6	48.5	17.1	17.1	7.1	11.4
ST8	III	54	84.3	53.7	22.2	18.5	1.8	5.5
ST5	III	69	95.8	7.2	--	1.4	--	92.8
ST3	II	77	97.5	1.3	5.2	7.8	1.3	84.4
ST9	II	79	100	5.1	3.8	12.7	--	88.9
ST10	II	64	100	12.5	12.5	10.9	3.1	73.4
Mean non-stutterers			99.3	38.9	1.4	2.7	2.0	55.3
Mean stutterers			93.7	24.8	9.9	9.2	4.4	55.4

no reasons to believe that as a group stutterers employ other physiological strategies for producing a specific auditory result than nonstuttering control subjects. The increase of the number of type 5 pressure build-up patterns goes completely at the cost of the frequency of the type 1 pattern ($F(2.18) = 17.29$, $p < .0001$). The condition of reduced articulatory effort cannot be distinguished from the normal speech condition. As far as the types 2, 3 and 4 patterns are concerned, it does not matter whether the utterances are produced normally, with a consciously practized gentle voice onset or with a deliberately reduced articulatory effort. Therefore, the remainder of this section will only be concerned with the proportion of type 5 patterns.

As can be seen from Tables 2 and 3 the effect of the manipulated conditions differs strongly for the individual subjects in nonstutterers as well as in stutterers. While from a perceptual point of view stutterers and nonstutterers manage to produce gentle voice onsets and to articulate with a deliberately reduced effort level after a short training, there seems to be no homogeneous pattern in the underlying physiological processes. Some subjects use type 5

Table 3. Relative frequency of types of pressure build-up for individual subjects in reduced articulatory effort condition. (cf. Table 1)

Subjects	Stuttering classication	Number of fluent utterances	% fluent	Type 1	Type 2	Type 3	Type 4	Type 5
Non-stutterers								
N4		78	100	100	--	--	--	--
N1		79	100	96.2	--	2.6	--	1.3
N2		80	100	100	--	--	--	--
N3		65	98.5	96.9	--	--	--	3.0
N5		76	97.4	97.4	2.6	--	--	--
N6		77	98.7	88.3	5.2	1.3	1.3	3.9
N7		79	100	94.9	1.3	1.3	2.5	--
Stutterers								
ST1	III	75	94.9	21.3	4.0	8.0	--	69.3
ST6	III	34	42.5	88.2	5.9	--	5.9	--
ST2	III	75	93.8	96.0	--	--	--	4.0
ST4	I	69	93.2	94.2	4.3	1.4	--	--
ST7	II	76	95.0	80.3	3.9	11.8	3.9	1.3
ST8	III	57	85.1	82.5	10.5	7.0	--	--
ST5	III	78	100	46.1	--	1.3	--	52.7
ST3	II	78	97.5	65.3	3.8	6.4	1.2	23.1
ST9	II	80	100	97.5	--	1.3	--	1.3
ST10	II	55	100	81.2	1.8	14.5	1.8	--
Mean non-stutterers			99.2	96.2	1.3	0.7	0.5	1.2
Mean stutterers			90.2	75.3	3.4	5.2	1.3	15.2

pressure build-up patterns in almost all gentle voice onset utterances (for instance the subjects N4, N5, ST4 and ST5), while others do so only occasionally (subjects N1, ST6 and ST8). Obviously, a specific perceptual speech output can be realized in different ways as far as the underlying physiological processes are concerned. It is interesting, incidentally, that there seems to exist a relation between stuttering severity and the ability to change articulatory behavior. Kendall's *tau*, computed for the relation between the classification as mild (1), intermediate (2) or severe (3) stutterer and the proportion of type 5 pressure build-up traces in the gentle voice onset condition is $tau = -.47$, $z = -1.894$, $p < .05$. This might be taken as an indication that severe stutterers are more difficult to train to change their phonatory and articulatory manoeuvres than mild stutterers and nonstutterers. Another question may be whether subjects with a high relative frequency of deviant patterns of pressure build-up in normal speech have greater difficulty in changing physiological processes. There is no relationship between the frequency of deviant patterns of pressure build-up and the frequency of the overgradual pressure build-up in the gentle voice onset condition (Kendall's $tau = -.111$, $z = -.447$, $p = .33$). The impression that there is no clear relation between the frequency of deviant patterns in the normal speech condition and the ability to perform in the manipulated condition is also obtained if one compares the subjects ST4 and ST7. In the normal speech condition 32% and 41% of their utterances have a deviant type of pressure build-up. Whereas subject ST4 produces a type 5 pattern of pressure build-up in all utterances in the gentle voice onset condition, subject ST7 does so only in 11%. Therefore, it seems impossible to predict the specific physiological results of a short and fairly unspecific training on the basis of a single physiological measurement. This result is not too surprising, given the very large number of degrees of freedom on the physiological level, which enables one to produce a given auditory effect in many different ways.

CONCLUSIONS

From the results of the experiments described in this chapter a number of conclusions can be drawn.

The first, and probably most important conclusion is that perceptually fluent speech utterances of stutterers are not always fluent on all relevant levels of speech production. From the data on subglottal pressure build-up it is quite obvious that in fluent speech stutterers significantly more often use unusual subglottal air pressure build-up patterns than do nonstutterers, despite of the very strict criteria for fluency. Thus we see that the physiologic processes, associated with or underlying utterances that seem to be completely fluent on the acoustical level, yet appear to contain a considerable proportion of deviant patterns, that might as well be called covert stutters. This finding, which corroborates previous observations of Freeman (1984), calls into question the outcomes of many other experiments in which perceptually fluent utterances of stutterers have been analyzed. A considerable portion of these allegedly fluent utterances might rather have been considered as physiological stutters and should have been analyzed separately from really fluent (both physiologically and perceptually) utterances.

The second conclusion which can be drawn is that both nonstutterers and stutterers manage to produce gentle voice onsets and to articulate with a deliberately reduced articulatory effort level after a short training in such a way that the performance is adequate from a perceptual point of view. In the gentle voice onset condition, both stutterers and nonstutterers frequently changed the underlying physiologic processes in the sense that they preferred a type 5 pressure build-up.

A third conclusion that can be drawn is that there are indications that the overall severity of stuttering is a better predictor of the difficulty the subject will encounter in performing specific phonatory manoeuvres than the amount of deviations in one of the underlying physiological processes in normal speech production. This illustrates that data obtained from a single process or single level in speech production are inadequate to predict the auditory quality of the speech output.

A last conclusion which can be drawn, is that the effects of the manipulated speech conditions are specific in that they cause different physiological results, which are, moreover, completely in line with our expectations. This implies that in therapy management specific strategies should be used at different levels in speech production and one should not rely too much on the hope that results of articulatory training will carry over to phonation and vice versa. If it is the case that stutterers do not form a homogeneous group in the sense that for some subjects the problems are mainly at the phonatory level and for others at the articulatory level, this finding may help to explain the fact that therapies that completely focus on a single level show widely diverging results, i.e., they succeed only for the subpopulation where the problems originate at the level addressed in the therapy and not for subpopulations where the main cause of the stuttering lies elsewhere.

REFERENCES

Adams, M.R. (1974). A physiologic and aerodynamic interpretation of fluent and stuttered speech. *Journal of Fluency Disorders, 1,* 35-47.

Adams, M.R. (1975). Clinical interpretations and applications. In L.M. Webster & L. Furst (Eds.), *Vocal tract dynamics and dysfluency.* New York: Speech Hearing Institute. 196-228.

Agnello, J.C. (1975). Voice onset and termination features of stutterers. In L.M. Webster & L. Furst (Eds.), *Vocal tract dynamics and dysfluency.* New York: Speech Hearing Institute. 40-71.

Azrin, N.H. & Nunn, R.G. (1974). A rapid method of eliminating stuttering by a regulated breathing approach. *Behavioral Research and Therapy, 12,* 279-286.

Berg, J.W. van den (1960). Direct and indirect determination of the mean subglottal pressure. *Folia Phoniatrica, 8,* 1-24.

Boves, L. (1984). *The phonetic basis of perceptual ratings of running speech.* Dordrecht: Foris Publications.

Conture, E., McGall, G. & Brewer, D. (1977). Laryngeal behavior during stuttering. *Journal of Speech and Hearing Research, 20,* 661-668.

Fourcin, A.J. (1981). Laryngographic assessment of phonatory function. In C. Ludlow & M. O'Connell (Eds.), *Proceedings of the conference on the assessment of vocal pathology.* ASHA report Nr. 11. Rockville: American Speech-Language-Hearing Association.

Freeman, F. (1979). Phonation in stuttering: a review of current research. *Journal of Fluency Disorders, 4,* 79-89.

Freeman, F. (1984). Laryngeal muscle activity of stutterers. In R. Curlee & P.H. Perkins (Eds.), *Nature and Treatment of Stuttering: New Directions.* San Diego: College Hill Press. 104-114.

Gregory, H.H. & Hill, D. (1980). Stuttering therapy for children. *Seminars in Speech, Language and Hearing, 1,* 351-365.

Koike, Y. (1981). Sub- and supraglottal pressure variation during phonation. In K.N. Stevens & M. Hirano (Eds.), *Vocal Fold Physiology.* Tokyo: University of Tokyo Press. 181-191.
Perkins, W.H. (1973). Replacement of stuttering with normal speech. II. Clinical procedures. *Journal of Speech and Hearing Disorders, 38,* 395-303.
Ryan, B.P. (1974). *Programmed therapy for stuttering in children, and adults.* Springfield: Thomas.
Shames, G.H. & Florance, C.L. (1980). *Stutter free speech. A goal for therapy.* Columbus: Ch. Merrill Publ.
Shapiro, A.I. (1980). An electromyographic analysis of fluent and dysfluent utterances of several types of stutterers. *Journal of Fluency Disorders, 5,* 203-232.
Schwartz, M.F. (1976). *Stuttering solved.* Philadelphia: Lippincott.
Van Riper, Ch. (1972). *The nature of stuttering.* Englewood Cliffs: Prentice-Hall.
Webster, R.L. (1978). *Precision fluency shaping program: Clinicians program guide.* Roanoke: Hollins Communications Development Corporation.
Wingate, M. (1976). *Stuttering theory and treatment.* New York: Irvington.
Yoshioka, H. & Löfqvist, A. (1981). Laryngeal involvement in stuttering: a glottographic observation using a reaction time paradigm. *Folia Phoniatrica, 33,* 348-357.

Chapter 17

A Speech Motor Control Perspective on Stuttering: Preliminary Observations

Anthony J. Caruso, Vincent L. Gracco and James H. Abbs

Most physiological investigations of stutterers' speech productions have focused on descriptive measures of muscular events and structural movements, air pressures and flows, and the resulting acoustic waveform during instances of stuttering. Specifically, during moments of *stuttering*, stutterers have difficulty producing: (1) proper onsets, offsets, transitions, and durations of muscle (in)activation prior to or during stuttering (Sheehan & Voas, 1954; Ford & Luper, 1975; Metz, Conture & Colton, 1976; Freeman & Ushijima, 1978; Shapiro, 1980; Stromsta & Fibiger, 1980), (2) appropriate degrees of muscle excitation (Sheehan & Voas, 1954; Ford & Luper, 1975; Freeman & Ushijima, 1978; Shapiro, 1980; Stromsta & Fibiger, 1980; McClean, Goldsmith & Cerf, 1984), and (3) appropriate timing of lip, jaw and tongue movements (Hutchinson & Watkin, 1976; Zimmermann, 1980b, 1980c).

More recently, physiological characteristics associated with stutterers' *fluent* speech have been investigated. In general, results of such research suggest that even during *fluency*, stutterers have difficulty producing (1) appropriate levels of muscle activity (Shapiro, 1980); (2) coordinated laryngeal activity (Shapiro, 1980; Conture, Rothenberg & Molitor, 1986); and (3) appropriate timing of jaw, lip, and tongue movement (Zimmermann, 1980a; Zimmermann & Hanley, 1983). Clearly, the *stuttered* speech of adult stutterers does not meet all of DeLong's (1971) requirements (proper muscle selection, precise timing, and appropriate magnitude of muscle activity) for coordinated structural movement. Moreover, the above results suggest that even stutterers' perceptually *fluent* utterances may be associated with aberrant neuromotor processes. Unfortunately, the nature of the underlying mechanisms associated with these physiological aberrations has not been thoroughly investigated. One way to study the neuromotor process associated with speech movement is to simultaneously record muscle activity and resulting structural movement for specific articulators (e.g., lower and upper lips). Recently, simultaneous recordings of EMG and movement from multiple structures and muscles involved during stutterers' (dis)fluent speech have begun (e.g., McClean et al., 1984); however, to date, such work has been descriptive in nature rather than exploiting experimental methods of motor control or motor neurophysiology.

Sensorimotor mechanisms underlying coordination patterns in normally fluent speech have been investigated using unanticipated perturbation techniques (Folkins & Abbs, 1975, 1976; Kelso, Tuller, Bateson & Fowler, 1984; Abbs & Gracco, 1984; Gracco & Abbs, 1985). Perturbation analyses involve testing of sensory contributions to control of particular motor acts by introducing unanticipated errors in lower lip, upper lip or jaw movement and examining the corrections that occur in response to that error. The remarkable finding in these studies is that compensations are seen in all of the multiple movements involved in a given speech gesture. For example, if a load is introduced on the lower lip immediately prior to or during a bilabial stop consonant (e.g., /p/), compensations are observed in the upper lip as well as the lower lip (Abbs & Gracco, 1984). Similarly, in other studies where jaw loads are introduced (Folkins & Abbs, 1975, 1976) during a combined jaw-lip speech movement gesture (e.g., production of /p/), compensatory responses are observed in both the upper and lower lips. Likewise, upper lip loads yield both upper and lower lip compensatory responses. In yet other experiments, jaw loads introduced during a jaw-tongue speech gesture (e.g. production of /z/) yielded compensatory responses in the tongue elevation muscles (Kelso et al., 1984). An interesting finding in these studies is that the particular pattern of sensorimotor responses to a perturbation are task specific. That is, when a perturbation is introduced on the lower lip during a bilabial closure for /aba/, responses are seen in both the upper and lower lips. By contrast, if the same perturbation is introduced on the lower lip during the lip elevation for /afa/, upper lip responses are absent; compensation is confined to the lower lip. These observations suggest that multiple speech movement coordination may be implemented via a set of sensorimotor linkages among the constituent parts of the speech production system. Further, these sensorimotor connections are only operational by virtue of the overall goals of the particular motor task.

Several related observations indicate that intermovement sensorimotor linkages revealed by perturbation analyses appear to reflect natural processes. First, despite some sizable movement perturbations (up to 15 mm), the speech utterance is not disrupted in any discernible way; that is, a listener cannot perceptually distinguish "loaded" versus "unloaded" speech productions of normal speakers. Secondly, consistently discernible compensatory responses occur to perturbations as small as 1.0 mm. Finally, compensations to the load *occur the very first time the load is introduced to the normal speaker*. Thus, it would appear that these sensorimotor compensations reflect "normal" processes of speech movement control rather than a learned strategy for dealing with the unanticipated perturbations (Abbs & Gracco, 1982). These results are consistent with the seemingly unremarkable observations that the lip, tongue, and pharyngeal movements are recognized for adequate speech when the jaw is fixed, as in pipe smoking (MacNeilage, 1970; Lindblom, Lubker & Gay, 1979). *Given these observations, one is led to the working hypothesis that stuttering reflects aberrations in sensorimotor control; that is, if normal intermovement coordination for speech is accomplished via sensorimotor linkages, the manifestation of discoordination suggests the need to evaluate these sensorimotor processes in stutterers.* Moreover, given the subtle physiological aberrancies associated with stutterers' *fluent* speech, one might speculate that aberrant neuromotor processes are present even during stutterers' perceptually fluent productions.

In this context, the objective of this research is to further develop our understanding of the sensorimotor processes associated with the disorder of stuttering. In the present study, the authors (1) observed upper lip and lower lip movements and simultaneous muscle activity during adult stutterers' *fluent* speech; (2) characterized the multiple actions of the sensorimotor mechanisms involved in orofacial speech movement coordination using unanticipated perturbation techniques; and (3) provided quantitative information concerning the response characteristics of these sensorimotor actions and associated aberrations thereof. Results of these preliminary observations provide a more concrete data set for judging the discoordination associated with stuttering and permit one to address recent theories suggesting potential sensorimotor aberrations underlying that discoordination (cf. Zimmermann, 1980c; Smith & Luschei, 1983; McClean et al., 1984).

METHOD

Subjects

Subjects for the present study were three adult stutterers and three normally fluent adult speakers. The mean age of the three adult stutterers was 28 (range: from 21 to 34), and the three normally fluent adults' mean age was 27 (range: from 22 to 35). Mean stuttering frequency for the three adult stutterers was 12 stutterings per 100 words spoken (range: from 6 to 16 stutterings per 100 words spoken). Mean stuttering duration was 750 msec (range: from approximately 100 msec to 1200 msec). None of the subjects included in this study had any history of language, hearing, neurological or speech problems (except for the stuttering).

Lower Lip Perturbations

Unanticipated perturbations were applied in an inferior direction, using a brushless dc torque motor (Aeroflex No. TQ34W-12). Details regarding the operational characteristics of the torque motor were described previously (Abbs & Gracco, 1984). The torque motor was designed to operate under force feedback control and to follow speech movements at tracking loads less than 5 grams. These small tracking forces did not produce sensation of movement restriction per subject report. Jaw movement was eliminated by having the subjects bite on a custom fitted bite-block.

Signals Recorded

Signals recorded included (1) displacement of the upper lip and lower lip (inferior-superior dimension) using (a) the displacement signal provided by the rotational variable differential transformer (RVDT; Pickering) coupled to the brushless dc torque motor (lower lip) and (b) cantilever beam instrumented with a strain gauge transducer (cf. Barlow, Cole & Abbs, 1983) firmly attached to a head stabilizing device (upper lip); (2) force output from the torque motor; (3) EMG from five perioral muscles (orbicularis oris superior (OOS), orbicularis oris inferior (OOI), depressor labii inferior (DLI), depressor anguli oris (DAO), mentalis (MTL)) using hooked-wire electrodes; and (4) a control signal which was used to specify both the magnitude of the force perturbation as well as the force rise time. EMG electrodes were placed as reported previously (cf. Abbs & Gracco, 1984). The bandwidth of the RVDT and the strain gauge transducer (dc to at least 40 Hz) exceeds the range of normal speech movements. All EMG signals were preamplified with a frequency range of 22 Hz to 20 kHz, a common mode rejection ratio of 110 dB, and an input impedance of 1000 MOhms. Additional amplification was obtained from Honeywell Accudata 135 amplifiers with filter settings of 50 Hz high pass and 2.5 kHz low pass. All signals were digitized on-line using a DEC PDP 11/44 lab computer. Myoelectric activity was digitized at 3500 sps, while movement and force signals were digitized at 500 sps.

Movement Task

Subjects were not aware of the purpose of the study and were instructed that this was a reaction time (RT) experiment. It should be emphasized that reaction time was not analyzed nor did the stutterers' tendency for slower reaction time (cf. Agnello, 1975; Adams & Hayden, 1976; Starkweather, Hirschman & Tannenbaum, 1976; Hayden & Jordahl, 1979; Reich, Till & Goldsmith, 1981; Watson & Alfonso, 1982) influence the primary measure of interest (that is, how stutterers compensated to an unanticipated perturbation to the lower lip). The subjects' task consisted of sustaining the vowel "ah", and upon hearing a tone (1000 Hz, 250 msec duration) to close their lips as rapidly as possible and generate a "p" sound. Once the sound was produced, they were to resume producing the vowel and respond again when the tone was heard. Effectively, subjects produced rapid lip closure from a static posture. The only demands placed on the subject regarding the task was that the "p" be generated in a manner that was unambiguous to a human listener. From an ecological perspective, the exact movements of the lips are subordinate to the acoustical goals of this natural, well-learned speech motor task. All stutterers produced *fluent* speech utterances during this task.

Perturbation Characteristics

Controlled loads of 250 msec duration with different magnitudes and rise times were used to produce a range of perturbation displacements and velocities. Two discrete force rise times (5 and 15 msec) and one level of force magnitude (35 gms) were used. These force magnitude/rise time combinations resulted in displacements and velocities within the range of normal lip movements for speech (cf. Sussman, MacNeilage & Hanson, 1973).

Introduction and Control of Perturbations

All aspects of the data acquisition procedure have been reported previously (Gracco & Abbs, 1985). Briefly, the experimenter controlled the onset of an auditory stimulus which served as a cue for the subject to respond. In parallel, the tone triggered the PDP-11/44 laboratory computer which digitized the physiological signals and periodically delivered the force perturbations to the lower lip. Perturbations were delivered randomly at an average frequency of 15% (viz., 15 perturbations/100 trials). The low percentage of perturbations was necessary due to concerns regarding adaptation/anticipation. Each perturbed (experimental) trial was digitized along with the immediately preceding control trial. These control/experimental pairs were used in statistical analyses of perturbation-related changes. The signals from all trials were recorded on FM tape.

Loads were applied prior to and during the initial phases of the major agonistic muscle contraction associated with the lip movements under investigation. Electromyographic activity from a muscle involved in the lower lip elevation movement (OOI) was monitored on an oscilloscope by the experimenter. By observing the muscle activity onset relative to the onset of the stimulus tone (the RT), it was possible, via the computer key-in delay, to deliver perturbations within a narrow range relative to activation of this muscle. Specifically, the target interval for the introduction of these loads was the 100 msec window centered on the onset of OOI activation (cf. Gracco & Abbs, 1985). Subjects were not informed of the possibility that speech movement might be perturbated.

Data Analysis

A total of 130 control-experimental pairs were obtained from the three stutterers and 300 trial pairs were obtained from the normally fluent subjects. Following the on-line data acquisition, each perturbed and control record was individually viewed on a DEC-VT100 Retrographics terminal. As reported previously (Gracco & Abbs, 1985), specific events were labelled and marked for subsequent analysis. Based on these event markers, computer programs were used to provide the following measures: (1) time of load onset relative to initiation of contraction in the lower lip elevation agonistic muscle (OOI), (2) lower lip displacement caused by the perturbation, (3) time of muscle activity onset for each of the muscles under investigation, and (4) peak displacement for both upper and lower lips. Peak movement displacements for each lip were calculated as the difference between the position of each lip immediately prior to movement onset and the maximum lip positions at closure. Similar analyses were conducted on the EMG signals (e.g., magnitude of change and latencies).

RESULTS AND DISCUSSION

Results indicate that all three stutterers displayed compensatory changes in labial EMG and kinematics in response to load perturbations; however, stutterers' responses to unanticipated loads were subtly different from normally fluent subjects. Similar to previously published reports of normally fluent speakers (Abbs & Gracco, 1984; Gracco & Abbs, 1985), stutterers' compensations were observed the first time a lower lip load was introduced. An attempt to randomly distribute loads ranging from +/- 50 msec re: OOI onset was made; however, approximately 80% of the loads occurred between 20 msec before to 20 msec after OOI onset. Specific results will be presented as follows: (1) compensatory response latencies, (2) muscle activity change with load, and (3) labial movement adjustments. Because previous speech perturbation studies have shown that compensatory responses are influenced by the time of load onset (re: muscle activity; Gracco & Abbs, 1985), responses from the control and experimental groups were matched as closely as possible.

Compensatory Response Latencies

Particular attention was focused on potential responses at latencies associated with the perioral reflex (12 to 18 msec), since it has been suggested that stuttering is associated with hyperactive brainstem reflexes (cf. Zimmermann, 1980c). Perturbations using rapid (5 msec) force rise times were used in an attempt to elicit perioral reflex responses.

Figure 1 displays representative ensemble averaged EMG activity associated with 15 loaded and 15 unloaded trials from one of the stutterers under investigation. Similar to previous reports in normally fluent speakers (Gracco & Abbs, 1982; Abbs & Gracco, 1984), there is no indication of hyperactive perioral reflexes in stutterers' *fluent* speech production. Moreover, this finding is in agreement with observations of Neilson, Andrews, Guitar, and Quinn (1979) and Smith and Luschei (1983) who reported that stutterers exhibited no evidence of hyperactive perioral reflexes during nonspeech tasks.

Latency values of compensatory actions were obtained using a previously reported technique (cf. Abbs & Gracco, 1984 for specific details). The digitized EMG signals were software integrated over 5 msec windows and manipulated with a computer algorithm that yielded latencies for individual loaded trials.

Figure 2 displays the latency values for four of the perioral (OOI, OOS, DAO, MTL) muscles for stutterers and normally fluent speakers. These latencies were obtained for loads applied in the time window ranging from +/- 20 msec re: the initiation of that

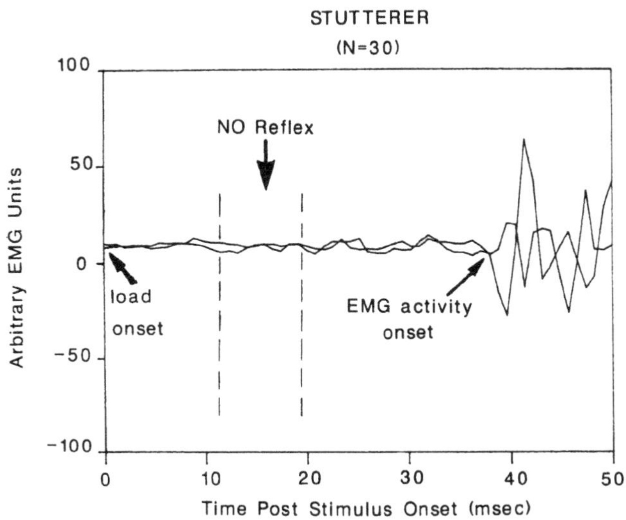

Figure 1. Ensemble averages of OOI activity associated with "p" for 15 control and 15 experimental (loaded) trials (for a total N = 30) from one stutterer. No indication of perioral reflex is present between 12 to 18 ms re: load onset.

muscle activity. Compensatory responses reflected in these latencies should be indicative of on-line/automatic sensorimotor control mechanisms since the time window does not provide sufficient time for the operation of intentional reprogramming or reaction-time responses. The latency values for loads in this interval were combined across the subjects studied. Stutterers' mean compensatory response latency of 92 msec (SD = 34) was significantly different ($p < .05$) from the normally fluent speakers' mean compensatory response latency of 79 msec (SD = 32). It is apparent that the responses are consistently longer in latency than those associated with the perioral reflex pathway, potentially implicating impaired supranuclear pathways in the disorder of stuttering.

Muscle Activity Change

In order to document the magnitude of stutterers' compensatory responses, the EMG signals for unloaded (control) and loaded trials were subjected to quantitative analysis and compared to normally fluent speakers. The EMG signals associated with lip closure for individual trials were rectified, digitized, and integrated providing an area under the curve index for each of the five muscles (cf. Abbs & Gracco, 1984). These values were then used to calculate a percentage of EMG change for loaded trials. It should be emphasized that the loads analyzed were introduced no earlier than 50 msec prior to the onset of muscle activity, thus minimizing the possibility that the measured load-induced changes reflected intentional responses. In other words, the responses displayed in

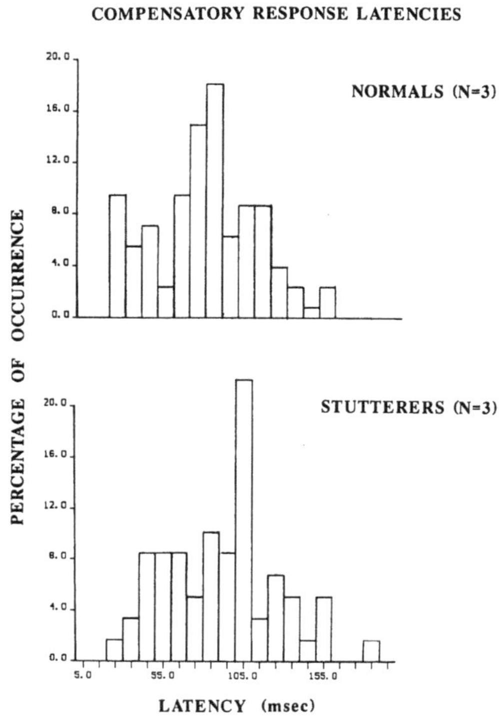

Figure 2. Stutterers' (N = 3) and normally fluent speakers' (N = 3) latency values for four perioral muscles (OOS, OOI, DAO, MTL).

Figure 3 are representative of the disorder of stuttering itself and not some strategy stutterers are using to initiate or maintain fluent speech. As is apparent in Figure 3, the normally fluent speakers showed increases in activity for all five muscles in response to the unanticipated lower lip loads. The stutterers likewise showed increases in activity for four labial muscles (OOI, OOS, DAO, MTL) in response to the unanticipated load; however, the magnitude of change was significantly smaller ($p < .05$) when compared to the normal speakers.

These results indicate that the stutterers' magnitude of increase in labial EMG activity is significantly reduced from normals in response to unanticipated loads during *fluent* speech production. Interestingly, the stutterers displayed no significant change in DLI activity in response to the load. It is tempting to suggest that this finding is in agreement with recent observations of McClean et al., (1984) and Stromsta and Fibiger (1980) demonstrating reduced levels of labial muscle activity associated with the disorder of stuttering; however, the use of different methodologies precludes us from strongly relating these apparently similar results. Be that as it may, this finding is intriguing since the disorder of stuttering is typically viewed as a "hypertense" behavior (cf. Van Riper, 1982). One might expect,

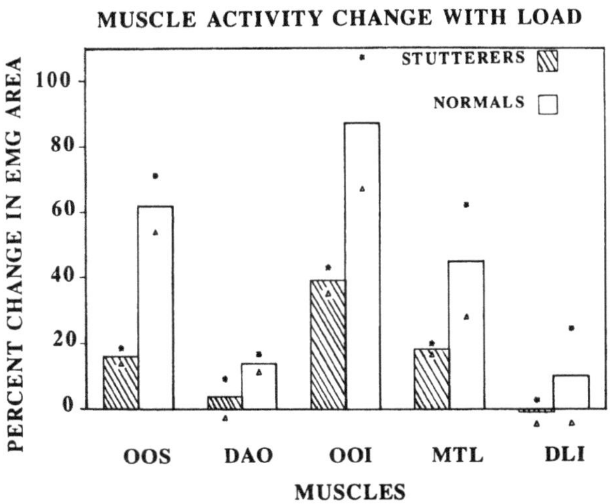

Figure 3. Percent increase in muscle activity for all five muscles with 35-g loads introduced during normally fluent speakers' (N = 3) and stutterers' (N = 3) fluent productions of "apa." One standard deviation above and below the mean percent increase for each muscle is indicated by '*' and '▵', respectively.

on that basis, that stutterers' responses to a load, even during fluent speech, would be associated with a greater increase in muscle activity as compared to the normally fluent group.

Labial Kinematic Adjustments

In order to evaluate movement adjustments in response to the induced error (unanticipated perturbation), the ratio of compensatory displacement (Xc; output) to perturbation displacement (Xp; input) or system gain (Xc/Xp) was calculated for each load trial. This ratio provides a normalized measure of compensation relative to the magnitude of the displacement error resulting from the load perturbation. A larger magnitude error generally results in greater compensations (Gracco & Abbs, 1985). These ratios were then averaged for loads occurring from 50 msec prior to OOI onset to 50 msec after OOI onset. It should be noted, however, that the majority of the loads (approximately 80%) occurred between 20 msec before to 20 msec after OOI onset. These output-input ratios, shown in Figure 4, reflect the degree to which the upper lip (UL) and lower lip (LL) acted to overcome the displacement perturbation. A total UL and LL ratio of 1.0 reflects perfect compensation, indicating the displacement perturbation was completely cancelled by the combined action of the upper and lower lips. It should be noted that later loads (from 0 to 50 msec after OOI onset) tend to be associated with smaller system gains (Gracco and Abbs, 1985). Stutterers demonstrated significant changes in displacement in response to the load; however, the total system gain for the normally fluent speakers was significantly different from the stutterers (.64 vs .38; $p < .05$).

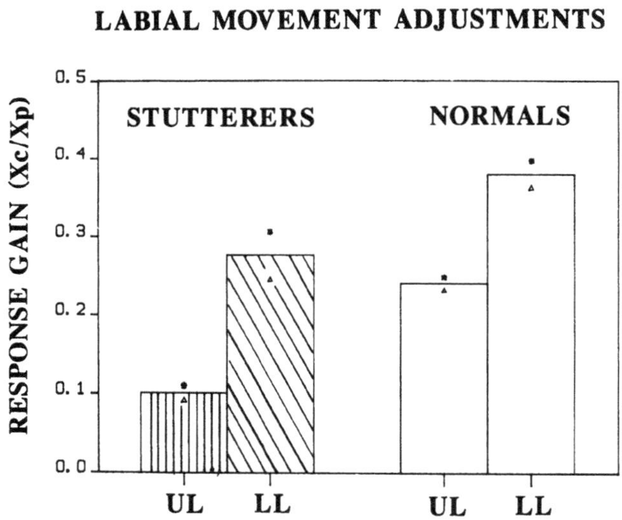

Figure 4. Upper lip (UL) and lower lip (LL) gain for stutterers (N = 3) and normally fluent speakers (N = 3). See text for discussion of the ratio of compensatory displacement (Xc; output) to perturbation displacement (Xp; input) or "system gain" (Xc/Xp).

In order to determine the response of each lip, individual gains were calculated for the UL and LL and displayed in Figure 4. It can be seen that the relative amount of compensation is larger for the UL for both stutterers and controls as is generally the case for later loads (Gracco & Abbs, 1985). However, stutterers' LL compensations were significantly smaller than the normals (.28 vs .39; $p < .05$). Similarly, stutterers UL compensations were significantly smaller than the normals (.10 vs .25; $p < .05$).

SUMMARY AND CONCLUSIONS

Present findings show that the adult stutterers sampled in this study responded (during their fluent speech) to unanticipated perturbations in a subtly different manner from individuals who do not stutter. That is, while the stutterers compensated for unanticipated perturbations, the nature of these compensations was generally different in degree rather than kind as compared to those of normally fluent speakers. Specifically, these subtle differences in response to the lower lip loads included: (1) consistently longer latency values of labial EMG activity, (2) smaller changes in levels of EMG activity, and, correspondingly, (3) smaller changes in magnitude of upper and lower lip movement. Interestingly, although stutterers compensated to the load on the very first time the load was introduced, the degree of compensation during the initial loaded trial was markedly smaller when compared to initial loaded trials of normally fluent speakers. On the other hand, the stutterers' responses to later loaded trials were more similar, but still different, from those of normally fluent speakers with more trials.

One possible interpretation of the present findings is that stutterers, at least those included in this study, are either at the lower ends of normal limits for speech motor control (cf. Conture et al., 1986) or have subtle neuromotor difficulties re: coordination for speech. It should be emphasized that the present study sampled *fluent* speech utterances that were considerably less motorically complex than conversational speech. Specifically, the present procedures allowed for: (1) reduction of a degree of freedom by fixing the jaw via a custom fitted bite block; and (2) reducing the rather rapid and intricate temporal constraints of conversational speech. Despite these simplifications, differences between stutterers' *fluent* speech and that of normally fluent speakers were found. Given both the nature of the unanticipated perturbation paradigm and the short response latencies (approximately 40 msec) typically associated with this task (cf. Folkins & Abbs, 1975, 1976; Lindblom, Lubker & Gay, 1979; Gracco & Abbs, 1982; Abbs & Gracco, 1984), it seems rather unlikely that the reported differences represent a strategy in the way that stutterers are dealing with the introduced errors. Moreover, it might be speculated that these neuromotor difficulties arise from supranuclear levels of the nervous system since no evidence of aberrant brainstem reflexes were found.

In general, present results are consistent with findings that respiratory (Baken, McManus & Cavallo, 1983), laryngeal (Shapiro, 1980; Conture et al., 1985), and supralaryngeal (Zimmermann, 1980 b) physiology during stutterers' perceptually fluent speech is subtly, rather than markedly, different from that of their normally fluent peers. In addition, results indicated that, similar to individuals who do not stutter, adult stutterers did not exhibit indications of hyperactive perioral reflexes during *fluent* speech productions - a finding similar to previous published reports of stutterers' *nonspeech* movements (Neilson et al., 1979; Smith & Luschei, 1983).

In conclusion, unanticipated perturbation analyses offer critical advantages in specifying sensorimotor aberrations underlying stuttering for various reasons. First, the measure obtained via this technique directly reflect neuromotor dysfunctions. Second, superficial subject strategies are circumvented, thus, results reflect the nature of the disorder of stuttering and not the stutterers' learned compensatory (either physiologically or psychologically) reactions to that disorder (cf. Caruso, Conture & Colton, 1986 for information concerning stutterers' reactions to speech disfluencies). Finally, adaptation or anticipation to this paradigm is minimized since perturbations were distributed randomly at a relatively low frequency of 15% (i.e. 15 perturbations/100 trials).

ACKNOWLEDGEMENTS

This work was supported by National Institute of Neurological and Communicative Disorders and Stroke Grants NS-07679 and NS-13274, and National Institute of Child Health en Human Development Grant HD-03352.

REFERENCES

Abbs, J.H. & Gracco, V.L. (1982). Motor control of multi-movement behaviors: Orofacial muscle responses to load perturbations of the lips during speech. *Society for Neuroscience, 8,* 282. (Abstract)

Abbs, J.H. & Gracco, V.L. (1984). Control of complex motor gestures: Orofacial muscle responses to load perturbations of the lip during speech. *Journal of Neurophysiology, 51,* 705-723.

Adams, M.R. & Hayden, P. (1976). The ability of stutterers and nonstutterers to initiate and terminate phonation during production of an isolated vowel. *Journal of Speech and Hearing Research, 19,* 290-296.

Agnello, J.G. (1975). Voice onset and voice termination features of stuttering. In L.M. Webster & L.C. Furst (Eds.), *Vocal tract dynamics and dysfluency.* New York: Speech and Hearing Institute.

Baken, R.J., McManus, D.A. & Cavallo, S. (1983). Prephonatory chest wall posturing in stutterers. *Journal of Speech and Hearing Research, 26,* 444-450.

Barlow, S.M., Cole, K.J. & Abbs, J.H. (1983). A new headmounted lip-jaw movement transduction system for the study of motor speech disorders. *Journal of Speech and Hearing Research, 26,* 283-288.

Caruso, A.J., Conture, E.G. & Colton, R.H. (1986). Speech physiology associated with young stutterers' stutterings. A paper submitted to *Journal of Speech and Hearing Research.*

Conture, E.G., Rothenberg, M. & Molitor, R. (1986). Electroglottographic observations of young stutterers' fluency. *Journal of Speech and Hearing Research, 29,* 384-393.

DeLong, M. (1971). Central control of movement. In E.V. Evarts, E. Bizzi, R.E. Burke, M. DeLong & W.T. Trach (Eds.), *Neurosciences Research Program Bulletin, 9* (1), 10-30.

Folkins, J.W. & Abbs, J.H. (1975). Lip and jaw motor control during speech: Responses to resistive loading of the jaw. *Journal of Speech and Hearing Research, 18,* 207-222.

Folkins, J.W. & Abbs, J.H. (1976). Additional observations on responses to resistive loading of the jaw. *Journal of Speech and Hearing Research, 19,* 820-821.

Ford, S. & Luper, H. (1975). *Aerodynamic, phonatory, and labial EMG patterns during fluent and stuttered speech.* Paper presented at the American Speech-Language-Hearing Association Annual Convention.

Freeman, F. & Ushijima, T. (1978). Laryngeal muscle activity during stuttering. *Journal of Speech and Hearing Research, 21,* 538-562.

Gracco, V.L. & Abbs, J.H. (1982). Temporal response characteristics of the perioral system to load perturbations. *Society for Neuroscience, 8* (part 1), 282. (Abstract)

Gracco, V.L. & Abbs, J.H. (1985). Dynamic control of the perioral system during speech: Kinematic analyses of autogenic and nonautogenic sensorimotor processes. *Journal of Neurophysiology, 54* (2), 418-432.

Hayden, P. & Jordahl, N. (1979). Stutterers' voice initiation times during conditions of novel stimuli. *American Speech-Language-Hearing Association, 21,* 693. (Abstract)

Hutchinson, J. & Watkin, K.L. (1976). Jaw mechanics during release of the stuttering moment: Some initial observations and interpretations. *Journal of Communication Disorders, 9,* 269-279.

Kelso, J.A.S., Tuller, B., Bateson, E. & Fowler, C. (1984). Functionally specific articulatory cooperation following jaw perturbations during speech: Evidence for coordinative structures. *Journal of Experimental Psychology (Hum. Percept.), 10,* 812-832.

Lindblom, B., Lubker, J. & Gay, T. (1979). Formant frequencies of some fixed mandible vowels and a model of speech motor programming by predictive simulation. *Journal of Phonetics, 7,* 147-161.

MacNeilage, P.F. (1970). Motor control of serial ordering of speech. *Psychological Review, 3,* 182-196.

McClean, M., Goldsmith, H. & Cerf, A. (1984). Lower-lip EMG and displacement during bilabial disfluencies in adult stutterers. *Journal of Speech and Hearing Research, 27,* 342-349.

Metz, D.E., Conture, E.G. & Colton, R. (1976). Temporal relationships among respiratory and laryngeal systems prior to fluent and stuttered utterances. *ASHA, 18,* 664. (Abstract)

Neilson, P.D., Andrews, G., Guitar, B.E. & Quinn, P.T. (1979). Tonic stretch reflexes in lip, tongue and jaw muscles. *Brain Research, 178,* 311-328.

Reich, A., Till, J. & Goldsmith, H. (1981). Laryngeal and manual reaction times of stuttering and nonstuttering adults. *Journal of Speech and Hearing Research, 24,* 192-196.

Shapiro, A. (1980). An electromyographic analysis of the fluent and dysfluent utterances of several types of stutterers. *Journal of Fluency Disorders, 5,* 293-331.

Sheehan, J. & Voas, R.B. (1954). Tension patterns during stuttering in relation to conflict, anxiety-binding, and reinforcement. *Speech Monographs, 21,* 272-279.

Smith, A. & Luschei, E.S. (1983). Assessment of oral-motor reflexes in stutterers and normal speakers: Preliminary observations. *Journal of Speech and Hearing Research, 26* (3), 322-328.

Starkweather, C.W., Hirschman, P. & Tannenbaum, R.S. (1976) Latency of vocalization: Stutterers versus nonstutterers. *Journal of Speech and Hearing Research, 19,* 481-492.

Stromsta, C. & Fibiger, S. (1980). *Physiological correlates of the core behavior of stuttering.* Paper presented to the XVIIIth IALP Congress, Washington, DC.

Sussman, H.M., MacNeilage, P.F. & Hanson, R.J. (1973). Labial and mandibular movement dynamics during the production of bilabial stop consonants. *Journal of Speech and Hearing Research, 16,* 397-420.

Van Riper, C. (1982). *The Nature of Stuttering.* Englewood Cliffs, New Jersey: Prentice-Hall, Inc.

Watson, B.C. & Alfonso, P.J. (1982). Comparison of LRT and VOT values between stutterers and nonstutterers. *Journal of Fluency Disorders, 7,* 219-242.

Zimmermann, G. (1980a). Articulatory dynamics of fluent utterances of stutterers and nonstutterers. *Journal of Speech and Hearing Research, 23,* 95-107.

Zimmermann, G. (1980b). Articulatory behaviors associated with stuttering: A cinefluorographic analysis. *Journal of Speech and Hearing Research, 23,* 108-121.

Zimmermann, G. (1980c). Stuttering: A disorder of movement. *Journal of Speech and Hearing Research, 23,* 122-136.

Zimmermann, G. & Hanley, J.M. (1983). A cinefluorographic investigation of repeated fluent productions of stutterers in an adaptation procedure. *Journal of Speech and Hearing Research, 26,* 35-42.

Chapter **18**

Labial Coarticulation in Stutterers and Normal Speakers: a Pilot Study

Ann-Marie Almé and Robert McAllister

Anticipatory labial co-articulation refers specifically to the early onset of features related to labiality, as, for example in the onset of rounding for rounded vowels. This particular example of anticipatory labial co-articulation has received considerable attention in recent research in normal speech production (Kent and Minifie, 1977). Some of this research has shown a temporally variable extent of anticipation related to the number of non-labial consonants preceding the rounded vowel (Benguerel and Cowan, 1974; Lubker, McAllister and Linker, 1979; Lubker, 1981). Other researchers have found relatively constant anticipation times (Gay, 1979; Bell-Berti and Harris, 1979, 1982). It has been suggested that inter-language differences may account for some of the differences in the results obtained in these various studies (Lubker and Gay, 1982). This is, of course, an important point since research in speech production is concerned primarily with underlying mechanisms. The need for separation of language specific variables and underlying mechanisms, therefore, is one motivation for part of the work presented in this chapter.

Anticipatory labial co-articulation, then, has been a topic of some interest in recent research in speech motor dynamics. Due to this interest there has been a considerable amount of data collected and its interpretation thoroughly examined. Therefore this research paradigm might be a good starting point for a physiological study of movement coordination in fluent and disfluent speech. It has been suggested that even perceptually fluent utterances produced by a stutterer can be associated with respiratory, phonatory and/or articulatory abnormalities in the coordination of speech gestures. Some studies have indicated that, as a group, stutterers may be motorically slower than normal speakers. Stutterers demonstrated longer durations of movement onset, slower VOT, increased latency of muscle activity and asynchrony between lip and jaw movements during fluent utterances compared to nonstutterers (McFarlane and Prins, 1978; Van Riper, 1982; Zimmermann, 1980). It has also been suggested that mild stutterers are more similar to normal speakers than are severe stutterers. In a recent investigation (Almé, 1984) on the psycholinguistic variables of stuttering and disfluency, a systematic difference was demonstrated between mild and severe stutterers. There was not only a difference in frequency of disfluencies but also with regard to type, loci and duration of stuttering events.

The purpose of this study is 1) to further define the temporal extent of anticipatory labial co-articulation through observation of the articulatory behavior of speakers of several different languages and 2) to compare co-articulatory behavior in normals and stutterers and thereby to demonstrate a methodological approach to studying co-articulation in a stuttering population. This pilot study is a first effort towards an ultimate goal of the description of the temporal and spatial characteristics of labial speech gestures in perceptually fluent and disfluent utterances of stutterers. We set out to test the following hypotheses:

A. The onset of the labial gesture for rounding is programmed in relation to the temporal extent of the non-labial duration preceding the rounded vowel.

B. The onset of the rounding gesture is temporally locked to the onset of the rounded vowel.

C. The stutterers would show a longer anticipation time than the normal speakers.

D. The mild stutterer's articulatory behavior will be more like the normal speaker's.

METHODS

Subjects

Two male stutterers and three female nonstutterers served as subjects. The stutterers and one female were native speakers of Swedish. The other female subjects were speakers of French and Danish.

None of the subjects had any history of audiological or neurological disorders.

Speech Sample

The speech material was made up of a group of words and phrases with the phonological structure: CVCnV(:)C. The French and Danish material was semantically meaningful and the Swedish material was composed of semantically possible but non existent compounds. Cn was a consonant string consisting of one to six non-labial consonants. The second vowel was a stressed rounded vowel. Each of the speech samples was pronounced in five randomly ordered sequences in a carrier phrase.

Instrumentation

Surface "paint on" electrodes (McAllister, Lubker and Carlson, 1974) were applied to the subjects' upper and lower lip at the vermilion border.

Labial movements in the anterior-posterior dimension (lip protrusion) were recorded via a custom made magnetometer system (Branderud, 1985). The generator coil attached to a frame extension from a helmet is located at ca. 1 decimeter in front of the mouth and is 9x5x4mm in size, while the sensor coils attached to the lips are 5x4x3mm in size.

Each subject was tested individually in a sound proof booth in the presence of one of the experimenters. A standard set of instructions was given. The subjects practised on the speech samples before the actual experiment.

EMG, movement and audio signals were recorded on five channels of a ten channel FM tape recorder. The signals were then a/d converted and stored on computer disc for analysis on a Data General Eclipse S/200 computer. The software package used was MIX written by Rolf Carlson and Peter Branderud.

Data Reduction

Four temporal measurements were made on each utterance:

1. Duration from onset of orbicularis oris superior EMG activity to acoustic onset of V2.
2. Duration from onset of orbicularis oris inferior EMG activity to acoustic onset of V2.
3. Duration from onset of upper lip movement (UL) to acoustic onset of V2.
4. Duration from onset of lower lip movement (LL) to acoustic onset of V2.

For each subject means and standard deviations were computed.

RESULTS AND DISCUSSION

As concerns the first of our hypotheses there seems to be at least a weak tendency in Figures 1 - 3 for anticipation time to be positively correlated to the number of intervocalic consonants in normals. This tendency is most clear in the EMG data for speakers of all three languages and for French and Swedish as regards the movement data. The decrease in anticipation times for the 6-consonant cluster is probably due to reduction of the cluster which could be auditorily observed during the data gathering experiments. The french speaker does not exhibit this reduction and presumably avoided reduction of this large consonant cluster. As for the stutterers, it appears that the mild stutterer, Figure 4, may exhibit this tendency for a positive correlation between anticipation time and number of intervocalic consonants. This lends some

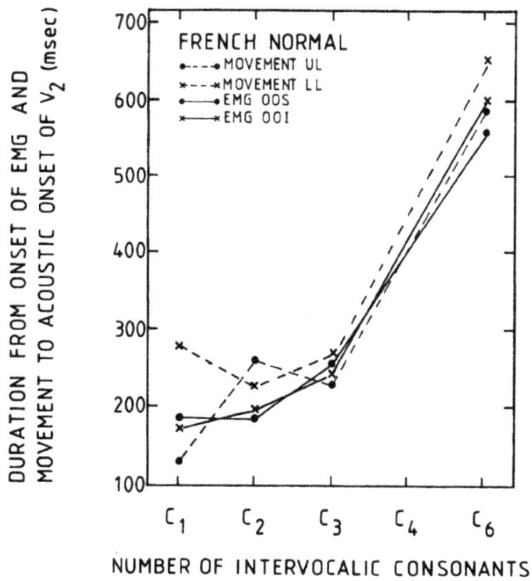

Figure 1. Anticipatory EMG and movement time related to the number of non-labial consonants preceding the rounded vowel in a French normal speaker.

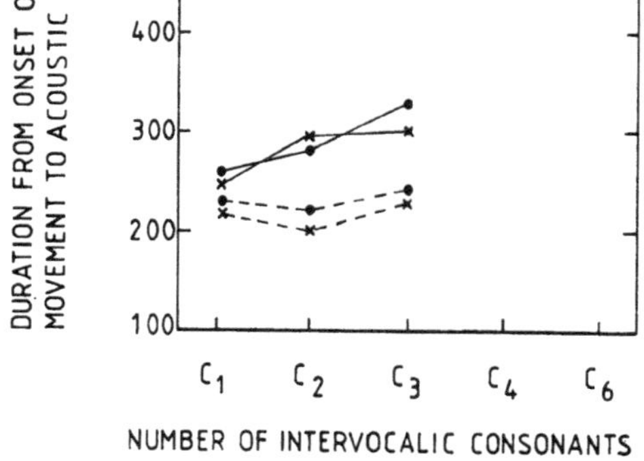

Figure 2. Anticipatory EMG and movement time related to the number of non-labial consonants preceding the rounded vowel in a Danish normal speaker.

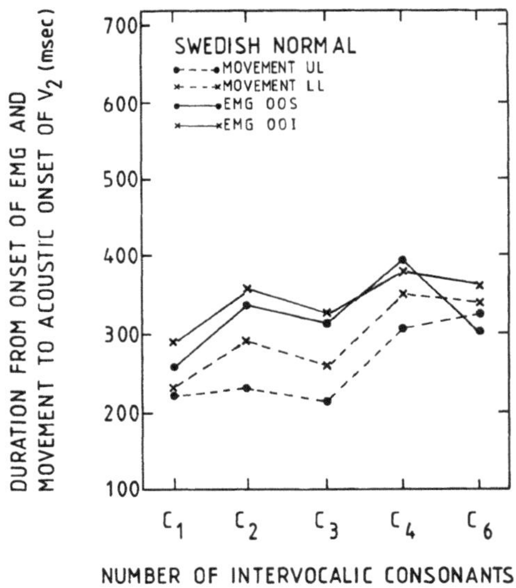

Figure 3. Anticipatory EMG and movement time related to the number of non-labial consonants preceding the rounded vowel in a Swedish normal speaker.

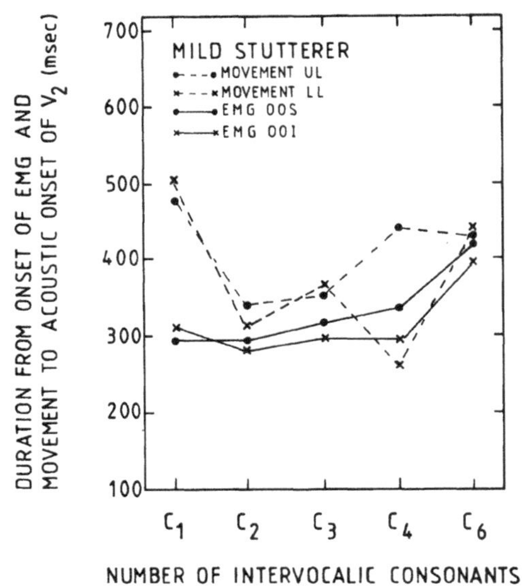

Figure 4. Anticipatory EMG and movement time related to the number of non-labial consonants preceding the rounded vowel in a Swedish mild stutterer.

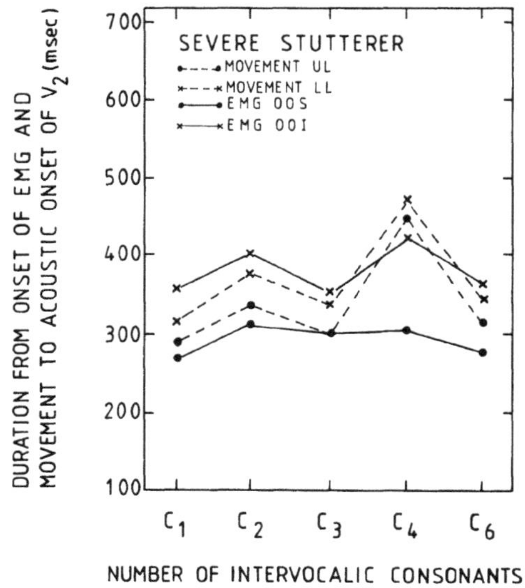

Figure 5. Anticipatory EMG and movement time related to the number of non-labial consonants preceding the rounded vowel in a Swedish severe stutterer.

support to the hypothesis concerning the mild stutterers similarity to the normal behavior when compared to the severe stutterer (Figure 5). Otherwise this hypothesis does not seem to be given much support by this data. There seems to be a tendency for the stutterers to have slightly longer anticipation times generally than the normals. All the normals' anticipation times fall approximately between 200 and 300 milliseconds whereas the stutterers exhibit times between 300 and 400 milliseconds. This result could be interpreted as supporting the hypothesis concerning the longer anticipation times for the stutterers which was suggested by the work mentioned in the introduction.

EMG activity should always precede movement. This may not always be the case as can be observed in Figure 1. When movement precedes EMG activity we can conclude that we have not been monitoring muscles that are initiating the labial gesture. While the french speaker shows considerable inconsistency in this respect the other two normal speakers are very consistent. The stutterers are, however, both quite inconsistent in this respect. They exhibit asynchrony between upper and lower lips and are obviously initiating the labial gesture in several different ways. While the evidence is far from adequate to make any strong statements about this observation, let us not forget that one of the purposes of this chapter is to explore the possibilities for comparison between the motor behavior of normals and stutterers. Let us venture the speculation that IF this would be found to be a consistent difference between normals and stutterers it may indicate some aspects of defective motor coordination in stutterers which could be a topic of further investigation. Further experimentation concerned with the dynamic properties of articulatory movements in different contexts for both mild and severe stutterers is needed. From our data one may conclude that our approach can be important not only as a potential elucidation of speech production in general but also of the nature of stuttering and in the long run of the clinical advantages of improved diagnosis and treatment of stuttering.

REFERENCES

Almé, A.M. (1984). Elicitation and perceptual judgement of disfluency and stuttering. In B. Lindblom *Experiments in Speech Perception.* Report III (Perilus III) from the Stockholm University Phonetics Research Seminar 1982-1983, 3-25.

Bell-Berti, F., & Harris, K. (1979). Anticipatory coarticulation: Some implications from a study of lip rounding. *Journal of the Acoustical Society of America, 65,* 1268-1270.

Bell-Berti, F. & Harris, K. (1982). Temporal patterns of coarticulation: Lip rounding. *Journal of the Acoustical Society of America, 71* (2), 449-454.

Benguerel, A.P. & Cowan, H.A. (1974). Coarticulation of upper lip protrusion in French. *Phonetica, 30,* 41-55.

Branderud, P. (1985). Movetrack - A movement tracking system. In B. Lindblom, *Experiments in Speech Processes.* Report IV (Perilus IV) from the Stockholm University Phonetics Research Seminar 1984-1985, 20-29.

Gay, T. (1979). Coarticulation in some consonant-vowel and consonant cluster-vowel syllables. In B. Lindblom & S. Öhman (Eds.), *Frontiers of Speech Communication Research.* New York: Academic Press. 69-76.

Kent, R.D. & Minifie, F.D. (1977). Coarticulation in recent speech production models. *Journal of Phonetics, 5,* 115-133.

Lubker, J., McAllister, R. & Linker, W. (1979). *Anticipatory labial coarticulation: Extent and influencing variables.* 98th Meeting of ASA, Nov. 1979, Salt Lake City, Utah.

Lubker, J. & Gay, T. (1982). Spatio-temporal goals: Maturational and cross-linguistic variables. In S. Grillner, B. Lindblom, J. Lubker & A. Persson (Eds.), *Speech Motor Control.* London: Pergamon Press. 205-216.

McAllister, R., Lubker, J. & Carlson, J. (1974). An EMG study of some characteristics of the Swedish rounded vowels. *Journal of Phonetics, 2,* 267-278.

McFarlane, S.C. & Prins, D. (1978). Neural response time of stutterers and nonstutterers in selected oral motor tasks. *Journal of Speech and Hearing Research, 21,* 768-778.

Van Riper, C. (1982). *The nature of stuttering.* (2nd ed.) Englewood Cliffs, NJ: Prentice Hall.

Zimmermann, G. (1980b). Articulatory dynamics of fluent utterances of stutterers and nonstutterers. *Journal of Speech and Hearing Research, 23,* 95-107.

Chapter 19

Acoustic and Electrophysiologic Correlates of Stuttering and Early Developmental Reactions

Courtney Stromsta

Observations made over the past thirty years will be presented in defense of the contention that over-inclusive definitions and descriptions of stuttering continue to confound theory, research, and therapy related to the disorder. At particular issue in this position chapter is whether phonatory disturbance is a correlate of stuttering or a consequential reaction to stuttering. The present discussion will focus on some attempts to verify longitudinal observations of speech behaviors found to precede phonatory-onset disturbance in stuttering children.

LONGITUDINAL SPECTROGRAPHIC STUDY

The results of a 10-year longitudinal spectrographic study (Stromsta, 1965) indicated that preschool children labeled as stutterers whose part-sound part-syllable repetitions were marked by abnormal formant transitions terminated by sudden arrests of phonation within phonemes were, with high probability, stuttering 10 years later. This type of speech disruption, marked by adequate initiation of phonation, is referred to as *intraphonemic disruption* and is considered to be the core behavior of stuttering - or primary stuttering - due to faulty coarticulation.

In contrast, preschool children labeled as stutterers whose whole-sound whole-syllable repetitions were not marked by intraphonemic disruptions were, with high probability, not stuttering 10 years later. Such children were judged to have been displaying excessive normal nonfluency.

During the longitudinal study, preschool children who exhibited intraphonemic disruptions were observed to initiate a typical progression of reactions within approximately six months after the advent of their unique repetitions. Along with but in contrast to the core behavior, the progression of reactions involved static positions of the vocal tract. The first reaction was prolongations of initial sounds characterized by adequate initiation of voiced or voiceless breathstream. Subsequently, static vocal tract positions were associated with difficulty, ultimately inability, to initiate voiced or voiceless breathstream, phenomena sometimes referred to as tonic blocks.

Whereas the core behavior of stuttering involved disruption of adequately initiated phonemes within their expected durations, the progression of following reactions involved static vocal tract positions which exceeded the expected durations of the involved phonemes. While prolongations involved other phonemes, in the case of prolonged voiced or voiceless stop plosives and affricatives, intraoral pressure was assumed to be minimized by lack of complete articulatory occlusion, thus allowing passage of breathstream and a transglottal pressure differential compatible with phonation. Subsequently, in concert with evidence of struggle and force, prolongations of voiced stops and affricatives, while showing adequate initiation of phonation, were arrested after approximately 300 msec by what appeared to be sustained articulatory occlusions, resulting in transglottal pressure differentials incompatible with phonation. In their early stage of development, the sustained and judged to be forceful occlusions were generally released after one or two seconds and then reformed again from one to several times before successful utterance. Later in development, the sustained occlusions for voiced stops and affricatives were maintained for longer durations, sometimes several seconds before successful utterance. It was during this stage of the development of reactions to the core behavior of stuttering that prolongations of voiceless stops and affricatives were observed to be arrested by articulatory occlusions, perhaps by generalization of the occlusions experienced previously for voiced stops and affricatives.

Characterized by individual differences concerning when it occurred, arrests of adequately-initiated prolongations of both voiced and voiceless stops and affricatives were followed by the onset of aberrant initiations of voiced and voiceless breathstream for stops and affricatives as well as for phonemes not requiring momentary articulatory occlusion. For the most part, it was only at this stage of development of reactions that comparisons of throat-microphone recordings of stuttering and nonstuttering children revealed aberrations of phonatory onsets in the stutterers. Intermingled with the advent of difficulty/inability in initiating voiced and voiceless breathstream was the onset of the myriad of differing complicating behaviors commonly referred to as secondary symptoms or accessory features of stuttering.

Before proceeding, an example may help to clarify the concept of intraphonemic disruption. Figure 1 is a spectrogram illustrating the core behavior of stuttering on the pronoun "I". Note (a) that the initial repetitions are characterized by adequate phonatory onsets as shown by the vertical striations, (b) that phonation is

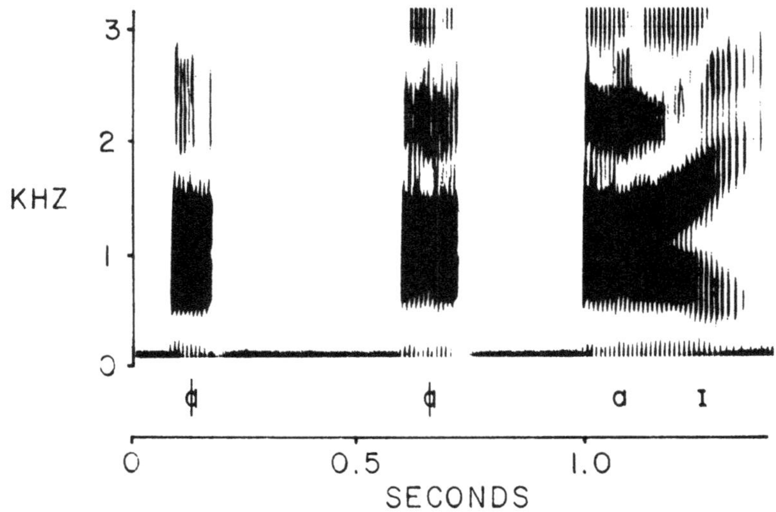

Figure 1. A sound spectrogram of basic stuttering of the pronoun I /ɑɪ/. The symbol /ɑ/ represents an abbreviated form of /ɑ/, the result of intraphonemic disruption which gave rise in this example to part-sound repetitions preceding transition into /ɪ/ and successful utterance of the word. See text for additional information.

arrested within the expected duration of /ɑ/ as indicated by vertical lines through the phonetic symbols, and (c) that the repetitions show an absence of formant transitions. In contrast, whole-sound whole-syllable repetitions characteristic of normal nonfluency are not arrested within phonemes and display normal formant transitions.

SOME EFFORTS AT VERIFICATION

Attempts to verify observations made during the longitudinal study have in large measure used adult stutterers willing to accept and tolerate detection procedures involving electrodes, pressure tubes, and so forth. Fortunately, many adult stutterers display a repertoire of speech behaviors that includes examples of repetitions and the progression of reactions that have been described. As such, examples from adults have been selected based on their spectrographic similarity to those used in the longitudinal study of preschool children. Verification attempts have been directed at several questions.

"Do intraphonemic disruptions - the core behavior of stuttering - involve faulty coarticulation?"

In a study by Stromsta and Fibiger (1980), electromyographic (EMG) activity indicating labial anticipatory coarticulation was detected during (a) core behavior repetitions and fluent utterances

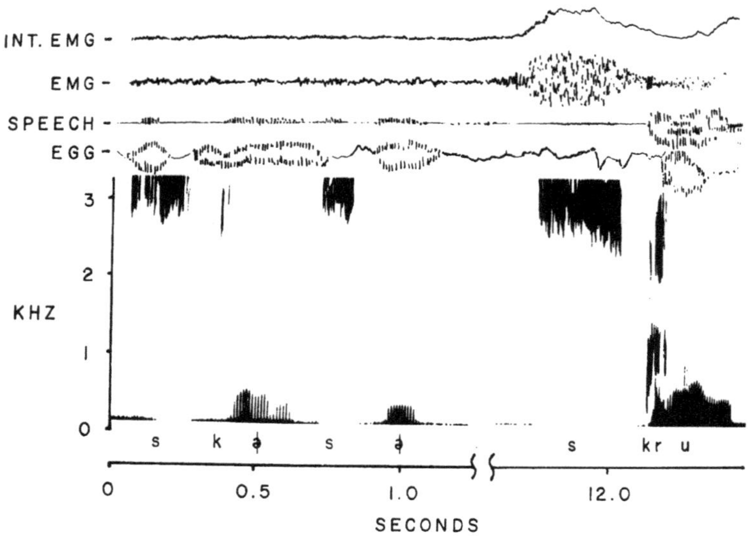

Figure 2. An example of repetitions involving intraphonemic disruptions which led ultimately to the successful utterance of *screw*. Only the two initial repetitions and the final successful utterance of the word are shown from a stuttering sample that lasted about 12 seconds. Note the relative lack of labial-muscle activity associated with the two initial repetitions - indicating lack of anticipatory coarticulation - as compared to the labial activity coincident with the initiation of the successful utterance of the word.

of 68 syllables containing rounded vowels from 10 adult stutterers and (b) the same syllables uttered by 8 adult nonstutterers. The results indicated that the core behavior repetitions of stutterers had significantly less anticipatory labial activity than (a) the successfully uttered syllables preceded by the repetitions and (b) the fluent utterances of the stutterers and nonstutterers. In other words, core behavior repetitions were characterized by faulty labial anticipatory coarticulation. Figure 2 illustrates faulty labial coarticulation associated with intraphonemic disruptions on the word *screw*. To be noted is that the top tracing showing integrated EMG indicates the relative lack of labial activity associated with the initial repetitions as compared to the labial activity coincident with the initiation of the successful utterance.

"Do intraphonemic disruptions involve adequate phonatory onsets?"

From data gathered in the forementioned study, analysis of the first 10 cycles of simultaneously recorded electroglottographic (EGG) signals showed no noteworthy differences in phonatory onsets between (a) core behavior repetitions of stutterers, (b) the following successfully uttered syllables of stutterers, (c) fluent utterances of stutterers, and (d) fluent utterances of nonstutterers. Statistically, a lack of association was shown to exist between the four listed categories and three criteria used to judge adequacy/inadequacy of laryngeal onset activities. Further analysis indicated

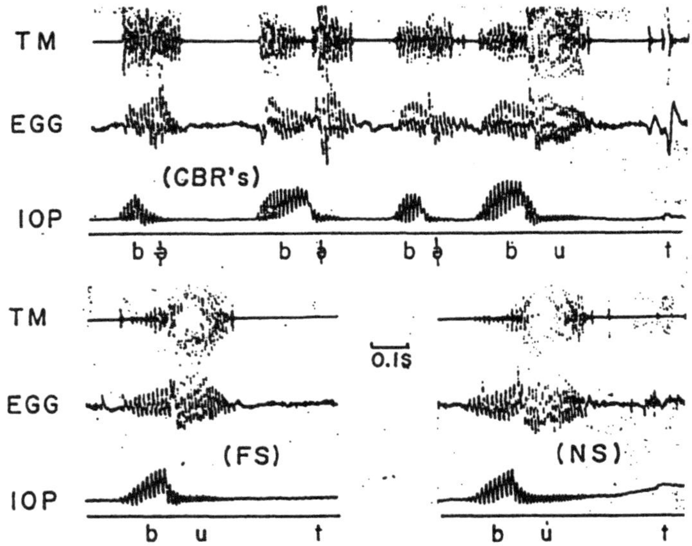

Figure 3. Throat microphone (TM), electroglottographic (EGG), and voice-modulated intraoral pressure (IOP) recordings of three core behavior repetitions (CBR's) and the following successful utterance of *boot*, and fluent utterances by the same adult stutterer (FS) and an adult nonstutterer (NS) on *boot*. Note the prephonatory 'spike' in EGG tracing of the stutterer's fluent utterance. See text for further discussion.

that prolongations of voiced initial sounds produced without undue force by the adult stutterers showed similarly adequate laryngeal onsets. Similar results have been reported by Borden and Baer (1983). Whereas their cycle-by-cycle EGG analysis indicated similar patterns of laryngeal activity onsets for fluent utterances of stutterers and nonstutterers, idiosyncratic strategies were used by stutterers in "breaking stuttering blocks".

Figure 3 displays throat-microphone (as used with children in the longitudinal study), electroglottographic, and voice-modulated intraoral pressure recordings of three core behavior repetitions and the following successful utterance as well as fluent utterances of the same adult stutterer and an adult nonstutterer on the word *boot*. The first and third repetitions, the following successful utterance, the fluent utterance of the stutterer, and that of the nonstutterer display similar phonatory onsets as shown in the EGG and intraoral pressure recordings. The irregularity seen in the EGG onset of the second repetition is not unlike those frequently displayed by nonstutterers. The 'spike' preceding laryngeal activity onset in the EGG tracing of the fluent utterance of the stutterer could relate to presetting of laryngeal muscles prior to phonation as described by Faaborg-Andersen (1964). Such prephonatory spikes were found in 49 of 74 EGG tracings involved in 28 comparisons of core behavior repetitions and fluent utterances, an example of which is shown in Figure 3.

"Does the transition from repetitions to prolongations have a plausible explanation?"

In our opinion, the transition from part-sound part-syllable repetitions to prolongations of initial sounds has no explanation other than those couched in conjecture. One possibility is that prolonging initial sounds avoids what would otherwise be repetitions; that in so doing, subconscious and/or conscious consequences of faulty coarticulation previously experienced in repetitions are circumvented; and that in their early stage of development, the duration of prolongations may serve as a learned/unlearned, perhaps reflexive, stalling maneuver during which the motor speech program awaits commands for appropriate movements to ensuing sounds.

"Is the duration of phonation before its arrest by intentionally sustaining articulatory occlusion in voiced stops and affricatives similar to the duration of phonation before its arrest in the same sounds prolonged by young stutterers during development of reactions to their core behavior repetitions?"

Recall from the discussion of longitudinal observations that as prolonged initial sounds became evident in young stutterers, it was observed that in conjunction with evidence of struggle and force in contrast to other phonemes, the previously prolonged phonation associated with voiced stops and affricatives was subsequently arrested after approximately 300 msec. It was hypothesized that such a time factor could be a function of static articulatory occlusions creating zero transglottal pressure differentials. To test this hypothesis, throat-microphone, intraoral pressure, and EGG activities were recorded simultaneously as three adult nonstutterers attempted to sustain phonation while maintaining complete articulatory occlusions associated with production of /b/, /d/, /g/, and /dʒ/ five times at what each subject took to be excessive respiratory force.

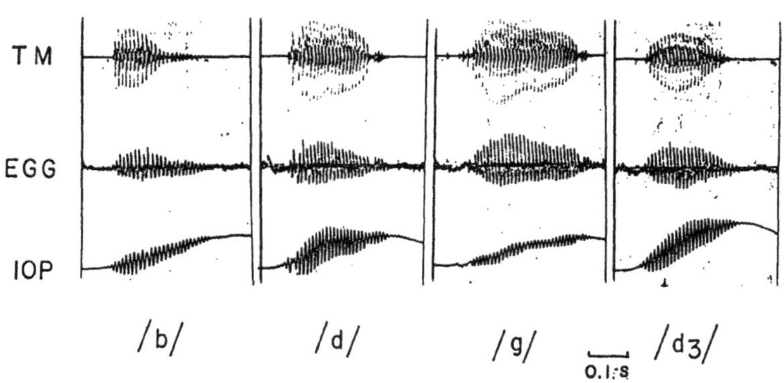

Figure 4. Throat-microphone (TM), intraoral pressure (IOP) and electroglottographic (EGG) recordings from an adult nonstutterer as he attempted to sustain phonation while maintaining complete articulatory occlusions associated with the production of /b/, /d/, /g/, and /dʒ/. The intraoral pressure signals were voice modulated.

Figure 4 shows a composite of tracings from one subject for the four phonemes. The voice-modulated intraoral pressure tracings were used to measure duration of phonation prior to arrest. The mean duration of phonation pooled for the four phonemes was 283 msec with a standard deviation of 22.6. Needless to say, comparing (a) phonatory durations prior to unintentional arrests obtained from stuttering children and (b) intentional phonatory arrests from nonstuttering adults is a tenuous approach. Nonetheless, the reasonable agreement between durations of 300 msec from children and 283 msec from adults lends some degree of credence to the hypothesis that adequately-initiated prolongations of voiced stops in the longitudinally observed stuttering children were arrested by articulatory occlusions associated with the advent of force at a particular stage of development of reactions to their core behavior of stuttering.

Added credence comes from a more direct approach based on 11 unintentionally arrested prolongations of voiced stops recorded from six adult stutterers. The tokens of this sample were judged as spectrographically similar to tokens obtained and so categorized while observing the development of reactions in stuttering children. EGG and voice-modulated intraoral pressure recordings from one of the adult stutterers are shown in Figure 5. An unintentional arrest of prolongation of /b/ followed by a shorter prolongation leading to utterance of the word *boat* is shown in (A); an intentional arrest of phonation on /b/ by maintaining articulatory occlusion is shown in (B); (C) illustrates the stutterer's fluent utterance of *boat*. The similarity between the EGG and pressure envelopes of the initial unintentional and the intentional arrests of adequately-initiated phonation characterizes the results obtained for the other 10 tokens. Also to be noted is their similarity to tracings for intentio-

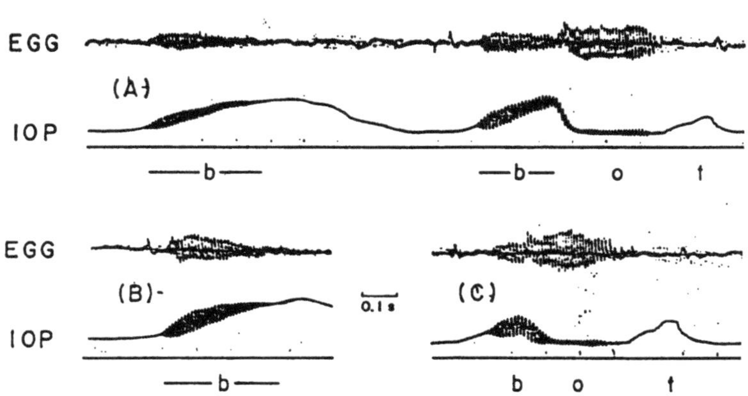

Figure 5. Electroglottographic (EGG) and voice-modulated intraoral pressure (IOP) recordings from an adult stutterer. An unintentional arrest of prolongation of /b/ followed by a shorter prolongation leading to successful utterance of *boat* is shown in (A). An intentional arrest of phonation on /b/ by maintaining articulatory occlusion is shown in (B). The stutterer's fluent utterance of *boat* is shown in (C). Note the prephonatory spikes associated with three of the four phonatory events.

nal arrests of stop plosives by nonstutterers shown in Figure 4. Phonatory onsets of the fluent utterances, as shown in (C), were compared to those of nonstutterers and judged to be without distinguishing differences. Figure 5 also displays prephonatory spikes associated with three of the four phonatory events.

"Are perceptually fluent utterances of stutterers characterized by aberrant laryngeal function?"

Meanwhile, the past two decades have brought forth another cycle of interest in aberrant laryngeal function being a primary correlate of stuttering. Numerous investigators, all of which have used advanced stage stutterers as subjects, have shown that voice reaction and voice onset times are longer in stutterers than nonstutterers. Other investigations have shown that initiation of perceptually fluent utterances of stutterers involve excessive laryngeal tension and failure of normal abductor-adductor reciprocity. Findings of the foregoing nature from advanced stage stutterers have had a significant - we believe questionable - impact on theory, research, and therapy of stuttering. Limiting our discussion to voice reaction time, our contention has been and continues to be that this form of aberrant laryngeal function is not a primary correlate of the core behavior of stuttering but, rather, a consequential reaction to it. In other words, how one views the involvement of laryngeal function in stuttering depends on what one is willing to accept in their definition of the disorder. In an attempt to clarify the issue, a study was undertaken (Stromsta, 1983) to determine if factors such as masking, practice, and experienced therapeutic intervention resulted in different effects on the laryngeal behavior of advanced stage stutterers as a function of their type of disfluencies.

Auditory masking is recognized as a fluency inducing agent in stutterers. However, a personal observation is that masking is considerably less effective in reducing core behavior repetitions than it is in reducing prolongations and tonic blocks. Therefore it could be hypothesized that masking may have different effects on reaction times of stutterers who characteristically exhibit repetitions as compared to those who have adopted alternative behaviors such as prolongations and tonic blocks. For example, if masking has more effect in normalizing reaction times of stutterers who characteristically exhibit prolongations and tonic blocks as compared to those who exhibit repetitions, it could signify, however remotely, that prolongations and tonic blocks are less innate in stutterers than are core behavior repetitions. On the other hand, since faulty initiation of phonation was not observed in the core behavior repetitions of preschool stutterers and because certain adults characteristically stutter in a similar manner, one could hypothesize that their phonatory reaction times would be equal to or even shorter than those of nonstutterers due to an 'everyday speech practice effect' of adequately initiating phonation more times per word than nonstutterers. Other adult stutterers who characteristically exhibit prolongations and tonic blocks might tend to have longer initiation times due to an 'everyday speech practice effect' of inadequately initiating phonation. Only contradictory evidence exists related to practice effects under experimental conditions. Whereas Adams and

Hayden (1976) observed the phonatory reaction times of adult stutterers to approximate those of nonstutterers after nine trials, Lewis et al. (1976) reported that throughout 30 responses, practice had only limited effect on improving voice reaction times in adult stutterers.

The study to be discussed involved 15 male adults ranging in age from 18 to 24 years. All had normal hearing and speech with the exception that 10 had stuttered since early childhood. Phonatory reaction times to a 500 msec light stimulus programmed to fire randomly anywhere between 3 and 6 seconds under no-masking and masking conditions were obtained from (1) five nonstutterers, (2) five core stutterers, those whose disfluencies were composed of at least 70% core behavior repetitions, and (3) five reacting stutterers, those whose disfluencies were at least 70% reactions defined as prolongations and tonic blocks. Whereas all reacting stutterers had experienced from one to two years of therapy emphasizing phonatory/respiratory manipulation, such was not the case for any of the core stutterers.

Subjects were instructed to phonate the schwa vowel as quickly as possible after the onset of the light stimulus. Each subject experienced three conditions presented in random order at one-day intervals, (1) no masking, (2) masking, and (3) nine massed no-masking trials. The masking and no-masking conditions each provided responses to three sets of 11 stimuli with a 30 second interset interval. The massed no-masking trials condition provided nine sets of 11 responses to stimuli with a 30 second interval between sets. All responses were recorded via a throat microphone as each subject monitored the level of their responses at approximately 85dB SPL. Masking was delivered via headphones at 95 dB SPL worn only during the masking condition. Phonatory reaction time was defined as latency between stimulus and response onsets and obtained from a Hewlett-Packard interval timer and printout system.

Group means for the no-masking and masking conditions are shown graphically in Figure 6. Figure 7 illustrates the group means for the nine massed no-masking trials. Under the no-masking condition, the mean reaction time of reacting stutterers was significantly longer (5% level) than those of nonstutterers and core stutterers. Under the masking condition, the mean reaction times of the three groups did not differ significantly. When exposed to nine massed no-masking trials, the mean reaction times of the three groups were not significantly different (5% level) following the fourth trial.

In general, the results indicate that core behavior repetitions should be differentiated from prolongations and tonic blocks for the purpose of formulating new hypotheses in our quest for understanding the basic nature of stuttering. The finding that adults exhibiting the core behavior of stuttering were not statistically different from nonstutterers in all conditions was not entirely unanticipated. In contrast, the finding that the mean reaction times for core behavior stutterers in nearly all conditions were numerically superior to those of nonstutterers was not anticipated. If replicated, such a finding when properly interpreted could provide salient leads for future research concerning the neurophysiological basis of stuttering.

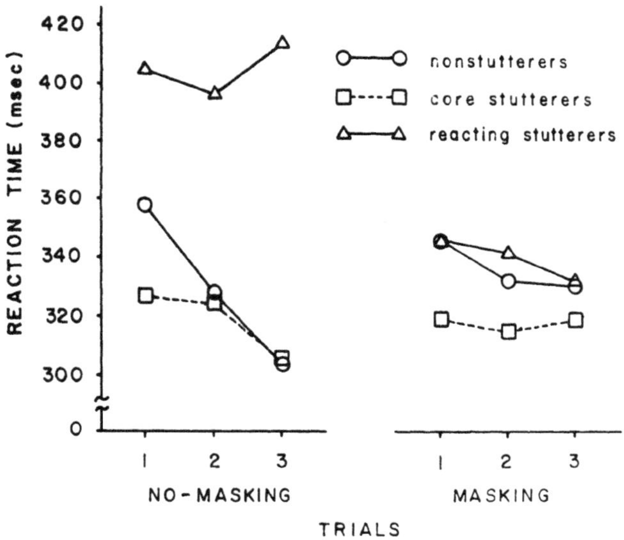

Figure 6. Mean reaction times in msec for the nonstutterers and both groups of stutterers in the no-masking and masking conditions.

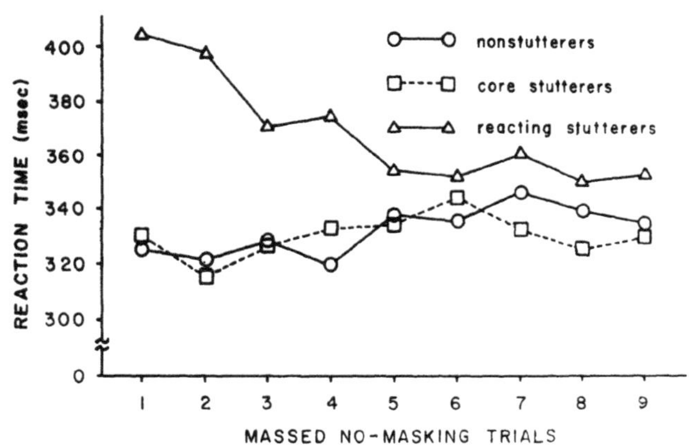

Figure 7. Mean reaction times in msec for the nonstutterers and both groups of stutterers for the nine massed no-masking trials.

DISCUSSION

The foregoing remarks point out that how one views the role of laryngeal activity onset in stuttering depends on what one is willing to accept in their definition of the disorder. Resolution of this issue would seem to be of prime importance. Let us assume for the moment something we believe to be true, that advanced stage stutterers characteristically minimize their innate core behavior repetitions by adopting a host of variable reactions including prolongations and tonic blocks. If this is true, then the continued unqualified use of advanced stage stutterers as research subjects in attempting to describe and define the basic nature of the disorder will continue to 'muddy the waters' of theory, research, and therapy of stuttering. Because of this, at least in our opinion, the literature of stuttering, while being a commendable source of information related to reactions to stuttering, verges on being vacuous concerning the acoustic and the neuromuscular output signals of the core behavior of stuttering.

REFERENCES

Adams, M. & Hayden, P. (1976). The ability of stutterers and normal speakers to initiate and terminate phonation during production of an isolated vowel. *Journal of Speech and Hearing Research, 19,* 290-296.

Borden, G. & Baer, T. (1983). Electroglottographic and acoustic waveforms of voice onset in stutterers. *Journal of the Acoustical Society of America, 74,* S115. Suppl. 1.

Faaborg-Andersen, K. (1964). In D.W. Brewer (Ed.), *Research Potentials in Voice Physiology.* New York: State University Press.

Lewis, J., Ingham, R.J. & Gervens, A. (1979). The effect of stimulus conditions and practice on voice reaction in stutterers and nonstutterers. *Asha, 21,* 693.

Stromsta, C. (1965). A spectrographic study of disfluencies labeled as stuttering by parents. *De Therapia Vocis et Loquellae, I,* 317-320.

Stromsta, C. & Fibiger, S. (1980). *Physiological correlates of the core behavior of stuttering.* Proceedings of XVIIIth IALP Congress, Washington, DC.

Stromsta, C. (1983). *Phonatory reaction time of stutterers as a function of masking and therapeutic intervention.* Proceedings of XIXth IALP Congress, Edinburgh.

Part Five

Acoustic Analysis of Speech Production

Overview

In the fifth part of this book a range of current studies using a broad scope of methods in acoustic analysis of the speech output are presented.

The first topic in this section concerns the use of acoustic methods in the evaluation of the outcome of stuttering therapy and the techniques facilitating the learning process during therapy. Unfortunately, the evaluation of stuttering therapy is very often restricted to the assessment of the disfluency percentage and speech rate. By means of more detailed acoustic analyses of the speech significant information can be added. In Chapter 20 Franken discusses the usefulness of a set of perceptual rating scales for the judgment of various dimensions of speech quality in connection with acoustic measurements. Perceptual and acoustical measurements proved to be sensitive and useful for measuring the effects of stuttering therapy on a number of relevant aspects of speech quality. An attempt to replace perceptual ratings, which are expensive and cumbersome, by acoustic analyses, which can be obtained automatically and efficiently, has only been partially successful. In the case of articulation scales, the perceptual ratings show a significant effect on the outcome of therapy, whereas the acoustic measures do not.

In stuttering therapy gentle voice onset seems to be an important fluency-generating target behavior. However, objective physical descriptions of voice onset characteristics in untreated and treated stutterers have not yet been obtained. In Chapter 21 Webster, Morgan and Cannon introduce a voice onset abruptness ratio which is derived from puls amplitude values during the onset of phonation. In their study they investigated the effect of increased syllable durations on voice onset during therapy, as well as alterations in voice onset charateristics in post-therapy speech. It could be demonstrated that the voice onset became significantly more gentle during the reduced velocity of speech movements. In post therapy utterances, however, despite the faster speech rate, there was a substantially larger improvement in the (learned) voice onset characteristics, compared to those associated with the shift from pre-treatment speech utterances to stretched syllable durations during the therapy.

During the last decennia, several instrumental training tools, based on the acoustic analysis of the speech signal, have been developed in stuttering therapy, to assist the stutterer in learning the concept and motoric patterns of easy voice onset. As described briefly in Chapter 21, Webster has developed an instrument, called the voice monitor, to facilitate gentle voice onset acquisition by clients participating in his Precision Fluency Shaping Program. This device, which is based on the analysis of the steepness of the rising slope of the audio envelope, evaluates voice onsets and demonstrates to the client whether or not a particular voice onset was appropriate for that portion of the tharapy. In Chapter 22 Agnello describes a computer program which helps the stutterer to develop the concept of easy voice onsets and is used in conjunction with the traditional Van Riper therapy. The idealized voice onset patterns of the stimulus words the stutterer has to read are defined by the computer program in advance and plotted on a TV screen. Stutterers attempt to match these idealized patterns and afterwards the computer gives a feedback indicating whether the stutterer achieved the ideal pattern or was too abrupt.

The second main topic in this part of the book concerns various aspects of speech rate as measured by acoustic measurements. In speech motor control the articulatory rate may certainly be considered to be an important variable in relation to disfluency. In Chapter 23 Amster and Starkweather firstly describe some relevant literature on this topic and a number of preliminary investigations on subsegmental duration, stress contact and tempo tracking which were done recently at Temple University. This is followed by a detailed discussion of an investigation on the articulatory rate of the speech of normal children, and an investigation into the relation between children's and parent's speech rate and children's fluency. A significant correlation between the articulatory rate and utterance length could be demonstrated via a clear tendency for the speech rate to be faster in older than in younger children. The rate of parent's speech seems to be an important variable in children's fluency. It could be demonstrated that the slowing down of the parents' rate of speech sometimes improved the children's rate of fluency dramatically. The fact that the relative rate and not the absolute rate may be of influence here is probably of great importance.

From speech physiological research one may conclude that stutterers are charaterized by difficulties in the timing and stabilizing of phonatory and articulatory movements. The Chapters 24, 25 and 26 are devoted to various aspects of variability in phonatory and articulatory rate on supra-segmental and segmental level.

In Chapter 24 Schäferskūpper and Dames describe an experiment in which the overall speech rate and articulatory rate, as expressed in syllable duration time are analyzed. They hypothesize that the timing during speech should be controlled on two levels: a global level - governing the overall speech rate - and a specific level - controlling the relationship between segment, syllable and larger entities of the speech act. Stutterers show longer reading times than nonstutterers but about the same articulation time. The stutterers made more and longer pauses which possibly enabled them to reduce the frequency of stuttering. It is suggested that the number and length of the pauses may be seen as a component of the mechanism controlling the overall speech rate.

In Chapter 25 Janssen and Wieneke show that stutterers as a group are more variable in the duration of voiced and unvoiced segments during normal oral reading. The authors hypothesize that various conditions, such as rhythmic reading and reading under DAF or with masking noise - which have been shown to induce fluent speech in stutterers - facilitate the production of speech and therefore reduce this instability. No significant differences were found under the fluency inducing conditions between groups. In general, the stutterers' mean variability scores did indeed decrease during the fluency enhancing conditions, except in the case of the DAF condition. The question if whether the greater variability may be considered to be a manifestation of general instability in stutterers or whether there are other reasons behind it was pointed out by Wieneke and Janssen in Chapter 26. By means of analysing the segmental variance, it is shown that the increased segmental variability of the stutterers could not be attributed to increased variations of speech rate nor to the presence of specific extremely variable segments in the stuttering group.

In all the previous chapters stuttering was approached from a speech production point of view. The well known effects of delayed auditory feedback suggest that other mechanisms may be involved, i.e. the monitoring of speech output. The next two chapters deal with this issue. In Chapter 27 Harrington presents a model to explain the disrupting influence that delayed auditory feedback has on normal speech. This model is then slightly adapted to a model of stuttering. Both models depend on the relationship between the time that the auditory perception of a syllable is expected and the time at which the production of the syllable is planned. It is suggested that a normally fluent speaker experiences a relative delay under delayed auditory feedback, while in the stuttering model, on the other hand, the expected time of perception of the vowel of a syllable is hypothesized to be early with respect to the time of production. This is considered to be the basis for explaining why delayed auditory feedback can improve stutterers' fluency, as the asynchronies between expected time of perception and the actual time of production are cancelled out.

Chapter 28, by Howell, El-Yaniv and Powell, presents very interesting data from four experiments, which cannot be explained by existing theories on delayed auditory feedback, including Harrington's model. Stuttering most frequently occurs at word onset, i.e. during the short interval in which the delayed auditory feedback is not yet heard. In the first experiment, delayed auditory feedback is compared with other forms of altered feedback without a delay. This feedback consists of a version of the speaker's own voice in which the frequency is shifted downwards by one octave. The latter form of feedback was found to be superior to delayed auditory feedback in enhancing stutterers' fluency. Frequency shifted feedback turned out to be very effective even if it was only presented during the very first 33 msec of speech onset. It also proved to be superior to a buzz masking noise and to forms of feedback that did not covary in pitch with that of the voice.

Detailed acoustic analysis of stutterers' disfluencies and the corresponding fluent tokens may give important clues as to whether supra-laryngeal articulation may be held responsible for stuttering or whether the control of phonation should be considered to be the main difficulty. The following two chapters both present evidence to support the second alternative. Howell, Williams and Vause draw this conclusion after three types of analysis, which are described in Chapter 29. First, a number of disfluent episodes were analysed acoustically and compared with the following fluent release of the intended vowel. There was little difference in the frequencies of the first three formants, but the disfluent vowels were shorter and had a lower amplitude. Subsequent perceptual tests showed that these vowels sounded like a "schwa", owing to their short duration and low amplitude, but were not articulated as such. This suggests that stutterers have problems in laryngeal or pulmonary control. This was corroborated via subsequent studies of phonatory control, by recording volume velocity waveforms at the glottis and simulating the measured properties with an articulatory synthesizer.

In Chapter 30, Harrington, describes the acoustic analysis of 200 monosyllables read by 36 stutterers. The spectograms suggest that the supra-laryngeal tract is shaped similarly at the onset of disfluencies as at the onset of fluent utterances. Electropalatographic analyses are offered to support this conclusion. The results of the experimental analysis also show that the 'vowel onglide' - the initial formant transitions - can be realized as part of the disfluency, but not the acoustic vowel 'target'. Instances of abnormal formant transitions are discussed. Like Howell et al. in the previous chapter, Harrington concludes that Van Ripers' articulatory theory on stuttering is not supported by the results of the experiments.

After the long series of preceding chapters on speech motor dynamics, the final chapter of the book, Chapter 31 by Bergmann, has special implications: the author tries to link speech motor dynamics with emotional processes. It appears that a connection can be made on the prosodic level. In two experiments the effect of accent structure and the importance of stressed syllables on the frequency of stuttering were demonstrated. Accent and stress clearly serve communication purposes. Bergmann describes some observations and the results of an experiment emphasizing the importance of the social and communicational aspects of a situation underlying stuttering. The final part of the chapter is concerned with the relation between stuttering, prosody and affect control. Stressed syllables possibly evoke stuttering because they are overcontrolled and, therefore, their quick and precise timing may be disturbed. Bergmann emphasizes that these ideas are only speculations, and that, we consider, is the best way to end this book.

Chapter **20**

Perceptual and Acoustic Evaluation of Stuttering Therapy

Marie Christine Franken

INTRODUCTION

Formal evaluations of the results of speech therapies are not carried out very often. Stuttering therapies form no exception to this rule. In general, such evaluations can have two goals, viz. to assess the results of a therapy for a given (group of) subject(s) after a certain amount of treatment time, or the identification of weaknesses in the therapy program. The lack of formal evaluations of speech therapies is at least in part due to the fact that few treatment techniques have been sufficiently refined so that a standardized form of treatment can be evaluated and a systematic feedback from evaluation to therapy becomes possible. Yet, there is a real and increasing need for formalized evaluations of speech therapies, if only to reduce the economic and emotional costs of ineffective therapies.

Also, those who intend to assess the effects of a therapy are severely hampered by the lack of a comprehensive and manageable measurement instrument. If such an instrument would be available, objective evaluation of its outcome would be much easier. However, the floating character of most therapies makes it very difficult to develop measurement instruments, because it is not really clear what must be measured. Neither is it clear what will be measured (e.g. the effect of the therapy as it is, or as it was, or chance effects of the interaction between therapist and client). In this study an attempt is made to break this circle. We will propose an instrument that is based on fairly general ideas with respect to the aims of therapies and the characteristic features of speech.

The ultimate aim of stuttering therapy should be: "restore or increase the stutterers' ability to speak normally in any situation" (Speech Foundation of America, 1960). In the few instances that an evaluation of stuttering therapies has been attempted, the measurements of speech performance have been mostly restricted to an assessment of the percentage of words or syllables stuttered and the syllable or articulation rate. However, programs for the treatment of stuttering frequently effect changes in the overall speech pattern, resulting in a situation where 'successfully' treated stutterers are relatively fluent, but their speech sounds slow, paced or monotonous and can be discriminated from the speech of nonstutterers (Martin, Haroldson & Triden, 1984). For this reason, the minimum evaluation data collected (fluency and rate) should be supplemented by assessment of a number of additional aspects of speech quality (Ingham, 1984).

When the evaluation is carried out with the intention to improve therapy practice (Ingham, 1984), then it will be obvious that overall descriptions of the speech quality will not suffice, but that elaborate descriptions of the speech quality before and after therapy are necessary.

It is the aim of this chapter to present practical instruments for a comprehensive evaluation of speech therapies. The first instrument to be described is a perceptual rating scale; the second is a set of global acoustic measurements. Both instruments have been tested on a large number of speech fragments of stutterers before and after therapy. Both instruments have proved to be capable of showing detailed and interesting effects of a stuttering therapy on the speech of the clients.

SPEECH MATERIAL

The work to be described here is based on speech samples from 21 clients, 17 adult males, 3 females and 1 male adolescent. Each client was recorded on three occasions, namely on the first day of the therapy, on the last day of the therapy and about six months after the end of the therapy. All recordings were made in the clinic, while the clients knew they were being recorded. The post-treatment measurements were always made by a clinician that had not participated in the treatment of the clients.

Use was made of spontaneous speech, produced while the clients gave their comments on the contents of a newspaper article. The first 30 seconds of the recordings were never used. From the remaining part of the recordings, 45 seconds of speech of the client was spliced on a master tape. This tape was then used both for the acoustic measurements and for the perceptual rating experiment. For the latter experiment the order of the speech samples was randomized, with the restriction that two samples of one speaker should be separated by a minimum number of samples of other speakers.

All clients went through a fluency shaping therapy, designed in accordance with the principles of the Precision Fluency Shaping Program of R.L. Webster (Peters and Kooiman, 1982; Webster, 1974, 1978). Fifteen clients were treated in the department of Speech Pathology of Nijmegen University; the remaining six were treated at the Logopedic Centre Hoensbroek. At both places the therapy was given by therapists who were especially trained for the job.

PERCEPTUAL RATINGS

The Raters and the Rating Instrument

The 63 experimental stimuli (21 speakers x 3 measurements) were rated by two groups of judges. Both groups consisted of first year students of logopedics, who may be considered as essentially naive listeners at the time of the experiment. One group consisted of 29 members, the other one of 17. Each group got the stimuli in a different order of presentation. This was done to control for possible speaker-dependent sequence effects upon listener ratings.

Ratings were given on 15 bipolar scales which are shown in Table 1. 14 Of these scales made up an instrument that was developed by Fagel, Van Herpt and Boves (1983) for judging the relevant aspects of normal speech. This instrument is supposed to represent seven dimensions of the perceptual space in which global perceptual ratings of speech can be described. These seven dimensions are interpreted by Fagel et al. as 'Melodiousness', 'Articulation Quality', 'Voice Quality', 'Pitch Level', 'Speaking Rate', 'Evaluation' and 'Potency'. To this instrument the scale 'natural - unnatural' was added. Because speech naturalness is an important

Table 1. The rating instrument consisting of 15 bipolar scales. Reliability-coefficients Ru for the mean of each the 15 rating scales of 46 raters for 63 speech samples.

Rating Scale	Ru
unpleasant - pleasant	.98
slow - quick	.99
low pitch - high pitch	.96
soft - loud	.93
husky - not husky	.72
broad - cultured	.97
expressionless - expressive	.97
monotonous - melodious	.97
slovenly - polished	.95
dull - clear	.95
weak - powerful	.95
shrill - deep	.95
dragging - brisk	.98
ugly - beautiful	.97
unnatural - natural	.97

consideration in recent treatment programs, Martin et al. (1984) and Ingham, Gow and Costello (1985) and Ingham and Onslow (1985a) have been using a scale of speech naturalness to study this aspect of the speech of stutterers. In the present study, the scale of speech naturalness was used to see how it behaves in a relatively elaborate rating instrument with respect to aspects of speech quality. It is of interest to know whether naturalness forms part of one of the seven factors just mentioned, or whether it constitutes an additional factor.

Results

Reliability. The listeners' ratings were first analyzed for their reliability. The total variance in the ratings is the sum of the variance due to the differences between the rated objects and the variance due to error of measurement. For determining the interrater-reliability, use was made of the Ru-coefficient, defined by Asendorpf and Wallbott (1979) (cf. Winer, 1971) as:

$$Ru = 1 - \frac{MSwithin\ items}{MSbetween\ items}$$

This form of the reliability-coefficient is based on the assumption that the variance due to the differences between the mean ratings given by the listeners is part of the error of measurement and does not represent a systematic source of variation, i.e., the listeners are not considered as a separate factor in an analysis of variance design. Table 1 displays the Ru-coefficients for each of the 15 rating scales that were used in this study. From the Table it can be seen that except for the scale 'husky - not husky' all scales proved to be highly reliable. Because of its wanting reliability the scale 'husky - not husky' was not used in the subsequent analysis of the data.

Factor Structure. Factor analysis (principal factoring with iteration, retaining only the factors with an eigenvalue > 1) of the scores of the remaining 14 scales resulted in a 5-factor solution, shown in Table 2.

The first factor has high loadings of the scales 'slow - quick', 'dragging - brisk', 'unnatural - natural', 'unpleasant - pleasant' and 'ugly - beautiful'. Thus it is clearly a combination of perceived speech rate and general evaluation. The second factor is an articulation quality factor contaminated with general evaluation, with high loadings of the scales 'slovenly - polished', 'broad - cultured' and also of the scales 'ugly - beautiful' and 'pleasant - unpleasant'. The third factor, with high loadings of the scales 'monotonous - melodious' and 'expressive - expressionless' can be identified as a voice dynamics factor. The fourth factor relates to voice pitch and static voice quality with high loadings of the scales 'low pitch - high pitch', 'deep - shrill' and 'dull - clear'. The last factor, with high loadings of the scales 'weak - powerful' and 'soft - loud' can be interpreted as the potency factor that always comes out of experiments employing the semantic differential (Osgood, Suci and Tannenbaum, 1957).

Table 2. Varimax rotated factors resulting from judgements of 46 listeners of 63 speech samples (spontaneous speech) from 21 clients on 14 bipolar scales.

Factor number	1	2	3	4	5
slow - quick	.77	.09	.18	.05	.27
dragging - brisk	.73	.15	.24	.05	.32
unnatural - natural	.54	.33	.33	-.05	.13
unpleasant - pleasant	.53	.47	.26	.06	.08
ugly - beautiful	.53	.54	.36	.04	.11
slovenly - polished	.21	.68	.20	.08	.15
broad - cultured	.07	.53	.06	-.10	.18
monotonous - melodious	.38	.22	.79	.15	.20
expressionless - expressive	.39	.28	.71	.14	.21
shrill - deep	.07	.13	.01	-.70	.05
low pitch - high pitch	.10	.01	.08	.68	.04
dull - clear	.07	.22	.16	.60	.34
weak - powerful	.28	.24	.20	.08	.70
soft - loud	.19	.14	.08	.06	.60

Proportion of variance explained 74.7%

Factor 1	64.2%
Factor 2	15.9%
Factor 3	7.7%
Factor 4	7.4%
Factor 5	4.8%
	100.0%

The factor solution in Table 2 represents much the same structure as found by Fagel et al. in that it produces factors with quite similar labels. With respect to the importance of the factors in terms of the proportion of variance accounted for, there are some dramatic differences. Fagel et al. found a very pure tempo factor, that accounted for not more than 3.8% of the variance. In the present solution tempo is contaminated with evaluation, and this factor accounts for more than 64% of the variance. This result confirms the well-known idea that speech rate is responsible for most apparent perceptual differences between speech samples obtained from a number of stutterers before and after therapy. In the study of Fagel et al. by far the largest amount of variance (viz. 72.3%) was explained by the voice dynamics factor, which only ranks third in the present solution. Apparantly, voice dynamics play a more important role in distinguishing between speech samples obtained from speakers who do not have any speech problems; if the speech material under judgement contains pathological speech, however, its role is likely to be taken over by the aspect that is most characteristic of the pathological speech. In both studies the articulation quality factor ranks second and the pitch/static voice quality factor ranks fourth, with comparable proportions of explained variance.

From Table 2 it can also be seen that the naturalness scale has its highest loadings on de first factor. Note, however, that it has nonnegligible loadings on the articulation quality and the voice dynamics factor too. The naturalness scale appears to behave in much the same way as the general evaluation scales. A similar behavior of these scales was already observed by Osgood et al., who found that the general evaluation factor must be considered as a 'cover factor', summarizing a number of distinguishable aspects of evaluation, like moral and esthetic evaluation; the more specific factors will appear as separate factors under appropriate conditions, i.e., with an appropriate combination of scales and stimuli. High loadings of the evaluation scales on a number of voice and articulation factors were also found by Fagel et al. and Boves (1984), who explain the finding by pointing out that the dissociation of the different aspects of general evaluation and their spread over the more specific speech related factors is due to the presence of a large number of scales in the rating instrument that refer explicitly to specific aspects of speech quality. Thus it seems that speech naturalness is a cover factor too, comprising a number of distinguishable aspects of speech, like rate, articulation quality, and voice dynamics. When used on itself the naturalness scale will probably yield valid and reliable ratings. However, the results may not be very instructive, because they will tend to be very global: there will be no direct way to determine whether perceived unnaturalness of a speech sample is due to either the rate being too high or too low, or the articulation quality being bad, or the dynamics being insufficient or exaggerated. The global information obtained by the naturalness scale may suffice if one has only to determine whether or not a specific client has met the therapy goal, if it is described in terms of overall naturalness. It may, however, not suffice as a source of feedback to the (researcher/)clinician about strategies to modify treatment or to investigate the nature of speech after the often observed relapse.

A rating instrument comprising a number of well-chosen scales covering the relevant dimensions of the perceptual space, on the other hand, may provide information that is sufficiently detailed to identify the weaknesses of a therapy program or the aspects where a specific client needs additional treatment, perhaps by means of a supplementary program.

Treatment Effects. Factor scores for each of the five factors were computed for the 63 stimuli and subjected to analyses of variance. The design was a single factor experiment with repeated measurements on the same subjects in three conditions (before, at the end of therapy and six months after completing therapy). Post-Hoc-Contrasts were computed according to the Student-Newman-Keuls procedure. The aim of these analyses was to obtain insight in the intended effects of the therapy as well as its possible side effects. The results are summarized in Table 3.

It can be seen that the average factor scores on the first (tempo/evaluation) factor drop slightly, but not significantly, in the condition just after therapy. Six months after therapy, however, the average factor scores are well above the levels in the first two conditions. Apparently, the fluency shaping program given to the clients attains its most spectacular measurable results only well after its ending. The fact that at the end of treatment, the average scores on the tempo/evaluation/naturalness factor are even slightly lower than before therapy suggests that, at least with a fluency shaping program, global naturalness ratings may not be a useful indicator of the need for continuation of the treatment.

Table 3. Results of analysis of variance on the factor scores of 21 clients, recorded on the first day of the therapy (1), on the last day of the therapy (2), and six months after the end of the therapy (3). The 5 factors correspond with the factor solution of Table 2.

Factor Number	Overall Signif.	Post Hoc Contrast 1-2	1-3	2-3	Condition Means 1	2	3
1	<0.01	@			-.19	-.28	.19
2	<0.05			@	-.23	0	0
3	<0.001		@		.14	-.31	.01
4	<0.001			@	.31	-.11	-.01
5	<0.05	@		@	.06	-.25	-.09

@ not significant at the 5% level

On the articulation quality and on the pitch level factor (factor numbers two and four, respectively) the condition before therapy differs significantly from the remaining two conditions, which do not differ among themselves. Perhaps the effect on the articulation factor can be interpreted as a side-effect of the target behavior of slow syllable speech (which is one of the major speech target behaviors in the Precision Fluency Shaping Program, Webster (1974)), in which the importance of reaching stable target articulation positions for all vowels is stressed. Also, the decreased frequency of stuttering after therapy, which leads to the impression of improved intelligibility, may have caused the impression of an improved articulation quality. The lower scores on the voice pitch/static voice quality factor just after therapy are supposed to be due to a reduced overall tension of the speech muscles, especially the laryngeal muscles, brought about by the therapy as a side-effect of the target behaviors of gentle voice onset and full breath and perhaps also as the effect of reduced anxiety.

The average scores on the voice dynamics and the potency factor (numbers three and five) show a V-type structure. Just after therapy the scores are significantly below the level before therapy, whereas in the condition six months after therapy the average scores have returned to a level that is only slightly below the level before therapy.

ACOUSTIC MEASUREMENTS

Even if perceptual ratings prove to be reliable and valid to yield useful information on the outcome of treatment for stuttering therapy, they remain extremely laborious. Therefore, we have attempted to find acoustic measures that can be obtained automatically and that might be able to replace the perceptual ratings. Table 4 gives an overview of the measures that were employed.

The numbers six to nine describe the global shape of the long-term average critical band spectrum of the voiced parts of the speech (Hammarberg et al., 1980). 'Neutral articulation setting' is

Table 4. The acoustic measurement instrument consisting of 13 global acoustic measures.

1. Utterance rate
2. Fo mean
3. Fo variation
4. Pitch perturbation
5. Proportion voiced
6. Level in first formant region
7. Spectral slope below F1
8. Spectral slope towards 1.5 kHz
9. Spectral slope towards 5 kHz
10. 'Neutral articulation setting'
11. Standard deviation of F1
12. Average intensity
13. Intensity variation

Table 5. Results of analyses of variance on the acoustic measurements of the speech samples of 21 clients, recorded on the first day of the therapy, on the last day of the therapy and six months after the end of the therapy.

Measure	Overall Signif.	Post Hoc Contrast 1-2	1-3	2-4	Condition Means 1	2	3	
1. Rate	.004	ns	.003	.001	2.11	1.95	2.68	s–s
2. Fo mean	.02	.025	.016	ns	126.9	120.0	121.5	Hz
3. Var(Fo)	.005	.008	.014	ns	20.2	13.9	16.7	Hz
4. Perturb.	.01	.007	ns	ns	.38	.50	.44	
5. % Voiced	.00	.000	.003	.001	43.2	67.4	58.0	%
13. Int. Var.	.00	.000	.027	.008	9.57	6.81	8.14	dB

defined as the Euclidian distance of the average frequencies of the first four formants of a speaker to the hypothetical neutral point of 500, 1500, 2500 and 3500 Hz in a four dimensional space (cf. Boves, 1984, where most of the other measures are also explained). Analyses of variance were carried out on the measurement results in order to find out if there are significant differences between the three conditions. Table 5 displays the results. Overall significance was found only for utterance rate, pitch perturbation, Fo mean, Fo standard deviation, proportion of voiced segments and intensity variation.

Therapy Effects

After therapy, utterance rate in terms of syllables per second speech production time (excluding pauses) has not changed as compared to the situation before therapy. Six months after therapy the utterance rate has increased considerably. This is completely in line with the results of the perceptual ratings. The proportion of voiced segments increases due to the therapy and although it is lowered somewhat six months later, it remains well above the level before therapy. This effect can be interpreted as a consequence of the target behaviors of stretched syllable speech and gentle voice onset. Pitch perturbation seems to increase due to the therapy, a result that cannot be explained. Average Fo is lowered as a result of the therapy and it remains at the lowered level six months later. The variation of Fo drops to a very low level just after therapy; six months later it has recovered somewhat but it has by no means returned to the level it had before therapy. A similar remark applies to the variation of the intensity. These last three effects correspond with the results of the perceptual ratings on the factors pitch level (#4), voice dynamics (#3), and potency (#5).

It is interesting to note that none of the spectral measures is significant. Apparently in its present form the acoustic instrument is not capable to register the effects of the therapy neither with respect to the mode of phonation nor of articulation.

CONCLUSIONS

From our work a number of preliminary conclusions can be drawn:

1. Both the perceptual and the acoustic measurements have proved to be sufficiently sensitive to measure effects of a stuttering therapy on a number of relevant aspects of speech quality. The comprehensiveness of the instrument has brought to light the fact that the stuttering therapy evaluated here succeeds in reducing the non-fluency of the speech of the clients without leading to a speech quality that cannot be discriminated from that of nonstutterers. This effect is very clear just after therapy, but it diminishes in the follow-up assessment.
2. The attempt to replace the perceptual ratings by acoustic measurements has been only partially successful. Especially in the case of the articulation scales the perceptual ratings show a significant effect of the therapy whereas the acoustic measures do not.

POSTSCRIPT

Although the instruments presented here have proved to be sensitive and useful (the perceptual instrument more so than the acoustic), still the work has led to the conclusion that it would be nice if even more detailed and specific information on the speech of the clients could be obtained, hopefully in an efficient and cost-effective way. This additional information should minimally include a description of laryngeal tenseness and voice onset. More detailed information is especially useful if it comes to improving a therapy, guided by objective knowledge about the success of specific parts of the treatment. As far as the perceptual ratings are concerned, we expect that the additional, more specific scales, can no longer be scored by naive listeners.

If a comprehensive measurement is to become really efficient so that it can be applied routinely, optimal use has to be made of automatic, acoustic procedures. It is clear, however, that much work remains to be done, before perceptual ratings can be replaced by acoustic measurements.

REFERENCES

Asendorpf, J. & Wallbott, H.G. (1979). Masse der Beobachterubereinstimmung: ein systematischer Vergleich. *Zeitschrift fur Sozialpsychologie, 10,* 243-252.

Boves, L. (1984). *The phonetic basis of perceptual ratings of running speech.* Dordrecht-Holland/Cinnaminson-U.S.A.: Foris Publications.

Fagel, W., Van Herpt, L. & Boves, L. (1983). Analysis of the perceptual qualities of Dutch speakers' voice and pronunciation. *Speech Communication, 2,* 315-326.

Hammarberg, B., Fritzell, B., Gauffin, J., Sundberg, J. & Wedin, L. (1980). Perceptual and acoustic correlates of abnormal voice quality. *Acta Otolaryng., 90,* 441-452.

Ingham, R.J. (1984). *Stuttering and behavior therapy.* San Diego, California: College-Hill Press.

Ingham, R.J., Gow, W. & Costello, J.M. (1985a). Stuttering and speech naturalness: some additional data. *Journal of Speech and Hearing Disorders, 50,* 217-219.

Ingham, R.J. & Onslow, M. (1985a). Measurement and modification of speech naturalness during stuttering therapy. *Journal of Speech and Hearing Disorders, 50,* 261-281.

Martin, R.R., Haroldson, K.H. & Triden, K.A. (1984). Stuttering and speech naturalness. *Journal of Speech and Hearing Disorders, 49,* 53-58.

Osgood, C.E., Suci, G.J. & Tannenbaum, P.H. (1957). *The measurement of meaning.* Urbana: University of Illinois Press.

Peters, H.F.M. & Kooiman, P.G. (1982). *Systematische spraakreconstructie voor stotteraars.* Nijmegen: Associatie systematische spraakreconstructie voor stotteraars.

Speech Foundation of America (1960). *On stuttering and its treatment.* Publication No. 1, Memphis.

Webster, R.L. (1974). *The Precision Fluency Shaping Program: speech reconstruction for stutterers.* Roanoke, Virginia: Communications Development Corporation, Ltd.

Webster, R.L. (1978). *Precision Fluency Shaping Program: clinician's program guide.* Roanoke, Virginia: Communications Development Corporation, Ltd.

Winer, B.J. (1971). *Statistical principles in experimental design.* New York: McGraw-Hill.

Chapter 21

Voice Onset Abruptness in Stutterers Before and After Therapy

Ronald L. Webster, Bryant T. Morgan and Maurice W. Cannon

In most research and clinical work on stuttering, recognition of stuttered speech is accomplished directly by an observer or observers. The observer is the instrument for identifying and quantifying characteristics of stuttered speech. Specific interests and perceptual skills of investigators determine the level of resolution attained in observation. Typically, resolution has ranged from global ratings of stuttering severity (Johnson, Darley and Spriestersbach, 1963), to frequency counts of a few particular types of disfluency (Williams, Darley and Spriestersbach, 1978) to more "molecular" levels in which numerous disfluency types are elaborated (L.M. Webster and Brutten, 1972). In spite of the diversity of events examined by different investigators, it seems clear that the focal features of stuttered speech involve aberrant properties of speech muscle activity, many of which are simply not readily available for direct, unaided human observation.

In the investigation of stuttering, as in other areas of science, descriptions of events improve and discoveries multiply as tools are developed that extend the resolution of observation and permit better quantification of what is being observed. Improved descriptions of aberrant motor activities during stuttered speech are now appearing.

Laryngeal activity during stuttering has been observed recently via several methods. Conture, McCall and Brewer (1977) used the fiberoptic endoscope to visualize and record behaviors of the larynx during stuttered speech. These investigators reported that at times during speech the larynx was inappropriately and unpredictably open and that at other times it was inappropriately closed. It was indicated that different types of disfluency were associated with different forms of laryngeal activity. Part-word repetitions were generally associated with abductory laryngeal activity during the time course of the perceived disfluencies while sound prolongations were generally associated with adductory laryngeal activity.

EMG measurements of intrinsic muscle activity were made with hooked wire electrodes during stuttered and fluent speech by Freeman (1977), Freeman and Ushijima (1978), and Shapiro (1980). The general findings were that stuttered speech was associated with higher levels of muscle activity than fluent speech, that coordination between agonist-antagonist muscles was reduced, and that sudden reductions in muscle activity occurred with the release of a stuttered word.

Articulatory responses during stuttered speech were examined with high speed cinefluorography by Zimmermann (1980). Stutterers showed frequent repositioning of articulators preceeding both fluent and disfluent utterances. Fewer synchronous relationships were found among articulators of stutterers in either fluent or disfluent utterances than for fluent utterances of a normal speaker. Relationships among articulators for perceptually fluent and disfluent utterances of stutterers were different from those found in fluent responses of a normal speaker.

While it might reasonably be expected that the disfluent speech of stutterers would be differentiated from the fluent speech of normal speakers along a number of physical continua (Van Riper, 1982), it is somewhat less obvious that the perceptually fluent utterances of stutterers would be physically differentiated from fluent utterances of normal speakers. However, a number of observations suggest that such differences exist.

Adams (1984) summarized a number of studies that indicated longer voice onset times occurred for fluent utterances of stutterers than for those of normal speakers. Freeman (1977) and Shapiro (1980) noted that perceptually fluent utterances of stutterers were often accompanied by disruptions in the usual coordination of laryngeal muscles. Conture (1984) suggested that electroglottographic wave forms might be different for fluent utterances of stuttering children when compared with those of fluent utterances from normal speaking children. Preliminary evidence was that the glottis was closed for approximately 70% of its cycle in the stutterer and only about 50% of its cycle in a matched comparison subject. Peters and Boves (1984) reported that subglottal air pressure build-up in fluent utterances of stutterers was often different from that observed in fluent utterances of normal speakers. In our laboratory, Bindewald (1978) found two conditions that generated fluent speech in stutterers were differentiated when frequency of voiced instances under 80 milliseconds in duration were examined. During white noise masking prior to entering therapy, the percent of voiced instances under 80 milliseconds in duration decreased compared with pre-entry scores. Posttherapy it was found that the frequency of voiced instances under 80 milliseconds increased and approximated those seen in the speech of normally fluent speakers. The interesting finding was that two different fluency generating conditions were differentiated in the vocal behavior of the stutterers.

The relatively subtle differences observed between fluent speech of stutterers and fluent speech of normals in basic research is quite meaningful. Patterns of lawfulness are starting to emerge. Further developments are likely to occur that will extend knowledge of speech motor behaviors in both stutterers and fluent speakers. It is also expected that improved observational resolution will be extended to the clinical arena.

My colleagues (in particular, Mauri Cannon and Bryant Morgan) and I at the Hollins Communications Research Institute have been concerned with how to assess, objectively and reliably, the extent to which certain fluency generating target behaviors are acquired by participants in our Precision Fluency Shaping Program (R.L. Webster, 1974). This treatment for stuttering is a tightly structured, systematic speech motor training program that deals with the reconstruction of behavior details involving respiration, voicing and articulation. In Table 1 an overview of the Precision Fluency Shaping Program is presented. Sequences of fluency generating speech targets are taught to clients, transferred to

Table 1. Overview of the Precision Fluency Shaping Program

PRECISION FLUENCY SHAPING PROGRAM
PART I ESTABLISHMENT OF BASIC TARGETS
Syllable durations (2 seconds) - Parallel clinic transfer Stabilizations of vocal tract shapes - Parallel clinic transfer Diaphragmatic Breathing - Parallel clinic transfer Gentle Voice Onset - vowels - Parallel clinic transfer Coordination of gentle voice onset - Parallel clinic transfer with articulatory activities for consonants
PART II CONSOLIDATION OF TARGETS
Syllable duration (1 second) - Parallel clinic transfer Targets used in combinations - Parallel clinic transfer Increased speech task complexity - Parallel clinic transfer (one-syllable, two-syllable, three-syllable words) Syllable duration (one-half second) - Parallel clinic transfer
PART III EXTRACLINIC TRANSFER OF TARGETS
Clinic Practice on short, self-generated sentences Syllable durations (one-fourth second) Telephone Transfer (one-message, two-message, three message calls) Shopping Centers (one-message, two-message, three message exchanges) Home activities program

extraclinic environments, and in most cases, are retained following completion of the program. Approximately 2,200 stutterers have participated in therapy at the Hollins Communications Research Institute.

Based on our clinical evaluation, one target behavior in particular, the gentle voice onset, has been observed to be of major importance in the establishment, transfer and continuing self-maintenance of fluent speech in stutterers. The Gentle Voice Onset Target is taught in therapy at three progressively reduced levels of exaggeration. These levels of exaggeration roughly parallel the three weeks of treatment. An instrument, the Voice Monitor, has been developed to facilitate gentle voice onset acquisition by clients participating in therapy. The device evaluates voice onsets, and signals to the client whether or not a particular voice onset or sequence of voice onsets was appropriate for that portion of therapy. In spite of the use of the Voice Monitor as a training tool in therapy, we still face a question about the extent to which clients possess control of the gentle voice onset following completion of treatment.

In the study described here, standard speech samples of one-syllable words initiated with vowels were taken at seven different times: 1) pretherapy; 2) at the point where stretched syllable speech was transferred to the clinic environment; 3) at the point where diaphragmatic breathing was transferred to conversations in the clinic; 4) at the point where the gentle voice onset was transferred to conversations in the clinic; 5) after the establishment of one-second syllable durations in clinic speech; 6) following the establishment of one-half-second syllable durations in clinic speech; and 7) posttherapy. To date, voice onset indexes have been derived for the pretherapy, two-second syllable duration, and posttherapy samples.

The questions with which we were concerned in this study were essentially as follows:

1. Do voice onset characteristics change as a function of dramatically increased syllable durations?
2. Do voice onset characteristics change with the establishment of correct, diaphragmatically controlled breathing?
3. Do voice onset characteristics change as a function of training in the establishment of the gentle voice onset?
4. Are voice onset characteristics changed with the reduction of syllable durations to one-second and again to one-half second?
5. Are altered voice onset characteristics evident in posttherapy speech?

Data are reported here that bear on questions number 1 and 5. That is, do voice onset characteristics change when syllable durations are dramatically increased, and are voice onset characteristics altered when posttherapy speech samples are examined?

METHOD

Participants

The participants in this research were ten male stutterers who were enrolled in the Precision Fluency Shaping Program: Speech Reconstruction for Stutterers (PFSP) at the Hollins Communications Research Institute. The participants ranged in age from 19 to 42 years, with a mean age of 33.7 years. Prior to the commencement of the therapy program this group of stutterers had a mean reading disfluency rate of 23.06%, with individual disfluency rates distributed between 4% and 74%. Post therapy disfluency rates ranged from 0% to 1.6% with a mean of .4%.

Apparatus

A Nakamichi 550 stereo cassette recorder was used to record the participants' one-syllable utterances. A Danavox 4145-57 sub minor earphone was altered to serve as a throat microphone. During recording, the throat microphone was situated at the central, front region of the neck near the base of the cricoid cartilage, and held in place by an elastic band.

Words printed 1.25 in. in height on 3 x 5 in. index cards were used to prompt the stutterers' utterances. All words consisted of one syllable with a vowel-consonant format. The words were specifically selected to represent a variety of combinations of the degree of constriction and the place of articulation for the initial vowel sound (Dew and Jensen, 1977).

Speech signals were digitized and stored in a Data Translation 2801 analog-to-digital converter in an IBM XT personal computer equipped with 512 kilobytes of random access memory and an Intel 8087 numeric co-processor. Analysis of the digitized signals was accomplished by means of an Interactive Laboratory System - Module 1 software package operating on the IBM XT Computer.

Procedure

Samples of the stutterers' speech were recorded prior to therapy, at specified points during therapy, and at the conclusion of their participation in therapy. At the time of each recording, the ten one-syllable words were randomly ordered by shuffling and were individually presented to the participant. Participants were instructed to view the word and then repeat it after it had been removed from view. The intertrial interval was approximately 20 seconds. If fewer than six fluent speech tokens were produced by a participant after the ten cards had been presented, the cards were re-shuffled and the presentation sequence was repeated. This process was continued until at least ten fluent utterances for each participant had been recorded.

An analysis was conducted of the first six usable utterances produced by each participant at each period of recording. A recorded utterance was considered to be usable if it had been judged fluent, if the speech signal was free of distortion or extraneous noise and if the associated peak recording level was within the range of -10 dB to +3 dB.

The speech signal was sampled at a rate of 5,000 Hz, digitized and subsequently stored on the computer hard disk. The ILS software was then used to determine the duration of each utterance and the length of the three intervals of time separating the first four pulses of the fundamental frequency of the speech signal. In addition, amplitude values were acquired for the three initial fundamental frequency pulses as well as the eighth, ninth, and tenth pulses.

The first pulse was defined to be that initial pulse that exceeded a threshold value of .1 volts, was differentiated from background noise (e.g., tape "hiss"), and generally corresponded in shape to the subsequently developed wave pattern. The pulse amplitude values (AV) were substituted in the following formula to establish an onset index value for each utterance:

$$\text{ONSET INDEX} = \frac{[AV(8)+AV(9)+AV(10)]-[AV(1)+AV(2)+AV(3)]}{[AV(1)+AV(2)+AV(3)]}$$

The Voice Onset Index was considered to be a quantitative representation of the relative abruptness with which voicing was initiated for the respective utterance. Since an abrupt voice onset would be one in which the voice rapidly increased in amplitude, the Voice Onset Index for such a word would be a relatively small one resulting from the difference of a large sum minus a comparably large second sum being divided by that large second sum. In contrast, the Voice Onset Index for a gentle voice onset would be the result of the difference for a moderately large sum minus a small sum being divided by that small sum, or a number larger in comparison to the Voice Onset Index of an abrupt utterance. The computed Voice Onset Indices were used to evaluate statistically changes in the abruptness of voice initiation that took place over the course of participation in therapy.

RESULTS

Mean voice onset indices for pretherapy, stretched syllable and posttherapy speech samples are shown in Figure 1. Voice onset scores were analyzed with one-tailed *t*-tests for correlated data (McGuigan, 1983). A significant increase in voice onset gentleness occurred for the stretched syllable mean when compared with the pretherapy mean ($t = -2.722$, $p < .05$, $df = 9$). The mean posttherapy voice onset index was significantly increased (indicating a more gentle voice onset) when compared with the mean for the stretched syllable speech sample ($t = -2.59$, $p < .025$, $df = 9$). Posttherapy mean voice onset gentleness was also significantly increased when compared with the pretherapy mean ($t = -3.026$, $p < .01$, $df = 9$).

The mean syllable durations in milliseconds for the pretherapy, stretched syllable and posttherapy speech samples are shown in Figure 2. The differences between mean syllable durations were

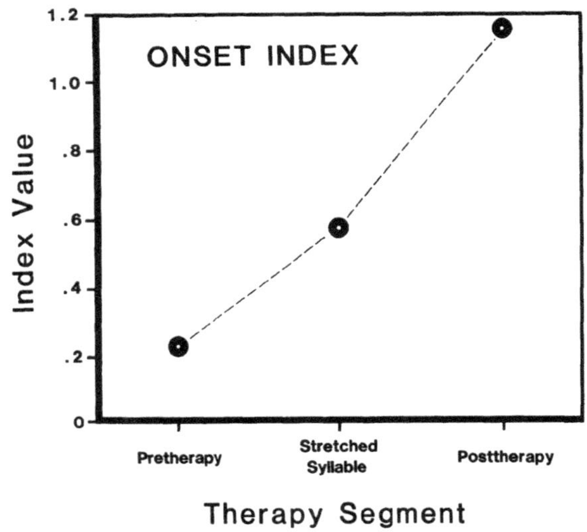

Figure 1. Mean voice onset index values as a function of period of observation.

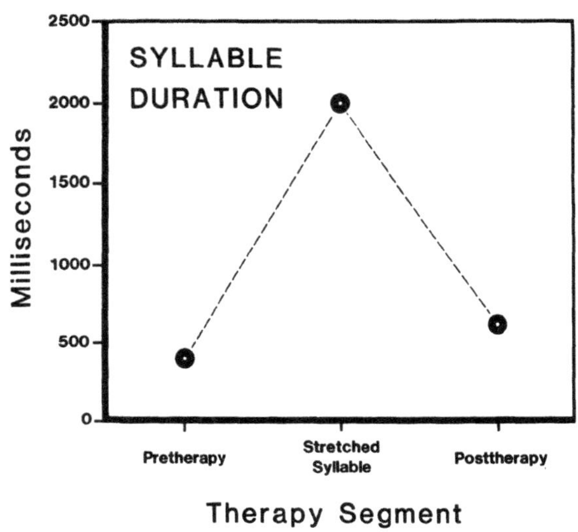

Figure 2. Mean syllable durations as a function of period of observation.

tested with two-tailed *t*-tests for correlated data. A significant increase occurred in syllable duration from the pretreatment to the stretched syllable condition (t = 31.80, $p < .001$, df = 9). Syllable durations were significantly shorter posttherapy when compared with the stretched syllable mean ($t = 28.92$, $p < .001$, $df = 9$). The posttherapy mean syllable duration was significantly longer than the pretherapy mean syllable duration ($t = 5.25$, $p < .001$, $df = 9$).

DISCUSSION

The data showed that the voice onset index increased significantly for stutterers at two-second syllable durations when compared with pretherapy utterances. That is, voice onsets became more gentle. It is not clear what factors account for increased gentleness of voice onsets associated with two-second syllable durations. A number of hypotheses appear to be relevant.

High levels of muscle tonus have been observed prior to stutterers' speech initiation (Van Riper, 1982). In addition, Zimmermann (1980) noted prepositioning of articulators prior to stutterers' initiation of fluent speech. If prepositioning of articulators is reduced with stretched syllable speech, it is possible that lower amplitude muscle movements may then be involved in speech initiation. No instructions were provided regarding articulatory prepositioning. However, instructions for the stretched syllable target did emphasize stabilizing vocal tract shapes for one second in the initial vowel position prior to making the transition to the next articulatory position. It is possible that the specificity of instructions regarding articulatory positioning for this target reduced muscle activity both prior to and during speech initiation.

The increased gentleness of voice onsets during two-second syllable durations could also be attributable to the fact that therapy participants were practiced in their use of extended syllable durations prior to the acquisition of speech samples used in data analysis. Overt stuttering was not perceived to occur with extended syllable durations. It is possible that reductions in emotional arousal associated with the reliable production of fluent speech may have decreased levels of muscle tension associated with speech initiation (Kent, 1984).

The simplest explanation for the increased gentleness of voice onsets with stretched syllable speech may be that muscle forces in articulation, voicing and respiration were reduced when exaggerated syllable durations were used. Reduced velocities of movement could have lowered physical force requirements for speech initiation. If this was the case, then voice onset gentleness could have been increased simply as a function of generalized, reduced tension of the intrinsic laryngeal muscles.

The increase in the voice onset index that occurred with the posttherapy utterances was substantially larger than that associated with the shift from pretreatment speech to utterances at two-second syllable durations.

While it may be premature to attribute voice onset gentleness improvements posttherapy to the intensive gentle voice onset training that occurred throughout the therapy program, it is likely that this is the variable that accounts for the observed posttherapy gentle voice onsets. However, it is possible that training in the use of diaphragmatic breathing may have had some impact upon properties of voice onsets. This question cannot be dealt with until the relevant data are analyzed.

It seems unlikely that the level of voice onset gentleness witnessed in posttherapy utterances can be attributed simply to the lengthening of syllable durations. In fact, syllables were substantially shorter posttherapy than with the two-second syllable durations used early in therapy, yet the voice onset index increased by approximately a factor of three over the increase observed in the pretherapy versus two-second syllable comparison. It will be interesting to observe the effects of diaphragmatic breathing upon the voice onset index. If no increases in the voice onset index occur, or if relatively small increases appear, then it can be more securely hypothesized that the specificity of voice onset training is responsible for the observed posttherapy effects.

The study indicates, at least for relatively simple utterances collected immediately following the completion of therapy, that the gentle voice onset was well represented. While clinical observations suggest that direct, careful training in the gentle voice onset is strongly associated with the effective transfer of fluent speech into everyday settings and long-term self-maintenance of fluent speech, it will be necessary to await the development of better instrumentation in order to evaluate *in vivo* speech samples from everyday settings.

The issue of the relative abruptness of voice onsets in stutterers compared with normally fluent speakers has not been dealt with here. There is, however, no *a priori* requirement for voice onset abruptness to be greater in stutterers than in normally fluent speakers. It is sufficient to observe a functional relationship between gentle voice onset training and the subsequent establishment and maintenance of normally fluent speech in order to justify the central position of this target in therapy.

It can be speculated that the effects of gentle voice onset training may be accounted for by a number of different mechanisms. Coordinative structures involved in speech could be parameterized by intensive training in therapy (Kelso, Tuller and Harris, 1983). It is also possible that background activity of motoneuron pools may be reduced by virtue of the magnitude and specificity of training in intrinsic muscle control (Zimmermann, 1981). Finally, there may be an alteration in the mechanisms by which the client controls motor behavior. The client may shift reliance on cues used for speech guidance away from auditory channels and toward proprioceptive sources (R.L. Webster and Dorman, 1971). Training in articulatory and respiratory targets may also involve the same mechanisms. Clearly, a good deal of research remains to be completed before the range of possibilities can be narrowed further.

REFERENCES

Adams, M.R. (1984). Laryngeal onset and reaction times of stutterers. In R.F. Curlee & W.H. Perkins (Eds.), *Nature and treatment of stuttering: New directions.* San Diego: College-Hill Press.

Bindewald, R.A. (1978) *Phonation times in stuttered speech: Before and after a fluency shaping program.* Unpublished Masters thesis, Hollins College.

Conture, E. (1984). Observing laryngeal movements of stutterers. In R.F. Curlee & W.H. Perkins (Eds.), *Nature and treatment of stuttering: New directions.* San Diego: College-Hill Press.

Conture, E., McCall, G. & Brewer, D. (1977). Laryngeal behavior during stuttering. *Journal of Speech and Hearing Research, 20,* 661-668.

Dew, D. & Jensen, P.J. (1977). *Phonetic processing: The dynamics of speech.* Columbus, Ohio: Charles E. Merrill.

Freeman, F.J. (1977). *The stuttering larynx: An electromyographic study of laryngeal muscle activity accompanying stuttering.* Unpublished doctoral dissertation, City University of New York.

Freeman, F.J. & Ushijima, T. (1978). Laryngeal muscle activity during stuttering. *Journal of Speech and Hearing Research, 21,* 538-562.

Johnson, W., Darley, F. & Spriestersbach, D. (1963). *Diagnostic methods in speech pathology.* New York: Harper & Row.

Kelso, J.A.S., Tuller, B. & Harris, K.S. (1983). A "dynamic pattern" perspective on the control and coordination of movement. In P.F. MacNeilage (Ed.), *The Production of speech.* New York: Springer-Verlag.

Kent, R.D. (1984). Stuttering as a temporal programming disorder. In R.F. Curlee & W.H. Perkins (Eds.), *Nature and treatment of stuttering: New directions.* San Diego: College-Hill Press.

McGuigan, F.J. (1983). *Experimental psychology: Methods of research.* Englewood Cliffs: Prentice- Hall.

Peters, H.F.M. & Boves, L. (1984). *Timing of aerodynamic and laryngeal functions in stuttering.* Paper presented at the Annual Convention of the American Speech-Language-Hearing Association. San Francisco, 1984.

Shapiro, A.I. (1980). An electromyographic analysis of the fluent and disfluent utterances of several types of stutterers. *Journal of Fluency Disorders, 5,* 203-232.

Van Riper, C. (1982). *The nature of stuttering.* Englewood Cliffs: Prentice-Hall.

Webster, L.M. & Brutten, G. (1972). An audiovisual behavioral analysis of the stuttering moment. *Behavior Therapy, 3,* 555-560.

Webster, R.L. (1974). *The precision fluency shaping program: Speech reconstruction for stutterers.* Roanoke, Virginia: Communications Development Corporation, Ltd.

Webster, R.L. & Dorman, M.F. (1971). Changes in reliance on auditory feedback cues as a function of oral practice. *Journal of Speech and Hearing Research, 14,* 307-311.

Williams, D.E., Darley, F. & Spriestersbach, D.C. (1978). Appraisal of rate and fluency. In F. Darley & D.C. Spriestersbach (Eds.), *Diagnostic methods in speech pathology.* New York: Harper & Row.

Zimmermann, G. (1980). Articulatory dynamics of fluent utterances of stutterers and nonstutterers. *Journal of Speech and Hearing Disorders, 23,* 95-107.

Zimmermann, G. (1981). Stuttering: In need of a unifying conceptual framework. *Journal of Speech and Hearing Research, 46,* 25-31.

Chapter 22

A Comprehensive Computer Program for Facilitating Fluency in Stutterers

Joseph G. Agnello

Van Riper (1973) has suggested that in order for a person with stuttering problems to correct such behavior, he must be made cognizant of the errors he produces while speaking.

An idealized speech production model is necessary for the individual to observe. Stuttering can be viewed as an error in articulation patterns.

Wingate (1964) has amply defined stuttering as repetitions and prolongations. Those incidences of stuttering which are so traditionally classified as "blocks" or "blocking" are recognized by Wingate as hesitations or silent intervals in the flow of speech. However, in much preliminary research, it has been noted that very rarely do individuals classified as stutterers exhibit within clinical or experimental settings the repetitions and/or the prolongations. Certainly in most experiments employing individuals diagnosed as stutterers, what often happens when the individual is required to orally read such a list of one or two syllable words, is that he rarely exhibits what might be construed as "stuttering".

What occurs is now popularly referred to as physiological stuttering and it is this so-called physiological stuttering that we have been able to note as an abrupt onset.

With the trained ear, or as one listens carefully and/or observes carefully, one can readily note what appears as hard glottal attacks; possibly even one or two vocal fry periodicities and/or oral muscular tension associated with excessive intra-oral air pressure. Individuals who stutter report most of their difficulty is in the initiation of speech. This trouble in initiation of speech has also been verified by research. It seems reasonable that one would therapeutically direct attention to this speech initiation problem.

In 1974, at the first Annual Conference on Vocal Tract Dynamics in New York, a microprocessor was reported, which served as bio-feedback as an aid for those with the problem of stuttering (Agnello, 1975). In this chapter a more advanced and much more sophisticated computer system is reported using both machine language to define an idealized speech onset pattern and to compare this idealized pattern to the input patterns of those individuals with a stuttering problem.

The first Speech Onset Comparator (SOC) reported in 1974 was a hard copy of a micro processing system. From that SOC unit, by going directly into the hybrid computer, we were able to obtain, from the adjusted speech wave forms, data on onset patterns from stutterers and nonstutterers. From such data we were able to observe that stutterers, as a group, have typically more abrupt ramps of the initial wave forms. Further, stutterers, as a group, typically make rapid transitions into the vowel peak when uttering a consonant plus vowel type word or syllable.

Further, when examining the acoustic pattern of stuttered speech, other aborations can be observed in the so-called fluent speech of stutterers. These aborations involve (a) hard glottal attacks; (b) abrupt air flow patterns where normally not expected; (c) usually a lowering of the second formant which would imply a constriction at the vocal fold level; (d) voice onset time of stutterers is typically longer than for nonstutterers. Also, the lack of smooth transitions reported by Stromsta in Chapter 19 of this book.

All of these above patterns plus the abruptness noted earlier are all subtle differences noted when stutterers are relatively fluent.

In a clinical setting, it is relatively easy to instruct a person with a stuttering problem to pronounce a series of words in a pre-determined fashion, whether this be stretched speech, snake speech, prolonged speech, easy on-set, pull-outs, gentle on-sets, breath controlled speech, slowed rate, prolonged vowels of prolonged consonants. All of these so-called techniques simply cause the individual to re-shape or reconfigurate his vocal tract and/or laryngeal tone creating an ameliorative effect or enhanced impression of "fluency".

It is this change of vocal tract configuration from the stereotyped pattern he has established over the years by habituation, that immediately gives the stutterer the enhancing feeling of fluency but any clinician with any reasonable experience knows this is only a temporary condition. Establishing fluency in the clinic and fluency in the laboratory is an easy task. It has been well established over the years, many quacks in the past and even some currently, have exploited this phenomenon and have seen it as a quick cure-all for stuttering. In order to counteract this strong pattern of abrupt onsets or subtle stuttering, it is necessary to have some kind of comprehensive learning experience focused on the initiation of speech that involves the comparison between the abrupt onset patterns and a more idealized onset pattern.

As noted earlier by Van Riper, an individual with a stuttering problem must be cognizant of the difference between his abrupt onset pattern and a more idealized pattern.

The idealized pattern of speech that we selected to be part of our Speech Onset Comparative System is based on three different patterns. These three patterns are not totally independent from the phonetic characteristics of the consonant plus vowel type words or syllables. Certain types of syllables of the consonant plus vowel characteristics have greater or lesser influence on the degree of abruptness of the onset pattern.

Listed in Table 1 are the various types of phonetic categories for all the words stored in the computer.

Table 1. Types of phonetic categories stored in the computer as specific test words. The programmer can make new lists, review a list, add words to old lists, change old lists, delete words, set up lists according to specific phonetic characteristics and–or onset pattern.

Computer Code Name	Phonetic Feature	Onset Pattern
MOLLY1	Fricatives (tʃ, ʃ, f, t,)	B
MOLLY2	Continuents–Glides (j,m,w,r,v,l,n)	C
MOLLY3	Plosives (k,p,t,d,b,g)	A
MOLLY4	Voiced Plosives + open vowels	A-
MOLLY5	Unvoiced Plosives + open vowels	A+
MOLLY6	One syllable -- random	R
MOLLY7	Voiced Fricative + open vowels	A+
MOLLY8	Common Sentence Starters	S
MOLLY9	"WH" Common Starters	WhB
MOLLY10	Nasal m,n	C
KIM1	Fricatives (d,z,dʒ,t)	B+
KIM2	Continuents–Glides (j,m,w,r,v,l,n)	C
KIM3	Plosives (k,p,t,d,b,g)	A
KIM4	Voiced Plosives + closed vowels	A
KIM5	Unvoiced Plosives + closed vowels	A
KIM6	One syllable -- random	R
KIM7	Voiced Fricatives + closed vowels	A-
KIM8	Unvoiced Fricatives + closed vowels	A
KIM9	Unvoiced Fricatives + open vowels	C
KIM10	Nasal m,n	C

These categories in the list shown in Table 1 are for the convenience of those knowledgeable in phonetics. Those lists of words with a particular phonetic composition such as an unvoiced plosive sound plus a particular vowel can be called out from the computer for the person who stutters to orally read. However, we have found that there are really only three basic onset patterns and some of these onset patterns are very much dependent on the nature of the syllable. For example, nasals "m" and "n" plus a closed vowel have a very gradual rise time whereas unvoiced plosives with an open vowel have a very abrupt rise time in normal speech. Those latter two types of syllables are the extreme from most gradual to most abrupt.

Listed in Table 2 are the lists of the types of phonetic syllables associated with the three basic patterns. Stored in the computer are approximately 3,800 syllables. Each syllable is coded accord-

Table 2. Three types of onset patterns associated with manner of production.

Phonetic Manner	Onset Pattern
Unvoiced Plosive	A
Voiced Plosives + Closed Vowel	A
Unvoiced Fricative + Closed Vowel	A
Fricative + Closed Vowel	A
Unvoiced Fricative + Open Vowel	B
Voiced Fricative + Open Vowel	B
Nasals + Vowel	C
Continuents + Vowel	C

Key
A = Abrupt
B = Midrange
C = Prolonged
These three criteria are defined in machine language as a power function–rise time.

ing to its phonetic characteristics, both for the vowel and consonant and they are also coded according to the schema mentioned in Table 2.

COMPUTER PROGRAM

There are basically two types of programs in this system. One program is in machine language and in this program the idealized onset patterns are defined by the computer.

In one earlier version of the computer programming, it was possible to have the computer differentiate between normal speech onset patterns and abrupt speech, repetitious type stuttering, hesitation, and prolongation. After extensive clinical applications of this program and others, we have found that it is not necessary to have the computer differentiate repetitious type stutterings versus hesitations. The far majority of stutterers and also their manner of stuttering, especially when speaking the simple syllable type task, 98% of the time, only exhibit the abruptness. Prolongation in certain types of syllables, for example "ma" is feasible whereas prolongation in a syllable like "fry" is not feasible. The degree of abruptness for any type of syllable can represent 95% of the problems that stutterers have when speaking relatively simple syllables in such laboratory tests.

If the stutterer does not match the idealized pattern, he is told by the computer that he either was too abrupt or he had too much of a prolongation.

The schema for showing the relationship between onset patterns as a function of voiced or unvoiced is illustrated in Figure 1. In Figure 1, we are illustrating the two syllables, "pa" and "ba".

The plosive "p" has far more pressure components than the plosive "b" and so consequently shown in the lower two figures of Figure 1, the onset pattern is somewhat more abrupt for "p" than for "b". This schema shown in Figure 1 can also be generalized to other such types of syllables like "ma" will certainly have a more gradual rise than the syllable "ka". All of these syllables in our selected vocabulary have been so coded that when such a word appears on the screen, the computer program knows the onset pattern the comparator has to match against the input pattern.

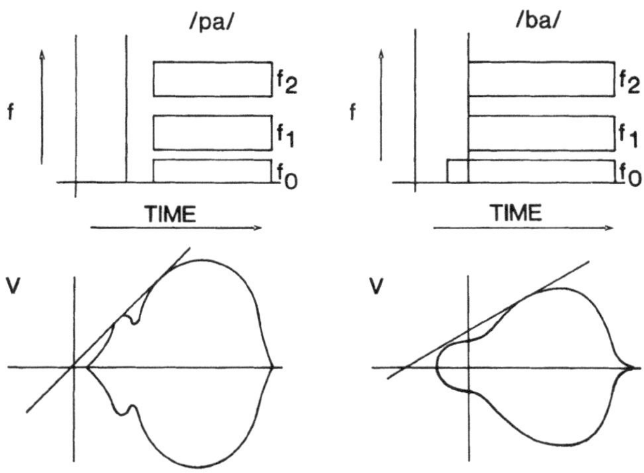

Figure 1. The relationship between voice onset time and slope onset pattern of the speech envelope.

In Figure 2, are the four types of stutterings that we were able to have the computer identify - abrupt, prolongation, hesitation and repetition. As mentioned earlier, only the degree between abruptness and prolongation was found practical for our computer to identify.

Listed in Figure 3, is our current computer program defined in machine language that allows us to make a comparison between the idealized pattern from one of the three lists of words to the idealized pattern built into our program.

STRATEGY FOR THERAPY

The previous section essentially defined how the computer, in machine language, made a comparison between the input or the spoken word from the stutterer to the idealized pattern.

In Figure 4, is our strategy for therapy. This was all defined in basic language within Figure 4, 5,000 words were coded in the computer. They were coded phonetically and they were also coded

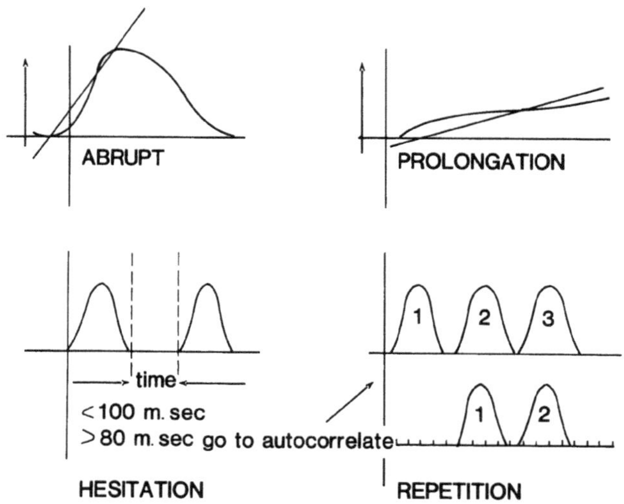

Figure 2. Four types of stuttering defined by the computer - abrupt, prolongation, hesitation and repetition. Repetition is identified by the computer through the process of autocorrelation. Hesitation is defined by the computer as any silent interval greater than 100 milliseconds.

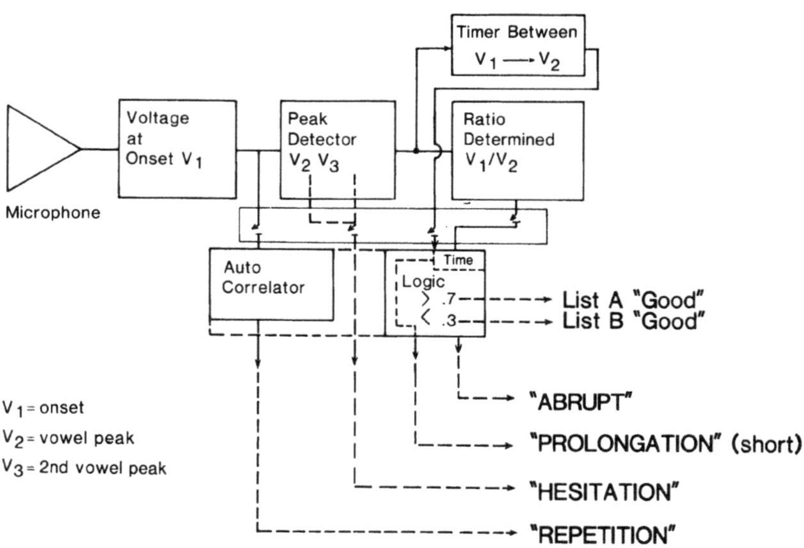

Figure 3. Flow chart illustrating the schema employed by the computer for estimating the slope values and identification of various forms of stuttering. This system is in machine language.

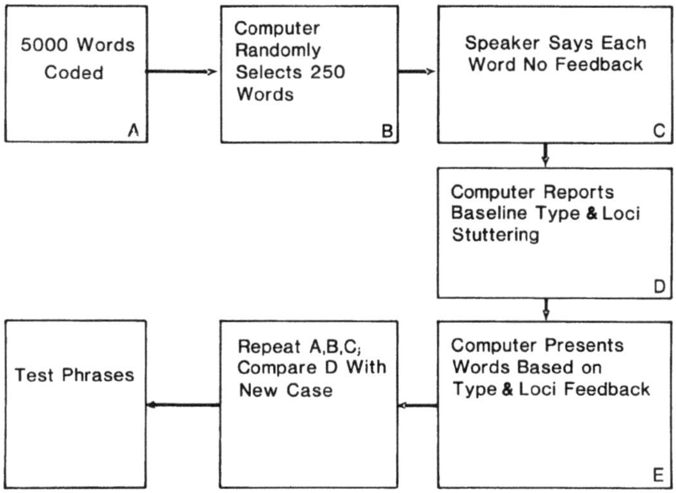

Figure 4. Overall program for the strategy employing basic computer language for the coding of all words and feedback system and the basic reporting of baseline and hit and miss record for each client.

according to the three criteria for onset patterns. The computer, at the initial session of therapy, randomly selects 250 words. The subject is instructed to speak each word. However, during this session he gets no feedback. The computer stores the type of onset he had. At the completion of saying these 250 words, the printer prints each word and also whether the stutterer was too abrupt, hit the ideal pattern, or was not abrupt enough. Essentially this is called base line data. Now the next task for the stutterer is to ask the computer to present to him words in lists of 50 from the least difficult to most difficult. The computer can extract this information from the base line data.

During this session when the stutterer says one word, after the completion of saying that word, he is instantly informed whether he matched the idealized pattern or was too abrupt or had too much prolongation. At the completion of this 50 word list, the computer prints out the results of each word and another list of words is called out by the computer and the subject continues to proceed until he has gone through all the extended lists presented by the computer.

We have found that after reading 8 lists of 50 words, we see a marked improvement, from 25 to 30 percent of the idealized criteria. After the 7th or 8th session, he is approximately at 75 to 90 percent criteria. The majority of our stutterers of more than 80 cases tested with this type of program, have been able to show typical learning curves with spontaneous recovery after an absence from the computer program. See Figure 5 for the learning curve for seven stutterers. Fifteen days of a trial/day for three weeks was the length of time on the computer. Further, less than 10% of our

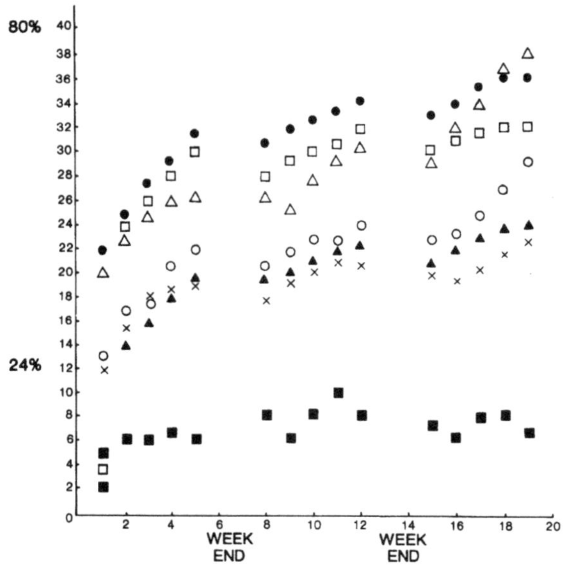

Figure 5. Learning curve for 15 trials over a 3 week period. Weekends of no practice on the computer illustrates spontaneous recovery. Six of the seven stutterers showed a typical learning curve.

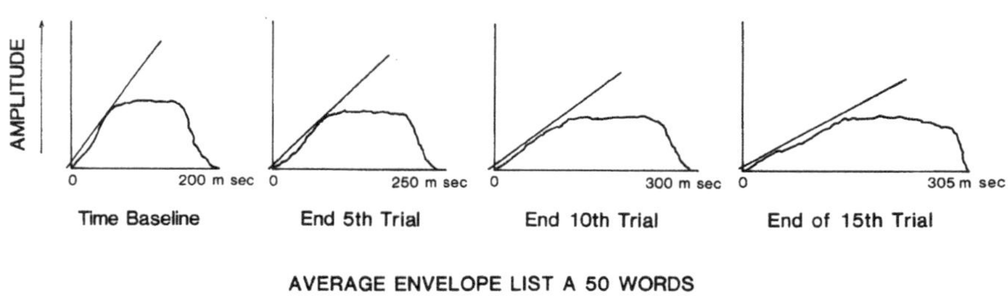

Figure 6. Illustrates the average envelope of the Speech Wave Form based on 50 words per each Wave Form.

stutterers have shown no improvement after extensive experience with the computer. The other 90% have shown gains after the 6th to 9th sessions anywhere from 70 to 95% criteria.

Figure 6, illustrates the onset pattern changes of one stutterer from baseline to the 15th trial. Each trial was the average of 8 lists of 50 words or 1600 words for the total learning session.

SUMMARY

In summary, there are three programs. One program is in machine language which defines the types of idealized onset patterns. The second program we have in our system in basic language is the vocabulary of word lists. The third program, and by the way all of our programs are related, is the task for the strategy program. We also keep a permanent record on disk of the individual's performance and are continually revising and improving all the programs.

One final note, this computer program is used in conjunction with the traditional Van Riper therapy. All of our stutterers experienced 75 hours of intensive group and individual therapy covering a 10 week period. They experienced approximately 10 hours on the computer program. Our task in therapy is to obtain the habituation of these onset patterns as well as dealing with the psychological components of the problem of stuttering.

REFERENCES

Agnello, J. & Wingate, M.E. (1971). Air pressure formants of stutterers and nonstutterers. *Journal of Fluency Disorders, 1,* 3-12.

Agnello, J, Wingate, M.E. & Wendell, M. (1974). Voice onset and voice termination times of child and adult stutterers. *Journal of the Acoustical Society of America, 56,* 362.

Agnello, J. G. (1975). Voice onset and voice termination features of stutterers. In L.M. Webster & L.C. Furst (Eds.), *Vocal tract dynamics and dysfluency.* New York: Speech and Hearing Institute.

Stromsta, C. (1965). A spectrographic study of disfluencies labelled as stuttering by parents. *De Therapia Vocis et Loquellae, 1,* 317-320.

Stromsta, C. (1986). Acoustic and electrophysiologic correlates of stuttering. In H. Peters & W. Hulstijn (Eds.), *Speech Motor Dynamics in Stuttering.* Wien/New York: Springer Verlag.

Van Riper, C. (1973). *The treatment of stuttering.* Englewood Cliffs, New Jersey: Prentice-Hall, Inc.

Chapter 23

Articulatory Rate, Stuttering and Speech Motor Control

Barbara J. Amster and
C. Woodruff Starkweather

INTRODUCTION

There is a close relation between the rate of speech and stuttering. Struggle behaviors, abnormally repeated and prolonged sounds, and other stuttering behaviors naturally slow the rate of speech. Correlations between judged severity of stuttering and speech rate have been significant - .76 (Sherman, Young, and Gough, 1958); .69 (Minifie and Cooker, 1964); .89 (Aron, 1967); .68 (Young, 1961); and .80 (Prosek, 1979). Similarly, the correlation between the frequency of stuttering behaviors and speech rate have also been significant - .88 (Bloodstein, 1944; 1974) and .86 (Sander, 1961).

It is evident that stuttering severity, whether measured by judges or determined by the frequency of stuttering behaviors, is related to the rate of speech production. Furthermore, if stuttering is related, either as cause or effect, to motor control and coordination as Zimmermann (1980) and others have suggested, the rate of speech may also be related if only by constraint to these same processes.

The possibility that speech rate and stuttering share common constraints of motor control suggests that speech rate may be related not just to stuttering but to the fluency of normal speech as well. Fluency has been defined as the absence of stuttering, but Starkweather (1980) suggested that fluency should be seen not just as the absence of disruptions in the continuity of speech but more broadly as the ease (lack of effort) with which speech is produced. He suggested also that both the continuity and rate of speech are measures of speech effort. Among the elements contributing to articulatory rate are the velocity of articulatory movements and the degree of coarticulatory overlap, both of which contribute to the duration of individual speech sounds. Umeda (1971; 1975) found that the duration of individual sounds fluctuates within the utterance according to syntactic structure, fluctuations that constitute minute variations in the rate of speech. These variations probably place some demand on the speaker's motor coordination, requiring individual movements to be made more rapidly and with greater overlap in order to shorten the duration of sounds, and yet the relative timing of movements must remain invariant so as not to exceed phonemic boundaries.

Several investigations provide evidence that link speech rate to motor coordination. Kent and Forner (1980) found that the duration of children's speech sounds diminishes and the variability of these durations also diminishes with increasing age. The authors interpreted these findings to be a reflection of children's increasing ability to control the temporal aspects of speech even as the rate of their speech also increases. Tiffany (1980) found a close correspondence between measures of motor control, such as diadochokinetic rate, and the normal rate of speech. He concluded that adults talk at a rate that is close to the limits of their motor ability. Starkweather (1980), in his review of normal fluency, came to a similar conclusion based on a different body of data. If speakers talk close to the limits of their ability and yet must still vary articulatory rate within utterances to reflect syntactic structure (Van Lancker, Canter, and Terbeek, 1981), it means that there are syntactic locations where the motor control of speech is taxed. As Starkweather (1980) pointed out, these locations are nearly the same as those at which stuttering occurs most often (Soderberg, 1966). There are also several therapies that rely on slowed rate (Webster, 1972; Curlee and Perkins, 1969; Gottwald and Starkweather, 1984), all of which have reported both successful outcome and efficiency. In addition Starkweather and Gottwald (1984) found that the amount of change in parents' rate was correlated significantly with the amount of change in their children's fluency. The amount of rate change in the children was also correlated with the amount of fluency change. These connections between the rate of speech, normal fluency, stuttering, and the motor control of speech production led to a number of preliminary investigations of various aspects of speech rate, which were conducted between 1979 and 1985 in the Temple University Speech Science Laboratory.

PRELIMINARY STUDIES

Study I

Starkweather and Myers (1979) wanted to find out how the extra time used by stutterers in voice onset and voice offset (Agnello, 1972; Hillman and Gilbert, 1977) was distributed within the intervocalic interval. From samples of oral reading in matched stutterers and nonstutterers, they excised a phrase ("the shape"), when it was judged to have been fluently produced. The recording was slowed to one quarter of its original speed and the intervocalic interval was extracted. Seven landmarks were located by a procedure with verified reliability, and the durations between adjacent landmarks were measured. The results showed clearly, and quite unexpectedly, that the extra time taken by the stutterers was located within intervals containing acoustic changes or transitions. None was located within intervals in which the acoustic signal was in a steady state. Since the duration of transitional subsegments depended on the velocity of vocal tract movement, while the duration of steady-state subsegments depended on the subjects sense of timing, it was concluded that the longer voice onset and offset times, and the generally slowed rate of stutterers' fluent speech, was associated with reduced velocity of movement of the speech mechanism.

Study II

Ingram's (1976) description of syllable reduplications in the first 50 words suggested the idea that children at this stage may lack the motor control to produce a destressed syllable, which demands faster movement. This speculation implied that poor motor control might also be responsible for excessive disfluency in children, since it is common precisely at the time when children stop reduplication and begin to produce destressed syllables. It seemed worthwhile to see if young stutterers and nonstutterers were different in their ability to achieve stress contrast. Accordingly, Holland and Starkweather (1982) examined samples of spontaneous speech from young children who stuttered and from nonstuttering children matched very closely for age (3 months), classroom placement, school achievement, sex, and socio-economic status. The pairs of speech samples from matched subjects were searched for words that could be matched for syllable structure, word length, stress pattern, position in the sentence, grammatical function in the sentence, and overall sentence length. Spectrograms of matched words were made and the duration of the stressed and unstressed vowels, overall word duration, and the proportion of the total word duration taken up by the vowels were measured.

The results were not entirely conclusive but were nonetheless interesting. Both groups showed an average difference of about 40 msec between the duration of the stressed and the duration of the unstressed syllables. There is no significant difference, indeed the two groups were almost identical.

In average word duration, however, the groups differed significantly. The nonstutterers' words were about 50 msec longer than the stutterers. Since stutterers tend to speak at a slower rate, their words should be longer, not shorter, so this result was unanticipated. Of course, measures were made on words that were selected with certain criteria in mind, not randomly, and perhaps words that stutterers tend to say faster were inadvertently selected. However, it is also possible that the 4-6 year-old stutterers in this study may have tended to talk faster than nonstutterers of the same age.

Accordingly, we measured the subjects' speech rate. Four stutterers were significantly faster speakers than their matched controls. Two stutterers were significantly slower speakers than their matched controls, and the rest showed no difference. These results indicated that some young stutterers may have faster speech than nonstutterers while others have slower speech. Unlike the older stutterer whose speech may be appreciably slowed by the presence of struggle behavior, it is possible that some young stutterers may actually talk faster. Later on, these children's speech may be slowed by increasingly abnormal patterns of struggling and tension.

When stress contrast is measured another way, there is a significant difference between the two groups. The nonstutterers' stressed syllables occupy a larger proportion of the total word duration than those of the stutterers. It is also evident that the proportion of the word occupied by the unstressed syllables is virtually equal between the two groups. Since both groups were able to demonstrate syllabic stress, it seems that the stutterers use a different strategy than the nonstutterers, one in which the stressed syllable is not lengthened. This suggests that the young stutterer may not be able to make the small reductions in speech rate (vowel lengthening) that are responsible, along with changes in intensity and frequency, for signalling stress and certain aspects of the syntax (Umeda, 1971; 1975; Van Lancker, Canter, and Terbeek, 1981). The result was contrary to our expectation. We thought that the child who stutters, lacking motor control, would be unable to speed up his articulatory movement in order to shorten the unstressed syllable. Instead, it appears that the child who stutters is less able to slow his articulatory movement momentarily in order to lengthen the stressed syllable.

Study III

The next study dealt with a person's ability to alter speech rate within the rhythmic constraints of language. When speech slows momentarily for syllable stress or a clause boundary, the rhythmic structure of the sentence (Martin, 1979) is otherwise maintained. These alterations in tempo while maintaining the rhythm of the language seemed to make a substantial demand on the speaker's motor control, and a comparison of stutterers and nonstutterers would be useful. But of course there was no information on how well normal speakers could do this. Consequently, we devised a tempo tracking task and administered it to a number of normal speakers. The subjects produced a speech sound - the syllable /ti/ ("tea") - simultaneously with a click. Driven by a computer program, the clicks began at a steady rhythm, with a half second between clicks. The first three intervals between clicks were equal in duration, but then the tempo changed. In one condition, the tempo increased to ten clicks per second within a total period of about three seconds. In the other condition, the tempo decreased at the same rate to a final tempo of one click every two seconds. Ten adult subjects, 5 males and 5 females, were asked to listen for the rhythm and to say the word "tea" at exactly the same time as the clicks. There were four practice trials before the actual task. The duration of the intervals between adjacent clicks (the interstimulus interval) and the corresponding intervals between adjacent syllables (the intersyllable interval) were both measured from visicorder and spectrographic records. Tracking ability was defined as the average difference between the interstimulus intervals and the corresponding intersyllable intervals.

The average difference between corresponding intervals was about 15 msec, and the largest average difference was a little less than 100 msec. There was a temporal error, or reaction time, effect that could be seen as a tendency for the subjects' tracking to continue at the same tempo momentarily just after the tempo began to change. This overshoot was larger in the decreasing condition than in the increasing condition, suggesting that it is somewhat more difficult for subjects to slow down than to speed up as they track a tempo. The average error was defined as the difference between each interstimulus interval and the corresponding (next) intersyllable interval. There was a significantly greater amount of error in tracking the decreasing tempo, attributable to the overshoot phenomenon, than in tracking the increasing tempo. This result recalled the earlier finding of Holland and Starkweather (1982) in which children who stuttered were less able than nonstutterers to slow their movement speed at stressed syllables.

INTRODUCTION TO MAIN STUDY

Since 1981, a clinical method of stuttering prevention has been used experimentally at Temple University (Gottwald and Starkweather, 1984). This therapy is based on the idea that young children whose speech is disfluent can be prevented from acquiring the disorder of stuttering by allowing their motoric and linguistic capacities for fluency to develop free from the influence of simultaneously increasing environmental demands for fluency. This model, which we call the "demands and capacities model", has been described elsewhere (Gottwald and Starkweather, 1984). The capacities for fluency fall into two categories - language fluency and speech fluency. Language fluency includes word-retrieval, syntactic planning, and pragmatic skill. Speech fluency can be measured in a number of ways, all of which reflect the child's speed motor control. Among the important measures are vocal and articulatory reaction time, length of utterance between pauses, pause duration, frequency and duration of discontinuities, and the child's rate of articulation.

Of these measures, the last is both important and problematic. It is important because rate is a primary indicator of fluency (Starkweather, 1980) and a sign of the speaker's degree of speech motor control. Rate measurements are a problem, however, because the rate of speech production reflects both speech fluency and language fluency. In spite of these problems, the articulatory rate of children at risk for stuttering are routinely assessed. Such an assessment, however, should be made by comparison with the rate at which normal children of preschool age usually produce speech, and this information has been lacking. The need for normative information on the articulation rate of preschool children was the motive for the following study.

Method

The senior author interviewed 120 normal preschool children, varying in age from 2;6 to 5;5, screening them for the presence of conditions or histories that might affect their rate of speech. During the interviews, most of which took place in the child's preschool setting, the examiner played with and encouraged the children to talk but made no attempt to influence their speech. The subjects lived in the greater Philadelphia area, and were for the most part the children of middle-class parents. All but one were white.

Ten utterances of at least two syllables in length were selected for each child. The method for assessing rate consisted of listening repeatedly to an utterance until its beginning and ending could be anticipated from the rhythm of the acoustic sequence, then starting and stopping an electronic stopwatch simultaneously with the beginning and ending of the utterance. Six measures were made for each utterance, and the average of the six was used as the metric. Utterances were defined as continuous strings of syllables, unbroken by pauses greater than 250 msec. This method had the advantage of using the human ear to locate the beginning and ending of meaningful utterances, which seemed more accurate than machine assisted methods, based solely on the presence or absence of an acoustic signal, and it also minimized reaction time effects[1]. The external reliability of the method was assessed by having another speech pathologist apply the same method to a 36-utterance sample of the whole. A reliability coefficient of .88 was obtained. Internal reliability was also assessed from the same 36-utterance sample and found to be .98.

Results

An analysis of variance, in which the main factors were the children's age and their rate of articulation, showed a clear tendency for speech rate to be faster for the older than for the younger children. However, the older children not only spoke more quickly, they also used longer utterances, and it had been reported (Lehiste, 1972; Huggins, 1978) that the rate of speech was correlated with the length of utterance in adults. An analysis revealed a substantial correlation (+.33) between the length of utterance and the rate of articulation in this preschool population. The data were then reanalyzed using an analysis of covariance, in which utterance length was the covariate. The results again showed a main effect for age, indicating that older children talk faster than younger ones, even when the influence of increasing length of utterance is removed.

Not found was a difference between the sexes in the rate of articulation. Previous investigators (Kowal, O'Connell, and Sabin, 1975) had found a sex difference in older children at certain ages. Nor was there any change in the variability of speech rate. Kent and Forner (1980) measured the duration of speech sounds in young children and found, as others before them, that variability in the duration of sounds decreases at the same time as the duration itself, suggesting that as children's speech rate increases, their precision of motor control does also. These data, based on 120 normal preschool children, showed no age-related change in the variability of articulatory rate.

Perhaps the most important observation in this study is the clear correlation between articulatory rate and the length of utterance in preschool children. This relationship is stronger for shorter than for longer utterances, the same pattern that Malecot, Johnston, and Kizziar (1972) observed for adults. This result suggests that one should not measure and report the rate of articulation without also reporting the length(s) of the utterance(s) being measured. In the clinic it is best to measure a variety of utterance lengths and report the rate for each separately as a profile of measurements. Such a profile is particularly important when assessing the articulatory rate of very young children who are likely to have short utterances. For older children, who have longer utterances and consequently less of a rate × length correlation, it might be simpler to select longer utterances for measurement. But the clinician should still report the length of the utterance in order for the rate measure to be comparable to normal rates.

FOLLOW-UP STUDIES

An interesting question based on these results is whether children who stutter show the same relationship between utterance length and rate of articulation. Since the presence of stuttering tends to slow the articulatory rate, and is also more likely to be present on longer utterances, the possibility that increased rate of speaking on longer utterances serves to precipitate stuttering needs to be examined. Other questions concerning the relation between rate and stuttering are also of interest.

One of the most important is the rate of the parents' speech. A number of dramatic improvements in children's fluency following a slowing of the parents' rate of speech have been reported (Gottwald and Starkweather, 1984). Gottwald and Starkweather (1985) examined the relation between reductions in parental rate of speech and improvements in children's fluency in the first ten families treated in the Temple University Stuttering Prevention Clinic. As part of the assessment procedure, each family plays together in a well-equipped playroom while video-taped samples of their behavior are collected for a period of 15 minutes. This play session introduces each session throughout the treatment phase. The first and the last of these play sessions were selected for analysis. The articulatory rate of parents and children was measured. The child's stuttering severity in each of these same sessions was also measured, using the proportion of speech time spent stuttering as the criterion measure. In this measure, the duration of each stuttering behavior is measured, and all such durations are summed, and the sum is divided by the total duration of the child's speaking time. The differences between the first and the last sessions were calculated for the parents' and the stuttering child's articulatory rate and for the child's stuttering severity. The correlation between the first-last difference scores for parents' rate was calculated. A significant (.05) correlation of +.63 was obtained, indicating that the amount of change in parents' speech rate is strongly related to the amount of improvement in the child's fluency.

The correlation between the extent of improvement in the child's fluency and the extent of change in the child's own rate of articulation was also assessed. Since the stuttering children's articulation rate tends to increase as the stuttering severity diminishes, it would not have been surprising to find increases in rate accompanying decreases in stuttering. Instead, we found again a positive correlation between changes in rate of articulation and stuttering severity. That is, those children improved in fluency the most whose speech rate increased the least during therapy. Consequently, it makes sense for clinicians to model slow rates of speech for stuttering children and to train parents to do likewise.

Another rate study was also carried out to see if it was the parents' absolute rate of articulation that influenced their children's stuttering or the relative rate of parents' speech, that is, the difference between the parents' and the child's rate. After all, some children are rapid speakers who do not stutter, and many children who do stutter have parents whose speech is not unusually fast, in absolute terms. But perhaps even the parents with slow speech talk enough faster than their children to stress the child's capacity for fluency. However, the concept of relative rate is new. There is very little known about the extent to which parents adjust their rate of speech in response to the development of their children. Snow (1972) observed that mothers adjust the complexity of their language according to their child's age, a phenomenon known now as "motherese". Phillips (1973) confirmed Snow's observations and found that motherese also included a tendency to use simpler vocabulary when talking to young children. Since the rate of speech is slower in younger children, it seemed plausible that mothers adjust the rate of their speech according to the child's age. Meyers and Freeman (1985) examined the rate of adults' speech when talking to children. They compared the rates of parents of stutterers with those of parents of nonstutterers, and found that the parents of stuttering children tended to talk faster than those of nonstuttering children. Unfortunately, there was no age breakdown in their study, and it was not possible to determine if the motherese effect included adjustments in speech rate.

Consequently, Hutt (1985) selected a sample of 12 families with no history of speech or language disorder and measured the differences between parents' and children's rate of articulation. Speech samples were taken from mothers and their children, six boys and six girls, at each of six age categories ranging from 30-65 months, as they talked in a free-play situation. The experimenter was absent from the setting, and the mothers were unfamiliar with the purpose of the study. The rate of speech (articulatory rate) was measured for six syllable utterances from these samples. A developmental pattern was evident in both boys and girls, in spite of the small sample size. No pattern of adjustment could be discerned in the mothers' rate. This does not mean, of course, that there is no such effect. The sample is too small to be used as a basis for general conclusions. It is nonetheless interesting to note that the developmental changes in the children seem more evident than corresponding adjustments in the mothers.

There was, however, a clear, and statistically significant difference, even in this small sample, between the boys' and the girls' speech rate, the boys being slower, which is not matched by a corresponding adjustment in the mothers. Consequently, there is a difference in the relative rate between the two sexes. Since other, more comprehensive studies of articulatory rate in children (Amster, 1984) have either failed to find a sex difference or have found significant differences only at certain ages (Kowal, O'Connell, and Sabin, 1975), it is unclear whether these results are generalizable. They do suggest, however, that future study in the area of relative rate may provide interesting information concerning stuttering and speech motor control.

CONCLUSION

This chapter has reviewed some of the relations between articulatory rate, speech motor control, and stuttering. It seems evident that such relations exist and that in general they indicate that the speed at which articulatory adjustments are made is a factor in the development and continuation of stuttering behaviors. There is no evidence from which to conclude that articulatory rate is the only factor related to stuttering development and continuation, nor is it the intention of this chapter to suggest that articulatory rate is conclusively or simplistically related to the onset of disfluency in very young children. Instead, it appears that changes in the rate of articulatory movements, perhaps most importantly attempts to slow an already rapid rate of articulation, as would occur, for example, on the first few stressed syllables of a long sentence, make fluency breakdown more likely and that a slower overall articulatory rate enhances fluency and makes recovery from stuttering more complete.

NOTES

[1] A recent study by Heuer and Meyers (1975) has found substantial error in visicorder and time/data generator methods of measuring rate. In addition, our attempts to validate the stopwatch method of measuring rate by comparing it with spectrographic records led us to conclude that judgements of the onset and offset of utterances taken from spontaneous conversational speech are more accurately made by ear, once the judge's reaction time is reduced by repeated listening and anticipation, than judgements made by measuring spectrograms.

REFERENCES

Agnello, J. & Wingate, M. (1972). *Some acoustical and physiological aspects of stuttered speech.* Convention address, ASHA.

Amster, B. (1984). *The rate of speech in normal preschool children.* Ph.D. dissertation, Temple University.

Andrews, G. & Cutler, J. (1974). Stuttering therapy: the relation between changes in symptom level and attitudes. *Journal of Speech and Hearing Disorders, 39,* 312-319.

Aron, M. (1967). The relationship among measurements of stuttering behavior. *Journal of the South African Logopedic Society, 14,* 15-34.

Bloodstein, O. (1944). Studies in the psychology of stuttering: XIX. The relationship between oral reading rate and severity of stuttering. *Journal of Speech Disorders, 9,* 161-173.

Curlee, R. & Perkins, W. (1969). Conversational rate control therapy for stuttering. *Journal of Speech and Hearing Disorders, 34,* 245-250.

Dixon, C. (1955). Stuttering adaptation in relation to assumed level of anxiety. In W. Johnson & R. Leutenegger (Eds.), *Stuttering in Children and Adults.* Minneapolis: Univ. Minnesota Press.

Gottwald, S. & Starkweather, C.W. (1984). *Stuttering prevention: rationale and method.* Short course, ASHA, San Francisco.

Heuer, R. & Meyers, S. (1985). *A Study of Methods of Measuring Speech Rate.* Convention address, ASHA.

Hillman, R. & Gilbert, H. (1977). Voice onset time for voiceless stop consonants in the fluent reading of stutterers and nonstutterers. *Journal of the Acoustical Society of America, 61,* 610-611.

Holland, T. & Starkweather, C.W. (1982). *Stress contrast in stuttering and nonstuttering children.* Poster session, ASHA.

Huggins, A. (1978). Speech timing and intelligibility. In J. Requin (Ed.), *Attention and Performance VII.* Hillsdale, NJ: Lawrence Erlbaum Assoc., Publishers. 279-297.

Hutt, D. (1985). *The relative speech rates of mothers and their children.* M.A. thesis, Temple University.

Ingham, R. & Andrews, G. (1973). An analysis of a token economy in stuttering therapy. *Journal of Applied Behavioral Analysis, 6,* 219-229.

Ingram, D. (1976). *Phonological Disability in Children.* New York: Elsevier.

Kent, R. & Forner, L. (1980). Speech segment duration in sentence recitations by children and adults. *Journal of Phonetics, 8,* 157-168.

Kline, M. & Starkweather, C.W. (1979). *Receptive and expressive language performance in young stutterers.* Convention address, ASHA.

Kowal, S., O'Connell, D. & Sabin, E. (1975). Development of temporal patterning and vocal hesitations in spontaneous narratives. *Journal of Psycholinguistic Research, 4,* 195-207.

Lehiste, I. (1972). The timing of utterances and linguistic boundaries. *Journal of the Acoustical Society of America, 51,* 2018-2024.

Malecot, A., Johnston, R. & Kizziar, P. (1972). Syllabic rate and utterance length in French. *Phonetica, 26,* 235-251.

Martin, J. (1979). Rhythmic (hierarchical) versus serial structure in speech and other behavior. *Psychological Revue, 79,* 487-509.

Minifie, F. & Cooker, H. (1964). A disfluency index. *Journal of Speech and Hearing Disorders, 29,* 189-192.

Meyers, S. & Freeman, F. (1985). Mother and child speech rates as a variable in stuttering and disfluency. *Journal of Speech and Hearing Research, 28,* 436-444.

Phillips, J. (1973). Syntax and vocabulary of mothers' speech to young children: Age and sex comparisons. *Child Development, 44,* 182-185.

Prosek, R., Walden, B., Montgomery, A. & Schwartz, D. (1979). Some correlates of stuttering severity judgements. *Journal of Fluency Disorders, 4,* 215-222.

Sander, E. (1961). Reliability of the Iowa Speech Disfluency Test. *Journal of Speech and Hearing Disorders,* Monograph Supplement 7, 21-30.

Sherman, D., Young, M.A. & Gough, K. (1958). Comparison of three measures of stuttering severity. *Proceedings of the Iowa Academy of Science, 65,* 381-384.

Snow, C. (1972). Mothers' speech to children learning language. *Child Development, 43,* 549-565.

Soderberg, G. (1966). The relations of stuttering to word length and word frequency. *Journal of Speech and Hearing Research, 9,* 584-589.

Starkweather, C.W. (1983). *Tracking a changing tempo.* Convention Address, ASHA.

Starkweather, C.W. (1980). Speech fluency and its development in normal children. In N. Lass (Ed.), *Speech and Language: Advances in Basic Research and Practice, 4,* 143-199.

Starkweather, C.W. & Myers, M. (1979). The duration of subsegments within the intervocalic intervals of stutterers and nonstutterers. *Journal of Fluency Disorders, 4,* 205-214.

Tiffany, W. (1980). The effects of syllable structure on diadochokinetic and reading rates. *Journal of Speech and Hearing Research, 23,* 894-908.

Umeda, N. (1971). Consonant duration in American English. *Journal of the Acoustical Society of America, 61,* 846-858.

Umeda, N. (1975). Vowel duration in American English. *Journal of the Acoustical Society of America, 58,* 434-445.

Van Lancker, D., Canter, G. & Terbeek, D. (1981). Disambiguation of ditrophic sentences: acoustic and phonetic cues. *Journal of Speech and Hearing Research, 24,* 330-335.

Webster, R. (1972). *An operant response shaping program for the establishment of fluency in stutterers: final report.* Hollins College.

Yairi, E. (1983). The onset of stuttering in two and three year old children: a preliminary report. *Journal of Speech and Hearing Disorders, 48,* 171-177.

Young, M.A. (1980). Comparison of stuttering frequencies during reading and speaking. *Journal of Speech and Hearing Research, 23,* 216-217.
Zimmermann, G. (1980c). Stuttering: a disorder of movement. *Journal of Speech and Hearing Research, 23,* 122-136.

Chapter **24**

Speech Rate and Syllable Durations in Stutterers and Nonstutterers

Paul Schäferskϋpper and Michael Dames

Recent research on stuttering has focused on time and timing aspects of general motor and speech motor control. For example, reaction time measurements have shown stutterers to be slower than nonstutterers (Adams & Hayden, 1976; Schäferskϋpper, 1981; Starkweather et al., 1984; Peters & Hulstijn, 1986; Watson, 1986).

Acoustic studies on the time structure of speech have been conducted on the subphonemic, the phonemic and the suprasegmental level. Subphonemically, voice onset time (VOT) measurements have led to conflicting results, suggesting that VOT needs to be correlated with suprasegmental influences on the time structure (Hillman & Gilbert, 1977; Watson & Alfonso, 1982; Healey & Gutkin, 1984).

The context-dependence of vowel durations in German words was studied by Reimann (1976). The stutterers investigated had shorter vowels relative to the duration of the whole word than the control subjects. But they altered vowel duration in the same way the control subjects did depending on what consonant followed. This context-dependent vowel length was also reported by DiSimoni (1974). For nonsense syllables DiSimoni found that the stutterers had significantly greater absolute vowel and consonant durations than the nonstutterers studied. In addition, the stutterers showed greater intraindividual variation in the duration of a given consonant. The electromyographic (EMG) and electroglottographic (EGG) studies by Wieneke and Janssen (1986) and Janssen and Wieneke (1986) reported elsewhere in this book are consistent with these acoustic findings.

In a study involving the repeated reading of sentences and paragraphs, Cooper and Allen (1977) reported that the amount of variation in reading time was greater for the stutterers than for the nonstutterers. These results have been confirmed by Bergmann (1986).

Taken together, these results show that there is a general timing abnormality in the speech of stutterers and not just problems such as repetitions or prolongations of speech segments. We therefore designed a study to determine whether stutterers also differ from nonstutterers with respect to speech timing in speech samples where stuttering is absent.

In stress-timed languages such as German, syllable durations systematically vary due to the word accent pattern, the location of the sentence stress, and the position of the word evaluated in a sentence (Lehiste, 1970; Nooteboom et al., 1978; Stock, 1980). Consequently, a certain variability in syllable durations within a paragraph reflects adequate speech performance. In our study we assumed that timing during speech is controlled on two levels, a global level governing the overall speech rate and a specific level controlling both the relationship between segment and syllable durations and that of segments and syllables to larger entities of the speech act. In order to evaluate the contribution of these levels to speech production in stutterers, we asked the following questions:

1. Do stutterers and nonstutterers differ with respect to speech rate during reading?
2. Do stutterers and nonstutterers differ with respect to syllable durations during reading?

METHODS

Acoustic Parameters

Speech rate is usually expressed as the quotient of the number of syllables divided by speaking time. With this procedure, similarities between stuttering and nonstuttering subjects may be masked by differences in the number and duration of pauses. To overcome this problem we included three time variables:

1. *Reading time (RT)*, defined as the time needed to read the whole text
2. *Articulation time (AT)*, defined as reading time minus the pauses between the phrases
3. *Syllable duration (t)*, with each syllable being assigned to one of the following speech rate categories:

fast rate:	$t<160$ msec	($t>6$ syllables/sec)
normal rate:	160 msec$\leq t<$330 msec	($t=3$ to 6 syllables/sec)
slow rate:	$t\geq 330$ msec	($t<3$ syllables/sec)

Subjects

Four adult stutterers and four age-matched controls without speech problems served as the subjects. The stutterers exhibited a wide range of stuttering during spontaneous speech, from very mild symptoms (S1) to extremely peculiar prolongations and repetitions of sounds (S2). They were chosen from an initial group of 15 subjects because they did not show either tonic or clonic symptoms on a reading task (with the exception of S2, who had two mild prolongations in this situation).

Procedure

Each subject read the German version of the IPA standard text "The northwind and the sun", which contains 140 syllables and all German phonemes. All recordings were taped.

A group of five phoneticians listened to the tapes and identified all stuttering symptoms. On the basis of these assessments the four stutterers were then selected for the study.

The recordings were digitized with a 20 kHz sample rate and analyzed under auditory and visual control. The beginning and end of the text, the pauses, and the syllable boundaries were marked on the digital copy by setting brackets of different types. The data were then analyzed with the chi-square test.

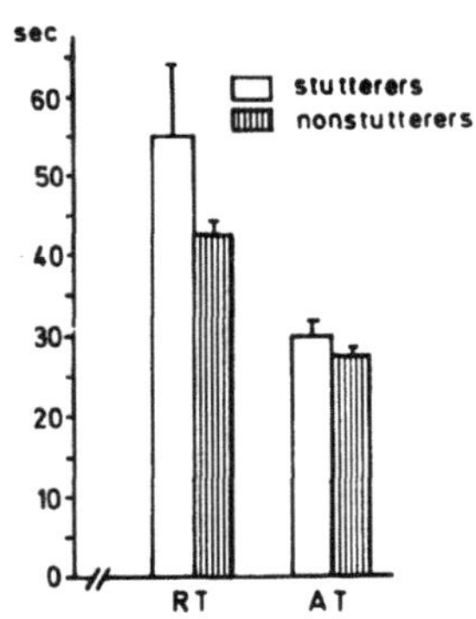

Figure 1. Shows the mean reading time (RT) and articulation time (AT) of four stutterers and nonstutterers.

RESULTS

Figure 1 shows that the reading time of the stutterers was about 1/3 longer than that of the nonstutterers, but the articulation time was about the same in both groups. Thus the stutterers needed more time for pauses than the nonstutterers.

Figure 2 shows the mean number of syllables spoken fast and normally. The stutterers spoke fewer syllables fast and more at a normal speech rate than the controls. The group differences are significant at the .01 level.

Table 1 shows that the number of slowly spoken syllables was about the same in both groups. Further, it shows that the group differences demonstrated in Figure 2 were also found for all subjects individually.

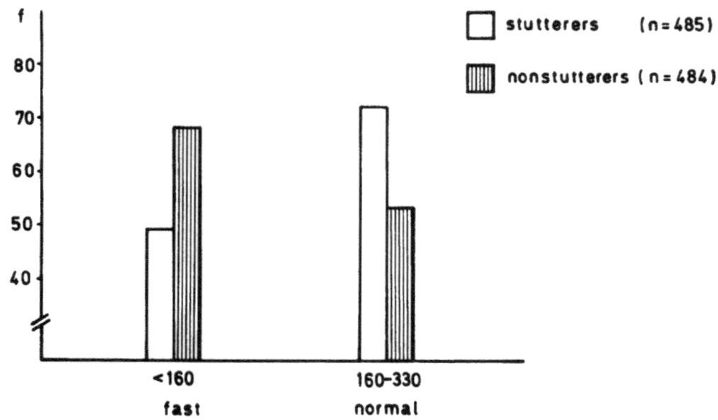

Figure 2. Shows the mean frequency of fast (t<160msec) and normal (160msec≤t<330msec) syllables in four stutterers and nonstutterers.

Table 1. Shows the frequency of fast (t<160msec), normal (160msec≤t<330msec), and slow (t≥330msec) syllables in stutterers (S1-S4) and nonstutterers (C1-C4).

	t<160 msec	160 msec≤t<330 msec	t≥330 msec	Total
S1	45	73	22	140
S2	52	67	18	137
S3	55	69	16	140
S4	43	81	14	138
S1-S4	195	290	70	555
C1	66	53	20	139
C2	70	54	16	140
C3	74	48	18	140
C4	59	60	21	140
C1-C4	269	215	75	559

DISCUSSION

In the present study we found that the stutterers had longer reading times than the nonstutterers but that the articulation time was about the same in both groups. The stutterers made more and longer pauses, which enabled them to reduce the frequency of stuttering markedly. The number and length of pauses may be one component of the mechanism controlling the overall speech rate. Allen (1973) and Cooper and Allen (1977) hypothesized a neural clock responsible for this time control. Our ideas about this mechanism are not so far-reaching. We merely want to emphasize that the overall speech rate is controlled independently of prosodic and linguistic timing. Our observation that the stutterers did not have a longer articulation time than the controls sheds some light on the possible structure of this mechanism. It appears that speech rate is regulated by the number and duration of pauses and by the speed of articulatory movements. In the first case, prosodic and linguistic timing are not affected because articulation is not involved in this process.

We also found that the stutterers spoke fewer syllables at a fast rate and more at a normal rate than the controls. In other words, the stutterers marked the durational differences between the different types of syllables less well, indicating that they were poorer at producing syllables of the appropriate duration (at least with regard to the fast syllables). We therefore conclude that our subjects are less flexible in articulatory timing. Cooper and Allen (1977) interpreted their findings of greater variability in stutterers as evidence of a defect in timing control, and this hypothesis is supported by DiSimoni's (1974) and Reimann's (1976) results and the physiologic studies of Wieneke and Janssen (see Chapter 26, this volume) and Janssen and Wieneke (see Chapter 25, this volume). Our own findings also lend support to such a hypothesis.

With reference to the slower vocal and manual reaction times they found in stutterers, Starkweather and his colleagues (1984) assumed a generalized slower reactivity for all types of motor behavior. But they also pointed out that "this does not completely rule out ...the possibility that these differences may be secondary to the disorder". Now this latter statement may also be true for all the other results on timing control in speech. But considering that stuttering itself may be seen as a speech timing disorder (see, for example, Van Riper, 1971), it seems very unlikely to us that the differences in speech timing control are reactions to stuttering or associated features. Consequently, the findings of Starkweather et al. (1984) can also be seen in the larger context of a generalized timing disorder characterized so far by three features: slowness, greater variability, and less flexibility.

The temporal organization of speech is part of the prosodic system, and one function of this system is to express emotional states (see, for example, Pike, 1945, and Stock, 1980). This function could be used to interpret the prosodic disturbance of stutterers as the expression of an emotional disorder. But from the behavior sciences it is known that we must differentiate carefully between expression and impression, with the latter being the perception and interpretation of the expressive behavior (Leyhausen, 1967). Expression and impression are two independent mechanisms with strong inborn components. Consequently, they are not always congruent, which can result in the misinterpretation of an observed expressive behavior. The problem then is that the impression may be very convincing to the observer because the biological component dominates, and thus there is hardly any chance of the misinterpretation being detected. Considering this fact, the psychological interpretation of stuttering may have the following structure: The expression of a pathophysiological behavior in stutterers (this is the defect in timing control) is interpreted by the observer's mechanisms of impression as the expression of a psychopathological state, resulting in the assumption of an emotional disturbance. The psychological theories of stuttering may thus be the result of a misinterpretation, which in turn is due to a biological mechanism for understanding the world.

In summary, the stutterers had longer reading times than the nonstutterers but about the same articulation time. We conclude from this that our subjects controlled the overall speech rate to reduce stuttering frequency. In addition, they tended to equalize their syllable durations. This result supports the hypothesis of a defect in timing control.

ACKNOWLEDGEMENTS

This research was supported by grant Po 121/5 from the Deutsche Forschungsgemeinschaft.

REFERENCES

Adams, M. & Hayden, P. (1976). The ability of stutterers and nonstutterers to initiate and terminate phonation during production of an isolated vowel. *Journal of Speech and Hearing Research, 19,* 290-296.

Allen, G.D. (1973). Segmental timing control in speech production. *Journal of Phonetics, 1,* 219-237.

Bergmann, G. (1985). Studies in stuttering as a prosodic disturbance. Submitted to *Journal of Speech and Hearing Research,*

Bergmann, G. (1987). Stuttering as a prosodic disturbance: A link between speech execution and emotional processes. In H.F.M. Peters & W. Hulstijn (Eds.), *Speech Motor Dynamics in Stuttering.* Wien: Springer Verlag.

Cooper, M. & Allen, G.D. (1977). Timing control accuracy in normal speakers and stutterers. *Journal of Speech and Hearing Research, 20,* 55-71.

DiSimoni, F.G. (1974). Preliminary study of certain timing relationships in the speech of stutterers. *Journal of the Acoustical Society of America, 56,* 695-696.

Healey, E.Ch. & Gutkin, B. (1984). Analysis of stutterers' voice onset times and fundamental frequency contour during fluency. *Journal of Speech and Hearing Research, 27,* 219-235.

Hillman, R.E. & Gilbert, H.R. (1977). Voice onset time for voiceless stop consonants in the fluent reading of stutterers and nonstutterers. *Journal of the Acoustical Society of America, 61,* 610-611.

Janssen, P. & Wieneke, G. (1987). Variability in the duration of physiological activity under fluency conditions. In H.F.M. Peters & W. Hulstijn (Eds.), *Speech Motor Dynamics in Stuttering.* Wien: Springer Verlag.

Lehiste, I. (1970). *Suprasegmentals.* Cambridge, Mass.: The MIT Press.

Leyhausen, P. (1967). Biologie von Ausdruck und Eindruck. *Psychologische Forschung, 31,* 113-176.

Nooteboom, S.G., Brokx, J.P.L. & Rooij, J.J. de, (1978). Contribution of prosody to speech perception. In V.J.M. Levelt & G.B. Flores d'Arcais (Eds.), *Studies in the Perception of Language.* Chichester: J. Wiley & Sons. 75-107.

Peters, H.F.M. & Hulstijn, W. (1987). Programming and initiation of speech utterances in stuttering. In H.F.M. Peters & W. Hulstijn (Eds.), *Speech Motor Dynamics in Stuttering.* Wien: Springer Verlag.

Pike, K.L. (1972). General characteristics of intonation. In D.D. Bolinger (Ed.), *Intonation.* Harmondsworth: Penguin Books. 53-83. (Reprint from 1945)

Reimann, A. (1976). Phonetische Untersuchungen über lautabhängige Vokallängen im Sprechen redegestörter Jugendlicher. *Die Sprachheilarbeit, 21,* 1-14.

Schäferskϋpper, P. (1981). *Stoerungen der zeitlichen Kontrollmechanismen in nicht gestotterten Aeusserungen von Stotterern.* Final report of grant Po 121/7 of the Deutsche Forschungsgemeinschaft.

Starkweather, C.W., Franklin, Sh. & Smigo, Th.M. (1984). Vocal and finger reaction times in stutterers and nonstutterers: Differences and correlations. *Journal of Speech and Hearing Research, 27,* 193-196.

Stock, E. (1980). Untersuchungen zur Form, Bedeutung und Funktion der Intonation im Deutschen, *Schriften zur Phonetik, Sprachwissenschaft und Kommunikationsforschung, 18,* Berlin: Akademie Verlag.

Van Riper, Ch. (1971). *The Nature of Stuttering.* Englewood Cliffs: Prentice Hall.

Watson, B. (1987). Coordination of prephonatory events in mild and severe stutterers. In H.F.M. Peters & W. Hulstijn (Eds.), *Speech Motor Dynamics in Stuttering.* Wien: Springer Verlag.

Watson, B. & Alfonso, P.J. (1982). A comparison of LRT and VOT values between stutterers and nonstutterers. *Journal of Fluency Disorders, 7,* 219-242.

Wieneke, G. & Janssen, P. (1987). Duration variation in the fluent speech of stutterers and nonstutterers. In H.F.M. Peters & W. Hulstijn (Eds.), *Speech Motor Dynamics in Stuttering.* Wien: Springer Verlag.

Chapter 25

The Effects of Fluency Inducing Conditions on the Variability in the Duration of Laryngeal Movements during Stutterers' Fluent Speech

Peggy Janssen and George Wieneke

INTRODUCTION

It seems to be a well documented fact that stutterers have slower phonatory and articulatory initiation times than normal speakers, even when they produce speech that is seemingly fluent (Adams & Hayden, 1976; Starkweather et al., 1976; Hillman & Gilbert, 1977; McFarlane & Prins, 1978; Cross & Luper, 1979; Prosek et al. 1979; McFarlane & Shipley, 1981; Reich et al., 1981; Hayden et al., 1982; Healey & Gutkin, 1984; Horii, 1984; Starkweather et al., 1984). However, evidence for this supposed neuro-motor dysfunction among stutterers stems, for the greater part, from studies with adult stutterers who were or had recently been in therapy at the time of data collection. Some researchers have, therefore, recognized the possibility that the stutterers' slowness may be attributed to coping behavior, that is, learned, adaptive, or in some instances maladaptive responses designed to avoid disruptions in the flow of speech.

It is our contention that the temporal variability in the initiation and execution of speech movements may be a less confounding measure of instability of the motor system than is speed. Although there is an inherent variability in speech production, the consistency of the motor output in repeated utterances of the same speech material provides an excellent opportunity to determine if there are meaningful differences in the motor control evidenced by stutterers and nonstutterers. In a previous study (Janssen et al., 1983) we investigated this matter and found that stutterers were more variable than normally fluent speakers in the initiation of phonatory and articulatory movements of perceptually fluent monosyllablic words. In contrast, the speed with which these movements were produced was more or less equal for both groups.

If stutterers, or at least a subgroup of stutterers, are characterized by having difficulty in stabilizing phonatory and articulatory movements, it may be hypothesized that any condition which facilitates the production of speech will reduce this instability. Conditions which have been shown to induce fluent speech among stutterers, such as whispering, choral reading, or rhythmic pacing, may be such conditions. Although the precise mechanisms underlying the effectiveness of these conditions are not yet fully understood, several authors (Perkins et al., 1979; Andrews et al., 1982) have suggested that the common element could be a simplification of the motor control task which may be achieved in a variety of ways. These considerations led to the present study. More specifically, we asked the following questions:

1. Is the difference that we found between stutterers and nonstutterers in the variability with which they initiate phonologically identical utterances also present in running speech?
2. If so, will this difference between stutterers and non-stutterers disappear under conditions which are known to induce fluent speech among those who stutter?
3. If so, can the greater variability be considered a manifestation of general instability in the stutterers' motor system, or should it be ascribed to noise factors, such as variations in speaking rate or the presence of specific variable segments due to, for instance, phonetic constraints?

In this presentation we will deal with the first two questions. Our second chapter (Wieneke and Janssen, this volume, Chapter 26) will address the third question.

METHOD

Subjects

The experimental subjects consisted of 19 stutterers, 4 females and 15 males. They were diagnosed stutterers who had not undergone therapy for their stuttering during the last five years. Nine of the subjects were subjectively diagnosed as severe, six as moderate and four as mild. Their age ranged from 16 to 40, with a mean age of 22 years. In the nonstuttering group there were 7 females and 13 males. Their age ranged from 16 to 40 years, with a mean of 20 years. The educational level of the subjects in the two groups approximated each other.

Procedure

Each subject read a series of four sentences that appeared one by one on a TV screen under computer control. This series was repeated ten times, or as many times as necessary to obtain ten perceptually fluent productions of each sentence. Fluency was defined in this study as speech that was free of any kind of disfluency and reading errors. The ten fluent productions of the four test sentences were collected under five conditions:

1. Normal oral reading.
2. Chorus reading, reading in unison with the experimenter.
3. Rhythmic reading, reading in time to the beat of a metronome. The metronome was set at 100 beats per minute.
4. Reading under delayed auditory feedback, with the delay set at 200 msec.
5. Reading with masking noise. For this condition the Edinburgh Masker was used.

In order to reduce the possibility of reading errors or disfluencies, the subjects were familiarized with the stimulus material and with the task in each condition by giving them practice trials before each condition. The order of presentation of the conditions was the same for each subject.

Instrumentation

During the experimental reading trials, vibrations of the vocal folds and the speech signal were recorded. Vibrations of the vocal folds were measured by means of an electroglottograph (F-J Electronics Type EG 830, output 25 Hz - 10 kHz) using surface electrodes placed on each side of the thyroid notch and recorded on an instrumentation tape recorder (Ampex FR 1300A). The speech signal was transduced by means of a microphone positioned approximately 20 cm from the subject's mouth and recorded on a second channel of the tape recorder.

Data Analysis

The current report has reference to only one test sentence. Measurements of the EGG-signal were made from paper transcriptions. The successive voiced and voiceless segments in each production of the test sentence in each condition could be easily identified on the basis of the presence or absence of vocal fold vibrations in the EGG-signal (see Figure 1).

Each voiced segment contained a voiced phoneme or phoneme cluster and each voiceless segment contained a voiceless phoneme or phoneme cluster and/or a pause. In this way for each subject in each condition a typical number of voiced and voiceless segments was obtained across the ten repetitions of the test sentence, as can be seen in Figure 1. However, due to different phonetic realizations of the sentence, there occasionally were differences in the number of voiced and voiceless segments that were identified across the ten repetitions of the sentence by one subject. Two irregularities could occur: (1) within a voiced segment containing two syllables a short pause was inserted resulting in an extra voiceless segment, and/or (2) a voiceless segment containing a short pause or a voiceless consonant was left out resulting in a contraction of two voiced segments. In dealing with the first type we followed the convention of taking the two voiced segments and the extra voiceless interval together and counting them as one voiced segment.

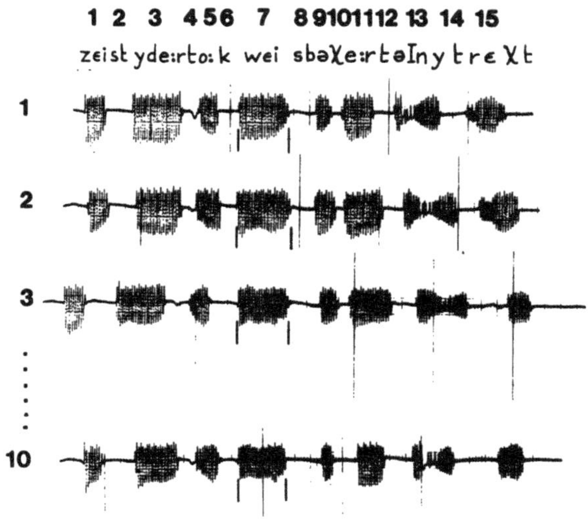

Figure 1. Graphic display of the first, second, third and tenth repetition of the test sentence "Zij studeert ook wijsbegeerte in Utrecht". The numbers displayed at the top correspond with the successive voiced and voiceless segments in the test sentence. The onsets and offsets of vocal fold vibration in the 7th sound segment are indicated by vertical lines.

When an irregularity of the second type occurred, the entire segment was excluded from the tally and disregarded from duration measurement.

Once each of the segments were identified the durations of the segments were measured and expressed in milliseconds. Measurement error was determined to be within 10 msec. The average value and standard deviation of each segment across the ten repetitions in each condition were computed for each subject. A relative measure of the variability of each segment across the ten repetitions was obtained by expressing the standard deviation as a coefficient of variation. The coefficient of variation that we used for this purpose was derived from the standard deviation by taking the square root of the variance in a segment divided by its mean. This relative measure was employed because there is a tendency for the variability of the duration of phonetic segments to vary with the mean duration of the segments. Finally, using this method, average intra-subject coefficients of variation were separately calculated for the voiced and voiceless segments in the test sentence. For each subject, in each condition, this yielded a variability score of the duration of glottal activity and a variability score of the duration of glottal inactivity.

To account for the slight deviation from normal distribution of the measured variables nonparametric tests were used to test for statistical significance of the data. Mann-Whitney U tests were used to determine if the stuttering and nonstuttering groups differed with respect to their variability scores. Wilcoxon matched-pairs signed-ranks tests were employed to assess within each group the significance of the differences between the normal oral reading condition and each of the four fluency-inducing conditions. Both analyses were carried out separately for the voiced and the voiceless segments.

RESULTS

Figure 2 presents the data with respect to the voiced segments. As may be evident from this figure, stutterers as a group were more variable during the normal reading condition than were the nonstutterers. Application of the Mann-Whitney U test (two-tailed test) revealed a highly significant difference ($z = 4.16$; $p < .001$). It is noteworthy, however, that under the fluency-enhancing conditions this between-group difference disappeared.

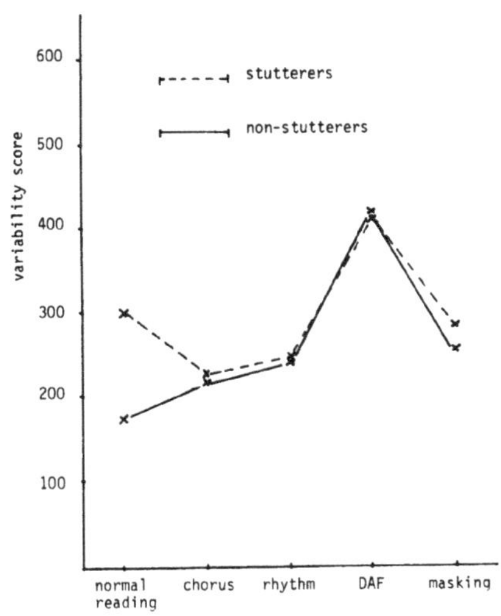

Figure 2. Mean variability in the duration of voiced segments during normal oral reading and four fluency-inducing conditions for the stuttering and non-stuttering groups.

Further analysis of the data of the sampled stutterers by means of Wilcoxon matched-pairs signed-ranks tests (two-tailed tests) indicated that stutterers' mean coefficients of variation decreased significantly during the choral reading ($T = 25$; $p < .01$) and rhythm ($T = 44$; $p < .05$) conditions, and increased significantly during delayed auditory feedback ($T = 38.5$; $p < .05$). No significant change was found for the masking condition. In contrast, the variability of the nonstutterers increased significantly under choral reading ($T = 42$; $p < .05$), rhythm ($T = 24$; $p < .01$), delayed auditory feedback ($T = 7$; $p < .01$), and masking ($T = 50$; $p < .05$).

Similar results were obtained for the variability in the voiceless segments. As figure 3 makes evident, stutterers were more variable than nonstutterers in all conditions. As tested by Mann-Whitney U tests the increased variability present among the stutterers was primarily accounted for by the normal reading ($z = 4.31$; $p < .001$) and, to a lesser degree, the choral reading ($z = 3.02$; $p < .01$) conditions. No significant between-group differences were found during rhythm, delayed auditory feedback, and masking.

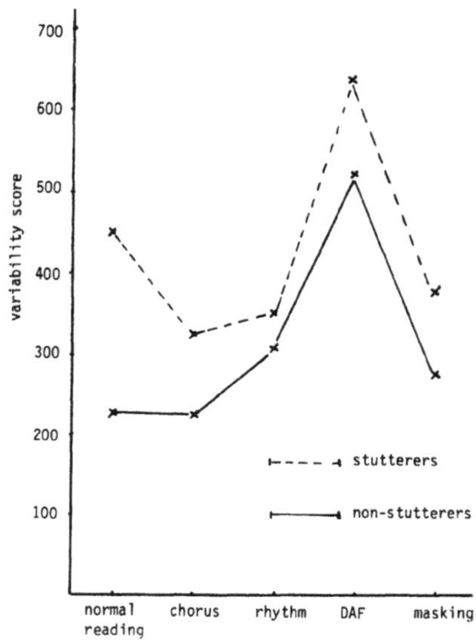

Figure 3. Mean variability in the duration of voiceless segments during normal oral reading and four fluency-inducing conditions for the stuttering and non-stuttering groups.

As tested by Wilcoxon matched-pairs signed-ranks tests it appeared that for the stuttering group there was a significant decrease in variability during the choral reading ($T = 27.5$; $p < .01$) and rhythmic ($T = 32$; $p < .01$) conditions. The increase during delayed auditory feedback and the decrease during masking was not significant. The nonstutterers, on the other hand, showed significant increases in variability during rhythmic speech ($T = 32$; $p < .01$), delayed auditory feedback ($T = 9$; $p < .01$), and masking ($T = 49.5$; $p < .05$).

It should be evident from these findings that the stutterers were more variable in the duration of their glottal activity and nonactivity during normal reading than were the nonstutterers and that this between-group difference disappeared under the fluency enhancing conditions.

Although the group differences that were observed during normal reading were highly significant, it is of interest to look at the individual performances of the subjects. This information is presented in Figure 4 which displays the frequency distributions of

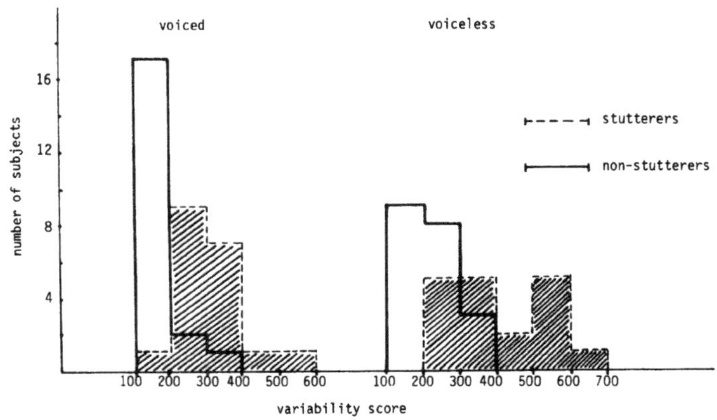

Figure 4. Frequency distribution of stutterers' and nonstutterers' variability scores during the normal oral reading condition. The numbers displayed on the horizontal axis are the boundaries of class intervals with a 100 msec range. The number of subjects falling within each class interval is shown on the vertical axis.

the variability scores of the stuttering and nonstuttering subjects. The left side of this figure illustrates the extent of overlap in the variability in the duration of the voiced segments. The right side shows the variability in the duration of the voiceless segments. Particularly with regard to the variability in the duration of the voiced segments, this figure clearly shows that there is a minimal amount of overlap between the two groups.

On the basis of these data, we have been led to conclude that the stutterers investigated in this study were characterized by greater variability in the duration of glottal activity and inactivity than were the nonstutterers. Whether these differences in variability can be attributed to an instability in the timing of the phonatory system or to noise factors, will be addressed in chapter 26 (Wieneke and Janssen, this volume).

REFERENCES

Adams, M.R. & Hayden, P. (1976). The ability of stutterers and nonstutterers to initiate and terminate phonation during production of an isolated vowel. *Journal of Speech and Hearing Research, 19,* 290-296.

Andrews, G., Howie, P.M., Dozsa, M. & Guitar, B.E. (1982). Stuttering: Speech pattern characteristics under fluency-inducing conditions. *Journal of Speech and Hearing Research, 25,* 208-216.

Cross, D.E. & Luper, H.L. (1979). Voice reaction time of stuttering and nonstuttering children and adults. *Journal of Fluency Disorders, 4,* 59-77.

Hayden, P.A., Jordahl, N. & Adams, M.R. (1982). Stutterers' voice initiation times during conditions of novel stimulation. *Journal of Fluency Disorders, 7,* 1-8.

Healey, E.C. & Gutkin, B. (1984). Analysis of stutterers' voice onset times and fundamental frequency contours during fluency. *Journal of Speech and Hearing Research, 27,* 219-225.

Hillman, R.E. & Gilbert, H.R. (1977). Voice onset time for voiceless stop consonants in the fluent reading of stutterers and nonstutterers. *Journal of the Acoustical Society of America, 61,* 610-611.

Horii, Y. (1984). Phonatory initiation, termination and vocal frequency change reaction times of stutterers. *Journal of Fluency Disorders, 9,* 115-124.

Janssen, P., Wieneke, G. & Vaane, E. (1983). Variability in the initiation of articulatory movements in the speech of stutterers and normal speakers. *Journal of Fluency Disorders, 8,* 341-358.

McFarlane, S.C. & Prins, D. (1978). Neural response time of stutterers and nonstutterers in selected oral motor tasks. *Journal of Speech and Hearing Research, 21,* 768-778.

McFarlane, S.C. & Shipley, K.G. (1981). Latency of vocalization onset for stutterers and nonstutterers under conditions of auditory and visual cueing. *Journal of Speech and Hearing Disorders, 46,* 307-312.

Perkins, W.H., Bell, J., Johnson, L. & Stocks, J. (1979). Phone rate and the effective planning time hypothesis of stuttering. *Journal of Speech and Hearing Research, 22,* 747-755.

Prosek, R., Montgomery, A.A., Walden, B.E. & Schwartz, D.M. (1979). Reaction time measures of stutterers and nonstutterers. *Journal of Fluency Disorders, 4,* 269-279.

Reich, A., Till, J. & Goldsmith, H. (1981). Laryngeal and manual reaction times of stuttering and nonstuttering adults. *Journal of Speech and Hearing Research, 24,* 192-196.

Starkweather, C.W., Hirschman, P. & Tannenbaum, R.S. (1976) Latency of vocalization onset: Stutterers versus nonstutterers. *Journal of Speech and Hearing Research, 19,* 481-492.

Starkweather, C.W., Franklin, S. & Smigo, T.M. (1984). Vocal and finger reaction times in stutterers and nonstutterers: Differences and correlations. *Journal of Speech and Hearing Research, 27,* 193-196.

Wieneke, G. & Janssen, P. (1987). Duration variations in the fluent speech of stutterers and nonstutterers. In H.F.M. Peters & W. Hulstijn (Eds.), *Speech Motor Dynamics in Stuttering.* Wien: Springer Verlag.

Chapter 26

Duration Variations in the Fluent Speech of Stutterers and Nonstutterers

George Wieneke and Peggy Janssen

INTRODUCTION

Previous investigations of the timing of speech motor responses of stutterers (Janssen et al., 1983; Janssen and Wieneke, this volume, Chapter 25) have indicated that stutterers were more variable in their segmental timing during oral reading than nonstutterers. The aim of the present study was to analyze further the measured durational variability in the speech of stutterers (Janssen and Wieneke, this volume, Chapter 25). An interesting question is, whether the greater variability can be considered a manifestation of general instability in the stutterers' motor system, or whether there are other reasons for it. We considered two possible reasons. Firstly the possibility that the greater variability evidenced by the stutterers was due to greater variability of speaking rate was explored. Secondly the possibility that the greater variability was due to one or more extremely variable segments was investigated.

METHODS

The experimental subjects consisted of 19 stutterers with a mean age of 22 years and 20 nonstutterers with a mean age of 20 years. Each subject read a series of four sentences that appeared one by one on a TV screen. The series of four sentences was repeated as many times as necessary to obtain ten fluent productions. The analysis in this chapter has reference to only one of the four sentences. During the experimental reading trials, vibrations of the vocal folds were measured by electroglottography (F-J Electronics EG830, 25-10000Hz). The duration of each voiced and voiceless segment in the ten repetitions of the test sentence was measured by hand from paper written records (accuracy 10 msec). The segments in each repetition of the test sentence were easily identified and means and standard deviations of the duration of these segments across the ten repetitions were calculated. In the stuttering group the average number of the voiced and voiceless segments in the test sentence was 16.3, in the nonstuttering group 15.3. The total number of segments were 309 for the stutterers and 306 for the nonstutterers. A relative measure of the variability of each segment across the ten repetitions was obtained by expressing the standard deviation as a coefficient of variation. The coefficient of variation that we used for this purpose was derived from the standard deviation by taking the square root of the variance in a segment divided by its mean. Details of the methods are described by Janssen and Wieneke (in chapter 25 of this volume).

RESULTS

Variations in Rate

Figure 1 has reference to the first of the possible reasons why the stutterers' timing was more variable. It shows a simulation of nine repetitions of a sentence containing five segments, when

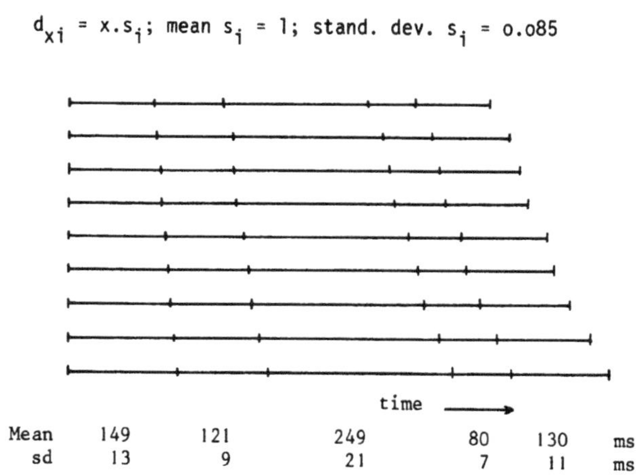

Figure 1. Segments generated by a model in which the variability is only due to variation in speaking rate. The formulas of the model are shown at the top: d(xi) = duration of segment x in the i° repetition; x = theoretical segment duration.

speaking rate is varied within a range of plus and minus 20%. The sentences are ordered according to their duration.

The variation of the total sentence duration is distributed proportionally over the five segments. The appropriateness of a simulation of the effects of variations in speaking rate as shown in figure 1 is demonstrated in phonetic experiments in which speaking rate was systematically varied (cf., Tuller and Kelso, 1984).

To quantify the influence of speaking rate on our measure of variability, we used a Spearman coefficient of correlation to establish the relation between the duration of each segment with the duration of the remaining sentence segments. In other words, we correlated the duration of the first segment with the sum of the durations of the second, third, fourth segment and so on. We also correlated the duration of the second segment with the sum of the durations of the first, third, fourth segment and so on. This procedure was repeated for each segment. If speaking rate is the source of variation then the correlation coefficient would be one. If instead the variation in the duration of the segments is due to random influences that were independent of speaking rate, the correlation coefficient would be zero.

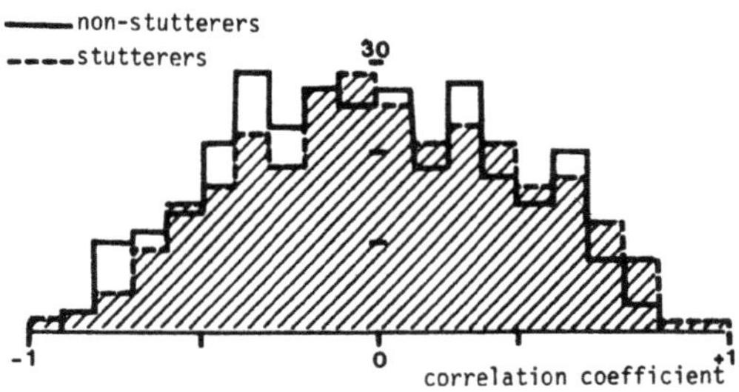

	median	positive significant	negative significant
non-stutterers	-0.05	5.7 %	10.1 %
stutterers	0.00	9.3 %	5.2 %

Figure 2. Histograms of spearman correlation coefficients between segment duration and corrected sentence duration for stutterers and non-stutterers.

The results that we obtained are depicted in Figure 2. The histograms shown here are based on segments which were present in seven or more of the repetitions of a subject. Also included in this figure are the medians and the percentages of statistically significant positive and negative values ($p \leq .05$, one tailed). Since the correlation coefficients are based on only seven to ten pairs of observations, the expected 90% range of the calculated coefficients for no correlation is about plus and minus .56. For both groups the median is close to zero, but the number of positive significant coefficients in the stuttering group was somewhat larger than the expected 5%. This increased number of positive significant values was interpreted as a slight shift of the central tendency of the distribution to positive values. Statistically it can be inferred that the ratio of the variance due to variations in speaking rate to the total variance is equal to or less than the mean value of the correlation coefficients. For example, when a correlation coefficient of .1 is found, a maximum of 10% of the total variance is due to the variations in the speaking rate. As we have pointed out already, the medians were close to zero for both groups. It may, therefore, be concluded that in both groups variations in speaking rate did not contribute substantially to the measured variance. Moreover, the small difference between the two groups cannot explain the about 100% increase of the mean variability in the stuttering subjects.

Segmental Inconsistency

The possibility that the stutterers' greater variability is a function of segmental inconsistency is addressed in Figure 3. Here, graphically illustrated, are two alternative possibilities for the shapes of the frequency distribution of the segmental variability of the two subject groups.

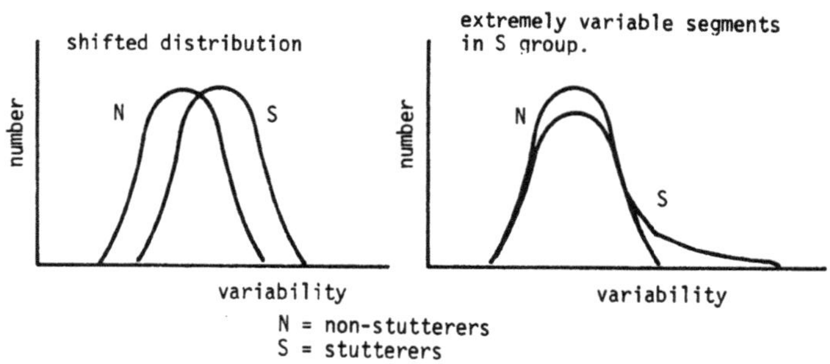

Figure 3. Two alternatives for increased variability in stutterers illustrated by the shape of the histograms of the variability among stutterers (S) and non-stutterers (N). For further explanation see text.

The increased variability evidenced by the stutterers may be brought about by either a shift in the distribution of the segmental variability towards increased values or by extreme values in some specific segments of the sentence that results because the stutterers anticipated a fluency break or a relatively difficult phonetic transition. To discriminate between these two possibilities, we used two tests. We examined the skewness of the coefficients of variation for each subject so as to determine presence of outlying values. It is evident that if the greater variability is a result of extreme values, skewness would be greater among the stutterers than among the nonstutterers.

As can be seen in Figure 4, intra-subject skewness is present for both the voiced and voiceless segments and for these categories combined. Clearly a positive skewness dominates, especially in the combined distribution.

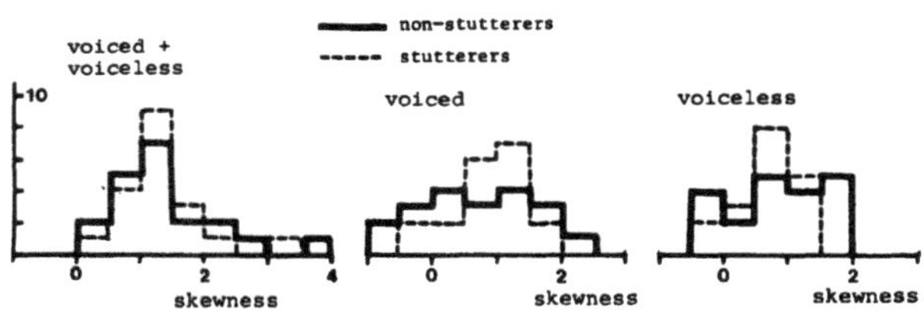

AVERAGE SKEWNESS

	voiced + voiceless	voiced	voiceless
non-stutterers	1.40	0.73	0.83
stutterers	1.36	0.90	0.80

Figure 4. Histograms of the skewness of the coefficient of variation of the segment durations in the sentence for 19 stutterers ans 20 non-stutterers. In the histograms at the right side the results for the voiced and voiceless segments are given separately.

Apparently, for both subject groups, a small amount of the segments shows an increased variability. However, the stutterers do not differ from the nonstutterers in this respect. The mean values are descriptively similar and when tested with a Mann-Whitney U test there are no significant differences; significance is not even approached.

The distribution of segment variability was evaluated in still another and more detailed way. It involved determining the subjects' variability ratio. This determination is illustrated in Figure 5, in which ten simulations of a sentence are given with five segments varying randomly in duration. In this theoretical example, the standard deviation of the durations are proportional to the square root of the duration according to:

$$sd_x = p_x * \sqrt{d_x}$$

d_x = duration of segment x
sd_x = standard deviation of duration of segment x
p_x = constant = coefficient of variation

On this basis, the coefficient of variation of the third segment is three times greater than that of the other segments. It follows that because of its greater variability, the duration of the third segment has much more of an effect on sentence duration than the duration of the other segments. As a result, the slope of the regression line of the segment duration on the sentence duration will be steeper for the third segment than for the other segments. The third segment can be distinguished in this way.

The variability ratio we used, was defined as the slope of the regression line of the segmental duration on the sentence duration, divided by the relative mean segment duration. Under the assumption that the segment durations are uncorrelated, the theoretical value is equal to the variance of the segment divided by the sum of the variances of all the segments in the sentence, normalized for the relative mean segment duration, according to the formula:

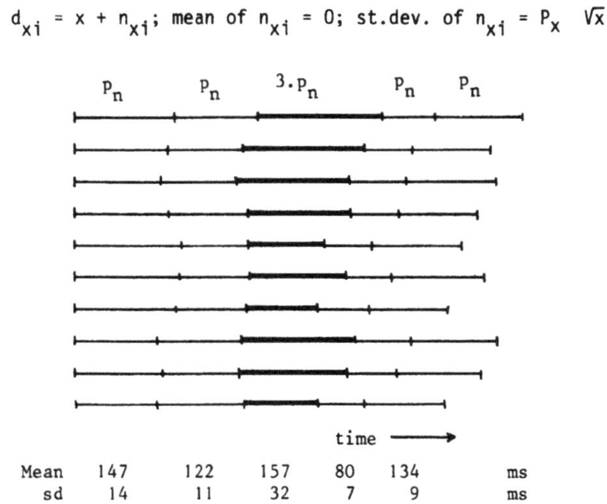

Figure 5. Segments generated by a model with random variability of the segments. The variability of the third segment (thick line) is three times that of the other segments. The standard deviation of the duration of a segment is proportional to the square root of the duration.

$E[vr_x] = (sd^2{}_x \,/\, \Sigma sd^2{}_i)/(d_x \,/\, d_s)$

$E[vr_x]$ = expected value of variability ratio
d_i = duration of segment i
sd_i = standard deviation of duration of segment i
Σ = summation over segments in sentence
D_x = segment duration averaged over repetitions
D_s = sentence duration averaged over repetitions

It follows from this that, if all segments have the same variability, the variability ratio is approximately one. However, if one of the segments is more variable than the other segments, as is the case in segment 3, the variability ratio is approximately the ratio of the squared coefficient of variation of the segment to the segmental mean, according to the formula:

$E[vr_x] \simeq (p^2{}_x \,/\, p^2{}_n)$

p_x = coefficient of variation of segment x
p_n = coefficient of variation of all the segments except segment x

Histograms were made of the variability ratios of the about 300 segments of the subjects in each group. The results are shown in Figure 6. Clearly, a small number of segments in both groups is much more variable than the majority of the segments. As a consequence of that, the maximum of the distribution is not equal to one but becomes smaller. The observed maxima of the histograms appeared to be about .5 for the stuttering group and about .7 for the nonstuttering group. The histogram is quantified at the bottom of figure 6.

The class interval is enlarged to 1.5, which is slightly larger than the value of the standard deviation, under the assumption that

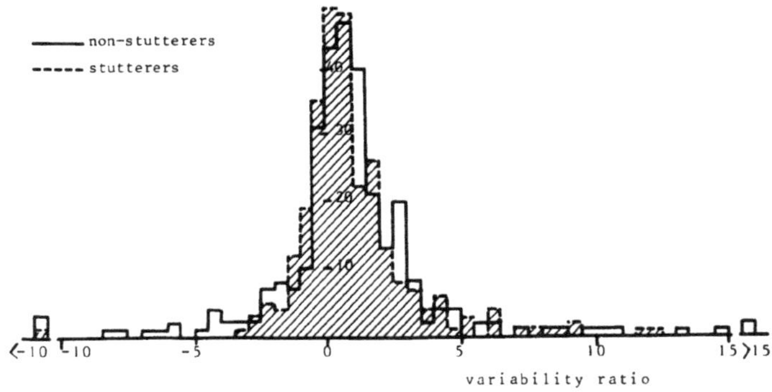

Number of values in the classes:

	-3.5	-2.0	-0.5	1.0	2.5	4.0	5.5		N=
non-stutterers	16	11	25	121	74	30	8	14	299
stutterers	1	9	35	132	61	19	10	12	279

Figure 6. Histograms of the variability ratios for all segments of the stutterers (hatched) area and non-stutterers.

all segments have the same variability. In the table, the outermost two classes on the right and left are outside the +/- 3 sigma range. For both groups, about 10% of the variability ratios are above or below these limits. Thus, a greater amount of extremely variable segments is present than would be expected by chance. However, the number of these segments is approximately the same for both subject groups. Yet, a comparison of the distribution in the classes of the two groups give a significant chi-square value with a p-value smaller than 2%. This result is almost exclusively due to the difference in the outermost left class. Here the variability ratios are smaller than -3.5 and 16 of the 17 values were specific to the nonstutterers. In fact, the histograms show that there was a smaller number of extremely variable segments among the stutterers than among the nonstutterers. Thus, the results of this test do not support the alternative hypothesis that the increased variability of stutterers is due to extremely variable segments. To the contrary, the results suggest that the segmental variability of the stutterers is substantially greater than that of the nonstutterers.

CONCLUSION

On the basis of the data of the present study we have been led to conclude that: speaking rate is not an important source of variability, and the increased variability that the stutterers evidence is not due to extremely variable segments. These findings seem to suggest that durational variability is a functional property of the speech motor system of stutterers.

REFERENCES

Janssen, P. & Wieneke, G. (1987). The effects of fluency-inducing conditions on the variability in the duration of laryngeal movements during stutterers' fluent speech. In H.F.M. Peters & W. Hulstijn (Eds.), *Speech Motor Dynamics in Stuttering.* Wien: Springer Verlag.

Janssen, P., Wieneke, G. & Vaane, E. (1983). Variability in the initiation of articulatory movements in the speech of stutterers and normal speakers. *Journal of Fluency Disorders, 8,* 341-358.

Tuller, B. & Kelso, J.A.S. (1984). The timing of articulatory gestures: Evidence for relational invariants. *Journal of the Acoustical Society of America, 76,* 1030-1036.

Chapter 27

A Model of Stuttering and the Production of Speech under Delayed Auditory Feedback Conditions

Jonathan Harrington

INTRODUCTION

The models of stuttering and speech produced under delayed auditory feedback conditions to be discussed in this chapter are based on some recent theories of linguistic rhythm (Martin, 1972; Shields, McHugh & Martin, 1974; Fowler, 1983). If, as has been suggested (Abercrombie, 1967; Donovan & Darwin, 1979), the perception of speech is rhythmic, a speaker must presumably control the intervals between the units of the rhythmic structure the listener perceives; in a stress timed language, such as English, these units are considered to be coincident with stressed syllables (Abercrombie, 1967). At the same time, suppose a listener is able to hypothesize the rhythmic structure intended by the speaker, based on his current perception of the relative time at which the units of the rhythmic structure occur in the speaker's utterance; in this case, the listener should be able to predict when *future* units of the rhythmic structure (i.e. stressed syllable in English) will be perceived (Shields, McHugh and Martin, 1974). The relationship between the units of a rhythmic structure encoded as part of the speech production plan and the listener's prediction of the time of occurrence of future units is fundamental to the model of delayed auditory feedback discussed below. In this chapter, it is suggested that delayed auditory feedback causes the speaker to predict the time of occurrence of a future (stressed) syllable in his own speech production which is at variance with the time at which the speaker has planned to produce the same (stressed) syllable. The attempted correction of this asynchrony is considered to be the source of the production of disfluent speech under DAF conditions.

The model of stuttering also depends on the relationship between the expected time of auditory perception of a syllable and its planned time of production. In addition, the model of stuttering is based on some theoretical and experimental work which suggests that rhythm is not simply focussed on stressed syllables in English, but on the relative time of occurrence of *vowels* of stressed syllables (Huggins, 1972; Allen, 1972; Tuller & Fowler, 1980; Fowler, 1983). This idea forms the basis for explaining why the vowel, in its entirety, is not realised as part of a stuttering disfluency when stutterers produce monosyllables in isolation (see Chapter 30; Wingate, 1977; Van Riper, 1982).

A MODEL OF THE PRODUCTION OF SPEECH UNDER DELAYED AUDITORY FEEDBACK

In the model of speech introduced under DAF conditions in Figure 1, a (fluent) speaker plans to produce two monosyllables, S1 and S2 such that S2 is produced *v* (arbitrary) units of time after S1 (box 1); since the speaker has planned to produce S2 *v* units of time after S1, the expected time of perception of S2 is also *v* units after S1 (box 2). It is assumed that the delay time in the delayed auditory feedback device is set to around 180 msec, since this is often cited as the delay which is most effective in disrupting the

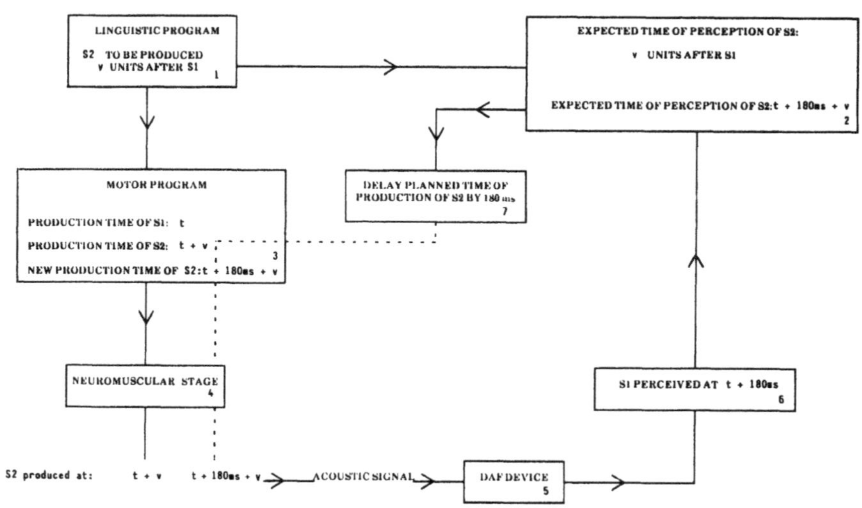

Figure 1. A model of the production of speech under delayed auditory feedback conditions when a (fluent) subject plans to produce two syllables, S1 and S2 at an interval of *v* (arbitrary units of time).

fluent production of speech (Black, 1951; Fairbanks, 1955). Since roughly six syllables are produced per second in connected speech (Lenneberg, 1967), S1 will be auditorily perceived at about the same time that S2 is produced.

Let the time of production of S1 be t units (box 3). In this case, S2 will have to be produced at $t + v$ if speech production is to be executed as planned (i.e. such that the S2 is produced v units after S1). Suppose, when the speaker begins to receive auditory feedback from S1, a prediction is made as to when S2 will be auditorily perceived. Since S1 is perceived at t + *180 msec*, the expected time of perception of S2 will be t + *180 msec* + v (box 2). Thus the plan for speech production specifies that the production time of S2 should be $t + v$, but its expected time of S2 is 180 msec earlier than expected, a correction of this asynchrony takes place (box 7) in which the time of production of S2 is delayed by 180 msec. If S2 is being produced at $t + v$ when this asynchrony with its expected time of perception occurs, delaying the time of production of S2 could be achieved by a prolongation of part of S2. Prolongation of syllables and a reduction in tempo are both reported characteristics of speech produced under DAF conditions (Black, 1951; Spilka, 1954).

A MODEL OF THE PRODUCTION OF STUTTERING

The model of delayed auditory feedback described above suggests that disfluent speech is caused by a *delay* in the expected time of perception of the syllable with respect to the time at which the speaker has planned to produce the syllable. If, as some have reported (Von Lotzmann, 1961; Goldiamond, 1965), delayed auditory feedback makes stutterers' speech production more fluent, the production of stuttering disfluencies may be caused by *premature* expected time of perception with respect to the planned time of production of a syllable. Informally, this would mean a stutterer expects to hear himself saying an intended syllable too soon relative to the time at which the syllable will be produced; the reason why DAF makes stutterers more fluent would then be because the asynchronies between expected time of perception and planned time of production are cancelled out.

Figure 2 shows a model of the production of stuttering in the context of a /CV/ target syllable. Two further assumptions are incorporated into this model which are implicit in the model of DAF described above. First, following Fowler, (1980), autonomous, coordinated strategies govern the production of consonants and vowels. In the model in Figure 2, coordination takes place at the motor programming stage which includes a specification that /C/ must be produced i units before /V/ for the production of /CV/ to be properly coordinated in time (box 3). Second, a prediction is made that /V/ will be auditorily perceived an arbitrary number of units of time (box 2) after the coordination of /C/ and /V/ at the motor programming stage.

Suppose the expected time of perception of the vowel is k units early with respect to the time of production of the vowel.

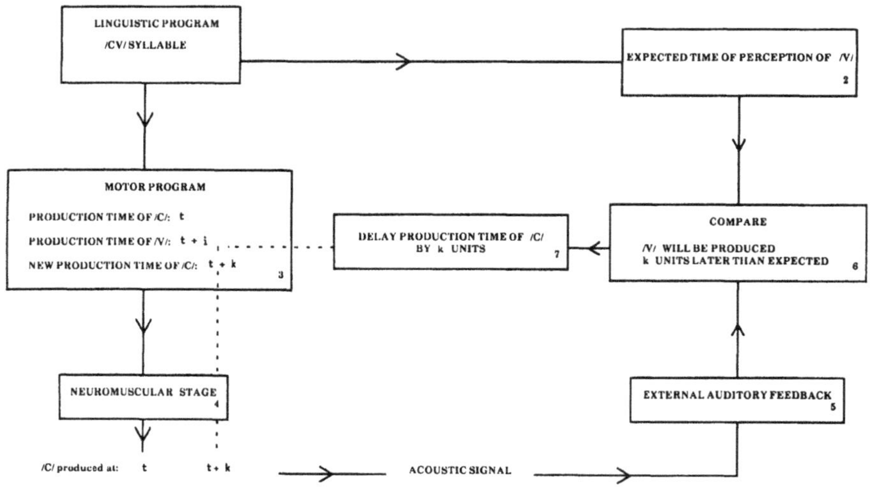

Figure 2. A model of the production of stuttering in the context of a /CV/ target syllable. The expected time of auditory perception of the vowel is *k* (arbitrary) units of time early with respect to the time at which /V/ will be produced. This can lead to a repetition of /C/ *k* units after the initial production of /C/; or else /C/ is prolonged by *k* units.

Thus, following the neuromuscular stage of speech production, a comparison is made between how much of the syllable has actually been produced and the expected time of perception of the vowel: this comparison (box 6) shows that the vowel will be produced *k* units later than expected. Such a conclusion leads to a recalculation and a delay in the time production of the consonant (box 7). This is because, if box 6 concludes that the vowel will be produced *k* units later than originally expected, box 7 will conclude that the vowel is going to be produced, not *i* units after the time of production of the consonant (as originally planned), but *i* + *k* units after the time of production of /C/. Thus, box 7 *incorrectly* concludes that the autonomous strategies governing consonant and vowel production are malcoordinated. The source of the production of the stuttering disfluency is the correction of this incorrectly detected malcoordination between consonant and vowel production strategies: to correct this apparent malcoordination, the time of production of /C/ will have to be delayed by *k* units. Suppose the consonant was being produced at time *t* when this 'error' is detected: in this case, the consonant will be produced once at *t* and then once again at *t* + *k*: the outcome, then, is a *repetition* of /C/. Alternatively, if the value of *k* is sufficiently small, the vocal tract might maintain the same configuration for *k* units: in this case, the result is a *prolongation* of /C/ by *k* units.

CONCLUSIONS

The model of stuttering can begin to provide an explanation for some of the conditions which are known to make stutterers more fluent as well as some of the characteristics of stuttered speech itself. Under binaural masking, a condition which is known to make stutterers more fluent (Cherry & Sayers, 1956; Conture, 1974), the auditory perception of syllables is eliminated. If a stutterer cannot hear his own speech production, it is unlikely that a prediction will be made of when future syllables will be heard. In this case, the frequency of stuttering should be considerably reduced, if the production of stuttered speech is caused by making an incorrect (i.e. early) prediction of the time of auditory perception of the vowel of the syllable. In metronome speech, the speaker plans to align the clicks with vowels of syllables (Tuller & Fowler, 1980; Fowler, 1983). Since the clicks occur at acoustically isochronous intervals, it should be possible to make a *correct* prediction of when future clicks occur. If a correct prediction can be made of the time of occurrence of future clicks, it should also be possible to predict correctly the time at which future vowels will be heard, since the goal in metronome speech is to align vowels with clicks. If a correct prediction can be made of the time of occurrence of future vowels, the frequency of stuttering should be considerably reduced, if the cause of the production of stuttered speech is premature auditory expectation of the vowel of the syllable. Finally, the model can account for the improved fluency when stutterers are subjected to delayed auditory feedback conditions since, in this case, the asynchronies between expected time of perception and actual time of production are cancelled out.

The model of stuttering accounts for both repetitions and prolongations. In addition, the model predicts that neither the vowel in its entirety, nor tautosyllabic, post-vocalic consonants, can be produced as part of the disfluency since the expected time of perception is focussed on the vowel of the syllable (and stuttered speech necessarily 'breaks off' before this point of rhythmic focus [1]). The model may also begin to explain the predominance of stuttering in the context of stressed syllables (Wingate, 1977). Following Abercrombie (1967), the perception of rhythm in English depends largely on the intervals between stressed syllables, and in a finger-tapping experiment by Allen (1972), in which subjects were asked to tap out the rhythm of an utterance, subjects placed their downbeats in the vicinity of vowels of *stressed* syllables. Translated into this present model, values of expected time of perception would only be assigned to vowels of stressed syllables, and this is why stuttering on unstressed syllables is less probable.

ACKNOWLEDGEMENTS

I am grateful to Francis Nolan, Bob Ladd and Jonathan Dalby for reading earlier drafts of this chapter and providing many helpful suggestions.

NOTES

[1] If equivalence can be assumed between the point of rhythmic focus, as defined here, and the term 'Perceptual Center', first used by Morton, Marcus and Frankish (1976) to mean a syllable's 'psychological moment of occurrence', the model would predict that a stuttering disfluency breaks off at the syllable's perceptual center. When speakers produce syllables in time to regularly repeating clicks of a metronome, the perceptual center of a syllable is coincident with the click.

REFERENCES

Abercrombie, D. (1967). *Elements of General Phonetics.* Edinburgh: Edinburgh University Press.

Allen, G.D. (1972). The location of rhythmic stress beats in English: an experimental study I. *Language and Speech, 15,* 72-100.

Black, J.W. (1951). The effect of delayed sidetone upon vocal rate and intensity. *Journal of Speech and Hearing Disorders, 16,* 56-60.

Cherry, C. & Sayers, B. (1956). Experiments upon the total inhibition of stammering by external controls and some clinical results. *Journal of Psychosomatic Research, 1,* 233-246.

Conture, E. (1974). Some effects of noise on the speaking behavior of stutterers. *Journal of Speech and Hearing Research, 20,* 661-668.

Donovan, A. & Darwin, C. (1979). The perceived rhythm of speech. *Proceedings of the Ninth International Congress of Phonetic Sciences, 2,* 268-274.

Fairbanks, G. (1955). Selective vocal effects of delayed auditory feedback. *Journal of Speech and Hearing Disorders, 20,* 333-345.

Fowler, C.A. (1980). Coarticulation and theories of extrinsic timing. *Journal of Phonetics, 8,* 113-133.

Fowler, C.A. (1983). Converging sources of evidence on spoken and perceived rhythms of speech: cyclic productions of vowels in monosyllabic stress feet. *Journal of Experimental Psychology: General, 112* (3), 386-412.

Goldiamond, I. (1965). Stuttering and fluency as manipulatable operant response classes. In L. Krasner & L.P. Ullman (Eds.), *Research in Behavior Modification.* New York: Holt, Rinehart & Winston.

Harrington, J. (1987). Coarticulation and stuttering: an acoustic and electropalatographic study. In H.F.M. Peters & W. Hulstijn (Eds.), *Speech Motor Dynamics in Stuttering*. Wien: Springer Verlag.

Huggins, A. (1972). On the perception of temporal phenomena in speech. *Journal of the Acoustical Society of America, 51* (4), 1279-1290.

Lenneberg, E.H. (1967). *Biological Foundations of Language*. New York: J. Wiley & Sons.

Martin, J. (1972). Rhythmic (hierarchical) versus serial structure in speech and other behavior. *Psychological Review, 79,* 487-509.

Morton, J., Marcus, S. & Frankish, C. (1976). Perceptual centers. *Psychological Review, 83* (5), 405-408.

Shields, J.L., McHugh, A. & Martin, J.G. (1974). Reaction time to phoneme targets as a function of rhythmic cues in continuous speech. *Journal of Experimental Psychology, 102,* 250-255.

Spilka, B. (1954). Some vocal effects of different reading passages and time delays in speech feedback. *Journal of Speech and Hearing Disorders, 19,* 37-47.

Tuller, B. & Fowler, C.A. (1980). Some articulatory correlates of perceptual isochrony. *Perception and Psychophysics, 27* (4), 277-283.

Van Riper, C. (1982). *The Nature of Stuttering*. (2nd edition) New Jersey: Prentice-Hall.

Von Lotzmann, G. (1961). Zur Anwendung variierter Verzoegerungszeiten bei Balbuties. *Folia Phoniatrica, 13,* 276-312.

Wingate, M.E. (1977). Immediate source of stuttering. In R.W. Rieber & J. Wollock (Eds.), *The Problem of Stuttering: Theory and Therapy*. New York: Elsevier, North Holland Inc.

Chapter 28

Factors Affecting Fluency in Stutterers when Speaking under Altered Auditory Feedback

Peter Howell, Nirit El-Yaniv and David J. Powell

INTRODUCTION

If the auditory feedback of a normal speaker is altered, speech control suffers. When, for example, a delay is introduced between when a sound is spoken and when it is heard (delayed auditory feedback, DAF), speech rate decreases and all types of speech error are made. The original explanation of these effects was that speakers normally monitor their auditory feedback in order to check that the speech is being produced correctly. Thus, when auditory feedback is artificially interfered with, speech control suffers.

In contrast to the poorer control in normal speakers when feedback is altered, speech control in stutterers improves. In line with the explanations originally proposed for normals, the stutterers were thought to have an auditory feedback monitoring problem in their speech which is rectified by altering feedback.

However, explanations of speech control which propose that normal speakers monitor auditory feedback have been critically assessed recently. For example, Howell, Powell and Khan (1983) have offered an explanation of how the disruptive effects of DAF arise which does not require that the altered sound is used as feedback. (See also Lane and Tranel, 1971 for a non-feedback account of the effects of amplifying and attenuating voice level.) If auditory feedback monitoring explanations of these effects do not apply to normals, it is unlikely that they account for the improvement that occurs in stutterers speech either.

The forms of alteration which have been shown to improve stutterers speech include DAF of the speaker's voice, a buzz masking noise (the Edinburgh masker), a metronome and the sound of one or several other peoples voices. One aspect shared by all these forms is that they involve presentation of a temporally-structured sound. Though this indicates the potential importance of this factor, there have been no systematic studies designed to establish what temporal structure a sound should have to produce best motor control in stutterers. In fact, some characteristics which would seem to be desirable from an a priori view do not figure in current forms of altered feedback.

For one thing, though the position in words where most speech problems occur is at onset (see, for example, Johnson and Brown, 1939, Hahn, 1942, Taylor, 1966 and Sheehan, 1974). However, certain of the altered feedback treatments listed above do not present any sound at onset. This applies to DAF and the Edinburgh masker (with the Edinburgh masker, triggering fails to occur with low amplitude, usually devoiced, sounds). Assuming that the sound that is presented has some local effect on speech control, it would seem advisable for signals to occur in this position.

One form of altered feedback which can be presented synchronous with speech is a frequency-shifted version of the speaker's own voice. In the experiments described below, speech is shifted down in frequency by an octave. In experiments 1 and 2, the effect of speaking under such frequency-shifted feedback are compared against DAF (Experiment 1) and the Edinburgh masker (Experiment 2). In each case, frequency-shifted feedback causes greatest reduction in disfluency.

Though these experiments show that it is desirable for the altered sound to occur at sound onset, they do not establish whether it is necessary to have the altered sounds on throughout words. This is tested in experiment 3 where the effect on fluency of having frequency-shifted feedback on right through a syllable is compared with having it at syllable onset alone. This shows that speech control is almost as good as if it is on throughout.

Timing information might also be given to the speaker by the pitch of a sound. The manufacturers of the Edinburgh masker state that this is one reason why their apparatus produces improved speech control. In the final experiment the effect of having an altered sound which covaries in pitch with that of the voice is assessed.

EXPERIMENT 1

In this experiment, number of disfluent episodes was measured in order to compare the effects on speech control of speaking under DAF with the effects of speaking under frequency-shifted feedback. It is expected that both forms of altered feedback will reduce disfluency rate but the reduction will be less under DAF because no sound is presented at the point where most disfluencies occur (sound onset).

Method

Subjects. Six stutterers were employed in the present experiment. Five were male. The number of blocks per hundred words during conversation ranged from 3 to 16 (mean 6.3/100).
Test material. The subjects were required to read a standard piece of prose under three conditions. The prose selected was the story of Arthur the rat.
Procedure. The three conditions in which the story was read were DAF, feedback shifted in frequency by an octave and normal auditory feedback (NAF) as a control.

When the stutterers had to speak under DAF, their voice was recorded by microphone. The output of the microphone was low-pass filtered at 4.5 kHz and the output of the filter was led to a computer which was programmed to operate as a delay line (the filter roll-off here, and throughout the present chapter was 48 dB/octave). The computer sampled the speech into a storage buffer at a 10 kHz rate. Output of the samples lagged behind their input so as to produce the required delay. When the end of the buffer was reached (either for sampling or replay), the program cycled round and reused the initial space (this part of the buffer having been finished with). In this experiment, speech was always delayed by 50 msec, this delay being chosen as Lotzmann (1961) has shown that it is optimal for the majority of stutterers. After the delay, the speech was low-pass filtered (again at 4.5 kHz) and played back to the stutterer at the same level as the stutterer had originally produced.

In the frequency-shifted feedback condition, recording of the original speech and playback to the subject were performed in more-or-less the same way as in the DAF condition (the only difference was in the cutoff frequency of the low-pass filter at output of the computer - see below). The principal difference was in the processing performed by the computer. Speech was shifted down in frequency by 50% (i.e. down an octave) as follows; the speech was digitized into the computer at a 10 kHz rate. In each 10-msec interval, the speech was only sampled for the first 5 msec. This 5-msec worth of speech was played out over 10 msec (i.e., twice the gap was left between successive samples so that the samples collected over 5 msec took 10 msec to play back). The cutoff of the low-pass filter at output was set at 2.2 kHz (i.e., at about half the value of the input samples to avoid aliassing caused by changing the output sample rate). The level of the output was adjusted to be the same as that the speaker originally used.

In the NAF control condition, the speech was digitized and output at the same sampling rate as used under DAF (i.e. 10 kHz) and low-pass filtered and its level set in the same way as under DAF too. The only difference was that no delay was introduced between when the samples were taken and when they were replayed.

The order in which the stutterers read the story under the three feedback conditions was counterbalanced across subjects to prevent adaptation effects. In all conditions, the subjects were instructed to read the story at as normal a rate as possible whilst attempting to maintain maximum fluency. Each reading was recorded on audio tape for analysis (performed after the experiment was completed).

Results and Discussion

The number of syllables that each stutterer was disfluent on was counted (counting repeated attempts at a syllable or when a sound was prolonged as one disfluent syllable). Sounds of more than 1 sec in duration were counted as prolongations in all experiments in this chapter.

The mean number of disfluencies across stutterers was 37 under NAF, 6.17 under DAF and 2.3 under frequency-shifted feedback. The difference between the number of disfluencies in the NAF and DAF conditions and between the NAF and frequency-shifted conditions were significant by sign test ($p < .05$ in each case). Additionally, the difference in number of disfluencies between DAF and frequency-shifted feedback was significant by sign test ($p < .05$). Thus these analyses show that fewer disfluencies occur when an altered sound is presented. However, there are differences in disfluency reduction between different types of altered feedback with alterations which present no sound at onset (DAF) producing a higher disfluency rate than sounds with no delay (frequency-shifted feedback).

EXPERIMENT 2

In the introduction it was mentioned that the sound produced by the Edinburgh masker does not start simultaneously with vocalisation. Moreover, evidence was reported in experiment 1 to show that DAF, which also has this characteristic, is not as satisfactory as frequency-shifted feedback which can be presented synchronous with speech. For these reasons it would be expected that the Edinburgh masker would have some of the disadvantages noted in connection with DAF too. In the present experiment, the effects on the speech of stutterers of shifting speech down in frequency by an octave are compared with those produced by the Edinburgh masker.

Method

Subjects. Six stutterers were employed in the present experiment. All were male. The number of blocks per hundred words ranged from 4 to 14 (mean 6.5/100). None reported having had any experience of using the Edinburgh masker.

Test material and procedure. The subjects were required to read the story of Arthur the rat under three conditions (NAF, Edinburgh masker, frequency-shifted feedback). Thus, the procedure was the same as that in experiment 1 except an Edinburgh masker was used rather than DAF. A portable version of the Edinburgh masker was employed. With this device, a neckband holds a pickup at the level of the larynx. The output of the pickup is led to an electronic circuit which senses when the speaker vocalises and delivers the masking sound down a plastic tube which can be secured into the ear canal by ear cuffs. The level of feedback from the Edinburgh masker was set so that when a speaker sustained a vowel at 70dB SPL the level of sound measured at the ear cuffs of the device was also 70 dB SPL. The manufacturers of the Edinburgh masker suggest that stutterers say "em" before they commence speaking in order to get the Edinburgh masker to trigger. This ploy was not mentioned to our stutterers nor did any of them discover it adventitiously.

Results and Discussion

Number of disfluent episodes was measured as in the first experiment. There were more disfluencies overall under NAF (an average of 13.7 per speaker) than with the Edinburgh masker (average of 2.7 per speaker) and fewest under frequency-shifted feedback (1.16 per speaker). The disfluency rate in the NAF condition was significantly higher (by sign test) than frequency-shifted feedback and the Edinburgh masker (both p's $< .05$). In addition, the disfluency rate was significantly higher in the Edinburgh masker condition than the frequency-shifted feedback condition. Thus, once again an altered sound which is delayed relative to the onset of speech produces a significantly higher disfluency rate.

EXPERIMENT 3

In the introduction, it was noted that stutterers tend to make speech errors in word-initial position. A question which naturally arises is whether it is sufficient for fluency enhancement to present sounds in this position alone. This hypothesis is tested in the present experiment by comparing the effects of frequency-shifting all speech with those of shifting the first 33 msec of each syllable only.

Method

Subjects. Six stutterers whose fluency varied from 5 to 18 disfluencies per hundred words in normal conversation were employed (the average disfluency was 7.3 words per hundred). Four were male.

Test material and procedure. The task for each stutterer was to read the story of Arthur the rat under three conditions. The three conditions were NAF, frequency-shifted feedback of all the speech and frequency-shifted feedback presented solely at word onset. The NAF and frequency-shifted feedback conditions were performed in the same way as earlier experiments.

The procedure for presenting frequency-shifted speech at onset was as follows. The technique depends on the intensity envelope being associated with syllable structure (Fant, 1959). The intensity envelope is at a maximum at the vowel nucleus and at a minimum at the margins of the syllable. The original speech was recorded and shifted in frequency as in earlier experiments. This has an intensity envelope the same as the original speech (thus, it delimits the syllables). In particular, its onset starts at the onset of a syllable.

The next requirement is to gate this off after the syllable has started. The offset gate was produced by obtaining the intensity envelope by a full-wave linear rectification of the original speech which was then low-passed at 50 Hz. This envelope was then inverted and delayed. All of these steps were performed with hardware giving negligible delays. The inversion was achieved with a purpose built inverting amplifier. Delaying of the gating waveform occurred by recording the output on a Racal FM tape recorder and replaying. Thus, the delay is specified by distance between the record and playback heads and the tape-speed setting. A delay of 33 msec was employed. Once the signal for gating the offset of the sound was obtained, this was multiplied with the frequency-shifted feedback and played back to the subjects in the same way as ordinary frequency shifted feedback. The net effect of these alterations is to present the frequency-shifted feedback for the first 33 msec of each syllable. The steps in constructing the frequency-shifted feedback at sound onset are summarised in Figure 1.

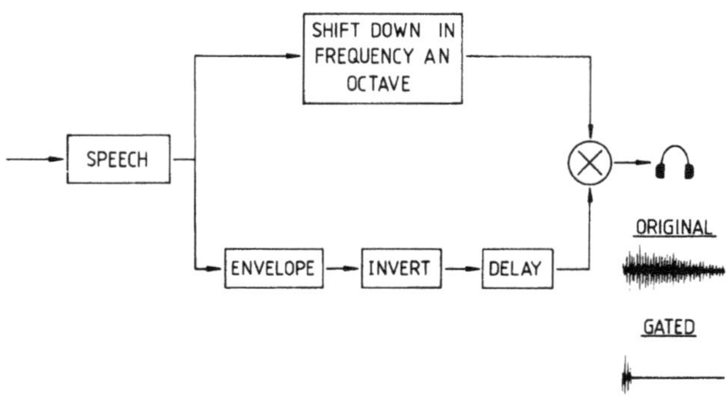

Figure 1. Summary of steps in constructing the feedback in experiment 3.

Results and Discussion

Disfluency rates were computed as earlier. Mean rates in NAF, frequency shift of onset alone and shift of everything were 17.16, 5.3 and 2.3 respectively. Sign tests showed that the difference between NAF and both forms of frequency-shifted feedback were significant ($p < .05$). A sign test showed that the difference between the onset-shifted and all-shifted conditions was significant too ($p < .05$). These results indicate that frequency shifting even part of a sound improves fluency although not as much as frequency-shifting all the sound.

However, even though the condition where just the onset of the sound was shifted was not as effective as frequency shifting all the speech, if this technique was included in a portable unit (similar to the Edinburgh masker) it might be preferred over frequency-shifting everything. The reasons for this are two-fold; first, it would restrict the stutterer's exposure to noise. Second, it might produce less reliance on the alteration per se and encourage rehabilitation without a device. We are currently investigating these.

EXPERIMENT 4

Dewar et al., (1979) state that it is helpful to stutterers to have the sound from the Edinburgh masker with a pitch which covaries with the pitch of the voice. This information is also supplied (right from sound onset) by frequency-shifted feedback. To assess whether this information is of use, we compare the effects on the fluency of stutterers of frequency-shifted speech which has a signal which covaries in pitch with a form that does not covary with voice pitch. If it is important to retain information about the voice pitch, a frequency shift which gives a signal covarying in pitch should produce better speech control than shifted speech which does not produce a pitch which covaries with that of the voice.

Method

Subjects. Eight stutterers performed the present experiment (seven male and one female). The number of blocks in spontaneous conversation per hundred words ranged from 5 to 9 with a mean of 6.25.

Test material and procedure. The story was, once again, that of Arthur the rat. The subjects read the story under four conditions. Two of these were the NAF and octave shift down in frequency employed in experiments 1 and 2.

The first of the other conditions was created as follows. Speech was sampled at 10 kHz into a buffer. The initial setting of the input buffer was that samples were collected over the first 25 msec of a 50 msec sampling epoch and this 25-msec-worth of samples was replayed over 50 msec (i.e., an octave shift down as earlier). At the end of the 50 msec epoch, the buffer needs refilling and output from the beginning of the buffer recommenced. Now, instead of collecting samples over 25 msec as on the first occasion, samples were collected over the first 20 msec. These are still output over 50 msec giving a downward frequency shift of more than an octave. At the end of this buffer, the input sampling period was altered again; this time reduced to 16.7 msec. This was again output over 50 msec. This process repeated another seven times with the sampling period at input being 14.1, 12.5, 11.1, 10.9, 8.3 and 7.6 msec (output period 50 msec in each case). This gives progressively more shift down in frequency up to almost three octaves. At the end of these ten cycles around the buffer (lasting a total of .5 sec), the buffer was reinitialized with its original settings (25 msec input period and 50 msec output period). This process carried on until this test condition was terminated. Thus, the shifts in frequency recycled at 2 Hz. In this condition the delays were longer than in the standard frequency-shifted feedback condition. This was unavoidable given the alterations we wished to make. It should be noted that the delays were never as large as those employed under DAF.

The other irregular frequency shift condition was produced in a similar manner except only five settings for sampling time at the input buffer were used (25, 20, 16.7, 14.1 and 12.5 msec). Reinitialization occurred more rapidly in this condition (4 Hz compared with 2 Hz in the previous setting).

Results and Discussion

Overall disfluencies showed that higher error rate occurred in the NAF condition (average of 13.25 words/100). The disfluency rates in the 2 and 4 Hz conditions were 2.75 and 4.25. Error rate was lowest overall in the frequency-shifted feedback condition (2.5 words per hundred). The difference between NAF and all other conditions was significant in each case ($p < .05$). The constant frequency shift condition only differed from the 4 Hz condition. Thus, there is some evidence that a sound with a pitch which covaries with the voice produces better speech control than a signal which varies at 4 Hz. It is unclear, at present, why the difference between the 2 Hz and frequency-shifted feedback condition occurs.

CONCLUSIONS

The experiments reported here show that in order to improve motor control in stutterers, it is important for altered feedback to be timed to occur synchronous with sound onset; an alteration which does present a sound at syllable onset (frequency-shifted feedback) is more effective than alterations which do not present a sound in this position (e.g., DAF or the sound presented via the Edinburgh masker). On the other hand, a sound presented only at the onset of a syllable is effective at reducing disfluency. It may also help if the pitch of the sound presented covaries with voice pitch.

Thus, these experiments, taken together, stress the importance of presenting a temporally-structured sound synchronized to syllable onset for improving fluency. The technique introduced here of frequency shifting a stutterer's feedback is well-suited to this requirement; a full clinical assessment is planned.

ACKNOWLEDGEMENTS

We would like to express our thanks to Celia Levy of the City Literary Institute, London and all the participants in the experiments for their cooperation.

REFERENCES

Dewar, A., Dewar, A.W., Austin, W.T.S. & Brash, H.M. (1979). The long-term use of an automatically triggered auditory feedback masking device in the treatment of stammering. *British Journal of Disorders of Communication, 14,* 219-229.

Fant, G. (1959). Acoustic analysis and synthesis of speech with applications to Swedish. *Ericsson Technics, 15,* 3-108.

Hahn, E.F. (1942). A study of the relationship between stuttering occurrence and phonetic factors in oral reading. *Journal of Speech Disorders, 7,* 143-151.

Howell, P., Powell, D.J. & Khan, I. (1983). The amplitude contour of the delayed signal and interference in delayed auditory feedback tasks. *Journal of Experimental Psychology: Human Perception and Performance, 9,* 772-784.

Johnson, W. & Brown, S.F. (1935). Stuttering in relation to various speech sounds. *Quarterly Journal of Speech, 21,* 481-496.

Lane, H.L. & Tranel, B. (1971). The Lombard sign and the role of hearing in speech. *Journal of Speech and Hearing Research, 14,* 677-709.

Lotzmann, G. (1961). On the use of varied delay times in stammerers. *Folia Phoniatrica, 17,* 276-310.

Sheehan, J.G. (1974). Stuttering behaviour: a phonetic analysis. *Journal of Communication Disorders, 7,* 193-212.

Taylor, I.K. (1966). The properties of stuttered words. *Journal of Verbal Learning and Behaviour, 5,* 112-118.

Chapter 29

Acoustic Analysis of Repetitions in Stutterers' Speech

Peter Howell, Mark Williams and Louise Vause

INTRODUCTION

A major focus of research has been on the question of why, in part-word repetitions in stuttered speech, the speaker terminates an attempt at an utterance and recommences one or more times. The difficulty the stutterer experiences at these points may occur because the articulators above the larynx are positioned incorrectly (e.g., Van Riper, 1971, 1982) or because stutterers experience difficulty in controlling phonation (e.g., Conture, McCall and Brewer, 1977).

Van Riper's view that repetitions occur because of a failure to position the supra-laryngeal articulators appropriately is based upon the observation that stutterers often appear to produce schwas in a sequence of repetitions even when some other vowel is intended. Since in standard articulatory phonetics, vowel quality is determined solely by the shape of the vocal tract above the larynx, the stutterer is producing an incorrect vowel and the stutterer stops speaking and recommences rather than continue the utterance and say it incorrectly.

Conture et al. (1977) reported that 60% of part-word repetitions were produced with the vocal folds abducted. The incorrect positioning of the vocal folds could arise because the laryngeal muscles are not contracting properly (as discussed by Conture et al., 1977) and, so, implies that a major contribution to the problem experienced by the stutterer is associated with control of the muscles within the larynx.

The following series of experiments was designed to assess these two explanations. Section I reports measurements which show that stuttered vowels have the acoustic properties of the following fluent vowel, not schwa. Perceptual experiments show the reason that the vowels sound like schwa is because of their low amplitude and brief duration. In Section II, the properties of laryngeal excitation in disfluent episodes are compared against those in fluent speech.

ACOUSTIC AND PERCEPTUAL ASSESSMENT OF ORAL ARTICULATION OF STUTTERED VOWELS

Acoustic Analyses

If the stutterer's problem is in the oral articulation of sounds and they produce schwas rather than the appropriate vowel to complete the utterance they intend (Van Riper, 1971, 1982), the formant frequencies of the vowel should be appropriate for schwa, not the intended vowel.

To test this, 30 disfluent episodes recorded from eight stutterers were analyzed. All of the disfluencies occurred on words spoken in isolation and they were spontaneous (not simulated stuttering). The words all consisted of an initial voiceless stop consonant followed by a vowel. In the material analyzed, the stutterers repeated the consonant and part of the vowel one or more times before completing the word successfully. The vowel before fluent release and the subsequent fluent vowel were selected for detailed analysis.

For the formant frequency analyses, the speech was recorded onto computer disc at a 10 kHz rate after low-pass filtering at 4.5 kHz. The second period of each vowel was iterated until there were sufficient samples for a 25.6 msec frame. Then the data were differentiated and a Hanning window applied. A model spectrum was calculated on the 256-point data frame using an eighth-order autocorrelation function. The formant frequencies were obtained by interpolating the model spectrum and picking the peaks (to the nearest 10 Hz).

The first three formant frequencies showed little difference between the fluent and disfluent productions. As a quantitative measure of this, discriminant function analyses were performed. The discriminant functions were set for the fluent vowels. When the disfluent speech was entered into these functions (i.e., the functions which were optimal for classification of the fluent vowels into their appropriate vowel category), 73.3% were still correctly classified as the same vowel as that of the following fluent vowel (not as schwa). This shows that the vowel the stutterers were producing were not schwas. Nor was there any tendency to use a position of the vocal tract nearer schwa than that of the fluent vowel; none of the disfluent vowels which were misclassified were categorized as more central (nearer schwa) than the vowel which was intended.

Although there was no difference between the formant frequencies of the fluent and disfluent vowels which could account for why the disfluent vowels sound like schwa, other differences did occur:

the disfluent vowels were shorter and lower in amplitude than the corresponding fluent vowels. Also, spectrographic analysis showed that the speech lacked normal formant transitions between the initial consonant and the following vowel (cf. Stromsta, 1965). Transitions would be absent if the stutterer was holding an abducted position of the vocal folds. This hypothesis is pursued in the next section. Before that, however, perceptual experiments are reported which were designed to test whether the duration and amplitude of the disfluent vowels could make correctly articulated sounds appear to sound like schwas. Our reason for testing this is that in other situations where vowels are brief and low in amplitude (e.g., in unstressed or fast speech), the vowels also sound more centralized. Thus these factors may also cause brief and low amplitude vowels in stuttered speech to sound like schwa.

Perceptual Tests

If duration and amplitude cause the stuttered vowels to sound like schwa, stuttered vowels should sound more like those intended and less like schwa if they are lengthened and increased in amplitude. Conversely, fluent vowels spoken by a normal speaker should sound more like schwa and less like the intended vowel when they are shortened and decreased in amplitude.

To test this, sequences of repetitions and the subsequent fluent word spoken by one of the stutterers used in the analyses were employed. The words all consisted of a single voiceless consonant followed immediately by a vowel. Sequences including five different vowels (/i/, /ɛ/, /a/, /u/ and /ʌ/) were available from this speaker. The repetitions before the fluent production were used in the test. The digital recordings used in the analyses were employed to construct the test stimuli. These same vowels spoken by a fluent speaker were also recorded to assess whether fluent vowels with low amplitude and brief duration tend to sound like schwa (these were recorded onto computer disc like the stuttered stimuli).

Two stimuli were employed derived in each case from the repetitions before fluent release; the first stimulus simply consisted of the original consonant. The second was prepared from the stuttered vowel so that it was the same length and amplitude as the fluently-produced vowel. This was achieved by iterating the second period of the stuttered vowel and scaling the vowel up in amplitude.

For the normal speaker, the initial consonant and the vowel of the normal-length utterance were taken. The vowel was spliced off and reduced in duration and amplitude to match the vowel in the corresponding stuttered repetition. This was then recombined with its consonant (these changes were performed to make the stimulus derived from the normal speaker equivalent to the original stuttered stimulus). This stimulus was then used to create a normal length and amplitude stimulus in the same way as with the stuttered stimulus.

Ten listeners performed the following perceptual test: all of the vowels were presented twice. On one occasion, the vowel was preceded by a criterion sound which had the same vowel as that the speaker originally intended. On the other occasion the vowel was presented, the criterion that preceded was schwa. The subject was required to judge how close the test item was to the criterion. The judgement was made using a seven-point rating scale (1 = no question that the vowels were different, 7 = no question that they were the same). Mean ratings for each subject, for each vowel preceded by schwa and intended vowel criteria were calculated. An analysis of variance on the ratings showed that the short, low-amplitude vowels (whether stuttered repetitions or truncated vowels reduced in duration and decreased in amplitude) were judged as closer to schwa and further from the intended vowel than when their amplitude and durations were made similar to those in normal speech. Since the vowels involved in this comparison had no other differences in their properties, this suggests that the original vowels had some of the intended quality but that this cannot be heard because of their low amplitude and duration.

In order to test the generality of this finding across stutterers, the speech of four additional stutterers who showed repetitions on the vowel /i/ were obtained (along with /i/ of the stutterer employed in the preceding experiment making five in all). The stuttered items were prepared in the same manner as in the previous experiment. Instead of using fluent vowels from a normal speaker as in the earlier experiment, the fluent vowel that followed the stuttering run was used as a control here. These latter vowels were prepared in the same way as the normal speaker's speech in the earlier experiment. The perceptual test was then performed as previously (again ten listeners were employed). The data confirmed the earlier findings: the short, low-amplitude vowels sounded more schwa-like and less like the intended vowel than these same vowels after lengthening and increasing the amplitude. Thus, the data again indicate that the amplitude and duration properties of the stuttered vowels cause them to sound like schwa.

There is no evidence, then, that these stutterers have problems in articulating the oral form of these vowels. Where the vowels sound dissimilar to those intended, this appears to be attributable to their short duration and low amplitude. It would appear then, that the stutterers were articulating these sounds appropriately. In the next series of studies, we examine whether the vowels in stuttered repetitions are phonated like the following fluent item.

PHONATION DURING REPETITIONS

To assess phonatory control during repetitions, volume velocity waveforms at the glottis were recorded. The acoustic properties of these disfluent waveforms are compared with fluent control material and several differences noted. Finally, an articulatory synthesizer is used to reproduce the gross differences between the fluent and disfluent phonatory signals (Ishizaka and Flanagan, 1972). The parameters of the articulatory synthesizer can be related directly to physiological control parameters and provides a means of comparing our results with physiological measurements obtained by others (e.g., Conture et al., 1977).

The volume velocity at the glottis was measured using a reflectionless tube (Sondhi, 1975). This consists of a long tube of constant diameter (approximately the same as the diameter of an unconstricted vocal tract) closed off at one end. A wedge of foam is located at the enclosed end and a microphone inserted through the sleeve of the tube, half way down. If the vocal tract is sealed tightly to this tube and a vowel with a neutral vocal tract shape is phonated into it, the resonances are damped down and the microphone registers the volume velocity at the glottis. The vowel that has a vocal tract configuration closest to the ideal neutral shape is /ə/. However, Hillman and Weinberg (1981) have shown that the volume velocity waveforms of vowels that have different vocal tract configurations can be recorded reasonably accurately with this technique. In particular, Hillman and Weinberg (1981) demonstrate that the method can be applied to measure the volume velocity at the glottis of the vowel /æ/.

Three stutterers were recruited to produce isolated /h/-vowel sequences. The /h/ was included as the transition from a voiceless to a voiced sound which increased the difficulty and made it easier to elicit repetitions; moreover, as /h/ is produced with a neutral vocal tract shape it conforms to the requirements necessary for recording glottal volume velocities in the reflectionless tube. The stutterers who were used were known, from previous measurements, to have a high incidence of repetitions in their speech. The disfluencies occurred spontaneously and the syllables were spoken less than 30 times each before a repetition occurred. Repetitions involving the initial /h/ and part of the following vowel for /ə/ and /æ/ were available for each stutterer. The repetition before the fluent production and the fluent production itself were employed for the analyses as in the earlier experiments.

There were several differences between the fluent and disfluent productions which occurred for each of the stutterers. The gross properties were that the repetitions were low in amplitude and short in duration compared with the fluent productions (this is, of course, consistent with the properties of the speech discussed earlier). Next, power spectra of each of the vowels were obtained. The original power spectra of the fluent speech and the repetition immediately preceding it are shown for each speaker in Figures 1 (/ə/) and 2 (/æ/). The power spectra show that the downward slope of the partials was greater in the disfluent vowels, indicating that for them energy is concentrated at the lower end of the spectrum.

The next step was to simulate the measured properties of the excitation source using a model which permits the laryngeal and pulmonary contributions to be estimated. For this work, an articulatory synthesizer based on Ishizaka and Flanagan (1972) was used to obtain the glottal volume velocity waveforms (see also the description by Boves, see Chapter 6). In particular synthesis of the vowels for which fluent and disfluent volume velocity waveforms were available (i.e., /ə/ and /æ/ were considered.

In the Ishizaka and Flanagan model, each vocal cord is represented as two coupled mechanical oscillators consisting of a mass, a nonlinear spring and some damping. The subglottal pressure sets them in motion and they modulate the flow through the glottal

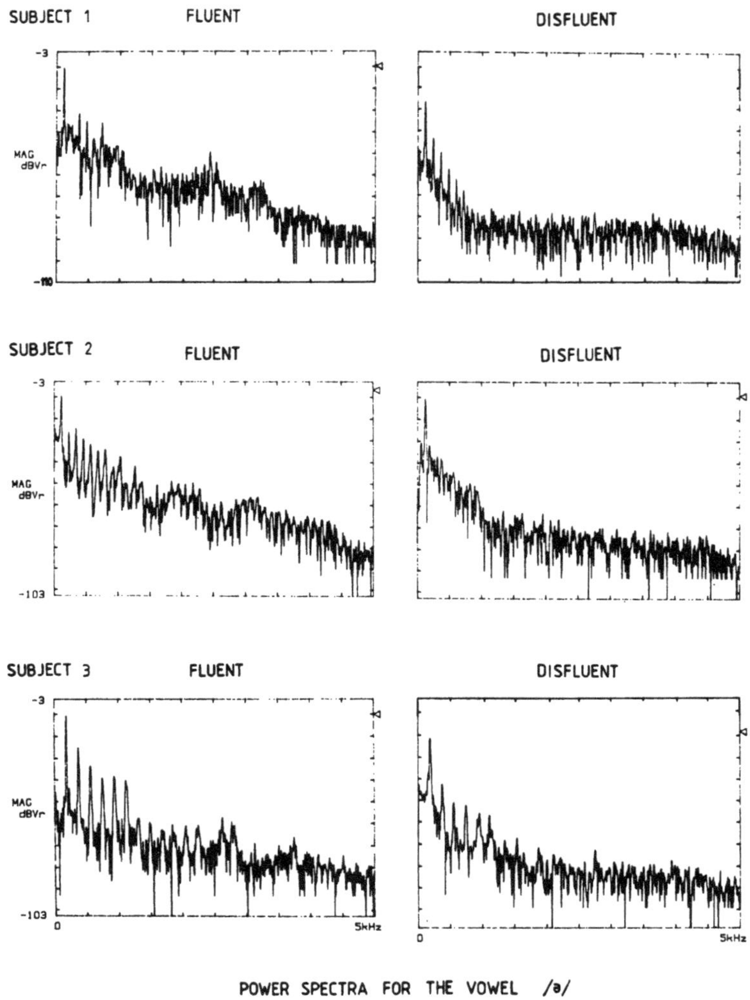

Figure 1. Power spectra obtained from recordings of three stutterers phonating the vowel /ə/ into a reflectionless tube. Examples of fluent and dyfluent phonation are given for each subject. The spectra were obtained using a 2 k point FFT with a Hanning window.

orifice as it passes into the vocal tract; simulated in the usual way as a set of right cylinders (4 and 5 sections were used for /ə/ and /æ/ respectively and their areas were taken from Hillman and Weinberg, 1981).

The whole mechanical model may be represented by an electrical analogue which can be implemented in a suitable computer program. By their very nature, details of the variation in glottal

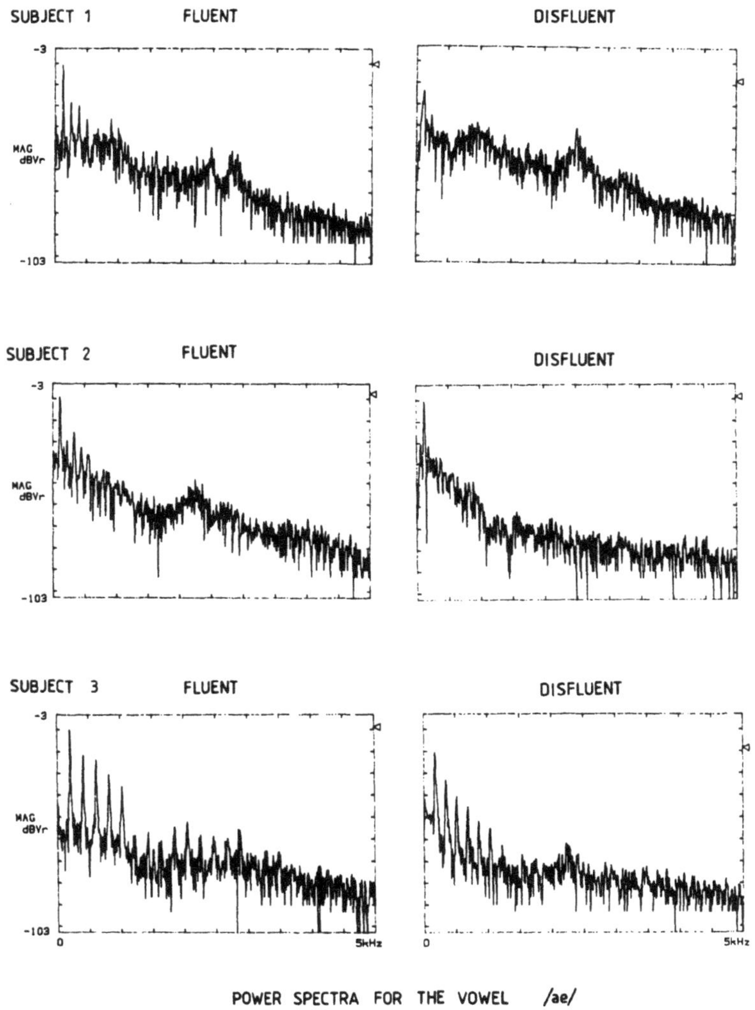

Figure 2. Power spectra obtained from recordings of three stutterers phonating the vowel /ae/ into a reflectionless tube. Examples of fluent and dysfluent phonation are given for each subject. The spectra were obtained using a 2 k point FFT with a Hanning window.

area, volume velocities and so forth may be obtained from a few initial parameters namely, subglottal pressure, P_S, the Q factor (simulating the tensing of the vocal cords by scaling the thicknesses and masses appropriately) and the glottal neutral area (A_{go}) which approximates the laryngeal adjustment.

In order to maintain compatibility with the data from stutterers, the vowels were synthesized at a 10 kHz rate. The stability of this model demands 25 kHz for /æ/ but this was later interpolated to the standard rate.

Examination of the original data showed that the interperiod times of the disfluent and fluent waveforms from the stutterers seem, to the resolution of the sampling rate, to be held constant and then increase towards the end of vocalisation. Similarly, the amplitude is constant and then tails off. In the initial section where the amplitude is constant, the period is constant to within 2%. These data were used next to establish the parameters for the fluent and disfluent syntheses. We concentrated on subject 3 for detailed consideration of parameters.

As implied above, both the fundamental frequency and amplitude of the glottal waveform may be influenced via the P_S, Q and A_{go} parameters. Since it is difficult to deconvolute these effects, it seemed that the best course of action was to attempt a physically and experimentally plausible combination of variations in these parameters for the syntheses. Our first step was to deduce possible values for the fluent syntheses.

Ladefoged's experiments applying impulses to subjects chest cavities suggests a fundamental frequency of about 1/4 Hz for the pulmonary system. This is much lower than required for period-to-period variation so it was assumed that P_S would be constant throughout the first half (50 msec as we decided to produce syntheses of 100 msec length) of the synthesis (corresponding to the steady-state part of the measured glottal waveform). The absolute value of P_S assumed for synthesis of fluent speech was 8 cm H_2O. Since variations in P_S cause variations in the fundamental frequency of the glottal waveform, the relationship observed by Ishizaka and Flanagan when applied to our data (i.e., the 2% fluctuation in the period in the constant amplitude section) implies a P_S constant to within 1/2 cm H_2O (unless the laryngeal adjustment is altered rapidly enough to cancel out any of these gross changes). If P_S is taken to be constant then, again since Q affects the interperiod times, Q must also be held constant during the steady state section. Q was set at 1 and A_{go} at .05 cm^2 for the fluent vowels.

During the decaying part of the waveform, it would seem likely that both Q and P_S reduce. Ladefoged's data offer an indication of the maximum rate of decrease in P_S - about .5 cm H_2O/msec with typical time constants of about 100 msec (that is to say, the time taken to reduce to about 1/4 of initial amplitude). The chosen, most computationally convenient, value was within this easily at .1 cm H_2O/msec. Thus, for the second half of the syntheses, the value of P_S reduced linearly from 8 cm H_2O to about 3.5 cm H_2O. Q, however, was kept constant (at 1) for simplicity (A_{go} was left unchanged at .05 cm^2 too).

Although the overall amplitude of the disfluent data was lower than the fluent, the shape of the envelope was in general similar to that of the fluent speech. The lower overall amplitude profile was reduced throughout by 1 cm H_2O. However, this reduction in P_S would cause a decrease in the period relative to the fluent data whilst no such difference was noted. The period can be readjusted by appropriate selection of the Q and A_{go} parameters. These are antagonistic as far as the value of the period is concerned since increasing Q increases the resonant frequency of the oscillations while increasing the value of A_{go} tends to increase the initial period of the glottal wave. Thus, for the disfluent syntheses, Q was increased by 20% over that used for the fluent and A_{go} increased to .06 cm^2. The settings used simulate a "locking open" of the glottis (as observed by Conture et al., 1977 in repetitions in stuttered speech). In the section where the amplitude was falling off, the P_S was reduced by 1 cm H_2O (as stated earlier). The values of Q and A_{go} were left at the same values as in the earlier part of the syntheses (at 1.2 and .06 respectively).

The synthesized examples show that the gross differences between disfluent repetitions and the subsequent fluent speech can be simulated by suitable adjustments of Q, P_S and A_{go}. In particular, these manipulations have the effect of reducing the overall amplitude of the disfluent speech whilst maintaining a constant period. Also, the drop-off rate of the partials is more rapid in the disfluent syntheses than the fluent, again as observed in the data. These effects are shown in the power spectra of the syntheses in Figure 3.

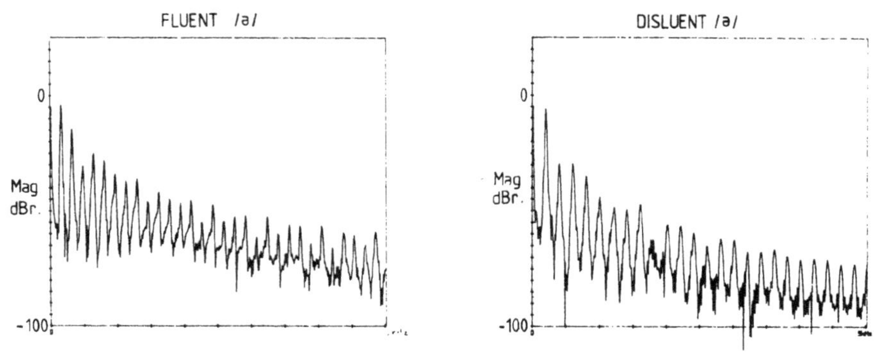

Figure 3. Power spectra of synthesized glottal volume velocities obtained with normal and abnormal laryngeal adjustments. Details of the syntheses are given in the text.

There are some difficulties in producing direct comparisons between the syntheses and measured data; for example, it can be noted that the partials in the power spectra of the fluent and disfluent data of the second subject are not well defined. This may be due to a difference between the laryngeal adjustment used by this speaker and the others; also, the P_S profile should perhaps be different and of course time-varying fluctuations in laryngeal adjustment will affect the spectrum.

Thus, it can be shown that the properties we have chosen to reproduce in our syntheses can be obtained by suitable choice of subglottal pressure, vocal cord tensions and glottal neutral area. These data offer some support for the view that these stutterers have problems in pulmonary and laryngeal control in their stuttered repetitions. Three qualifications need to be made concerning this conclusion; first, the data currently available is sparse. Second, we have only attempted to reproduce gross characteristics of the excitation waveform of the stutterers. Finally, the parameters that we have manipulated to reproduce the fluent and disfluent waveforms may not be the only configuration that can produce these characteristics. Nevertheless, the findings suggest that laryngeal and pulmonary control are not comparable between disfluent repetitions and fluent productions by stutterers. The question remains whether this has a causative or symptomatic role.

ACKNOWLEDGEMENTS

The first two authors are supported by the Medical Research Council of the United Kingdom. Additional assistance from Adrian Fourcin and the Laryngograph trust is gratefully acknowledged.

REFERENCES

Boves, L. (1987). Acoustical analysis and physiological parameters. In H.F.M. Peters and W. Hulstijn (Eds.), *Speech Motor Dynamics in Stuttering.* Wien: Springer Verlag.

Conture, E.G., McCall, G. & Brewer, D.W. (1977). Laryngeal behavior during stuttering. *Journal of Speech and Hearing Research, 20,* 661-668.

Hillman, R.E. & Weinberg, B. (1981). Estimation of glottal volume velocity waveform properties: A review of some methodological assumptions. In N.J. Lass (Ed.), *Speech and Language: Advances in Basic Research and Practice.* New York: Academic Press.

Ishizaka, K. & Flanagan, J.L. (1972). Synthesis of voiced sounds from a two-mass model of the vocal cords. *Bell Systems Technical Journal, 51,* 1233-1268.

Sondhi, M.M. (1975). Measurement of the glottal waveform. *Journal of the Acoustical Society of America, 57,* 228-232.

Stromsta, C. (1965). A spectrographic study of disfluencies labeled as stuttering by parents. *De Therapia Vocis et Loquellae, 1,* 317-320.

Van Riper, C. (1971). *The Nature of Stuttering.* Englewood Cliffs, N.J.: Prentice-Hall.

Van Riper, C. (1982). *The Nature of Stuttering.* 2nd edition. Englewood Cliffs, N.J.: Prentice-Hall.

Chapter **30**

Coarticulation and Stuttering: an Acoustic and Electropalatographic Study

Jonathan Harrington

In Van Riper (1982) a claim is made that the production of a disfluency is phonetically *dissimilar* to the onset of fluent production of the target syllable [1]. For example, a stuttering disfluency in the context of [kʰeitl] (*Katy*) might be [k̟ʰə] [k̟ʰə] [kʰə] (orthographically represented by Van Riper (1982: 435) as "kuh" "kuh" "kuh") rather than [k̟ʰe] [k̟ʰe] [k̟ʰe]. Van Riper (1982: 415) explains this phenomenon as a 'disorder of timing', and suggests that the presence of the perceived schwa in syllabic repetitions may be due to a failure in coarticulation. The most explicit statement of the implications of a 'failure in coarticulation' and the 'presence of the perceived schwa' for the realisation of the disfluency are made in Van Riper (1973):

On words beginning with an "h" such as "he" the stutterer will at first realise that his mouth is shaped for the schwa vowel. (Van Riper, 1973: 329-330).

By analogy, it could be proposed (not suggested by Van Riper) that possible disfluencies in the contexts of target syllables [çu] and [c̠ʰi] (*Hugh* and *key*) might be [h] and [kʰ] respectively, rather than [ç] and [c̠ʰ], since [h] and [kʰ] are the allophonic realisation of /h/ and /k̄/ in the context [-ə].

Wingate (1977: 49), on the other hand, discusses stuttering as a phonetic transition defect:

Whether we observe a repetition or prolongation, the difficulty is typically not manifested in the articulatory postures essential to that sound, but instead in moving on to the succeeding one. Under Wingate's interpretation, a disfluency might be realised as a production from the (acoustic) onset of the target syllable, up to a certain point in the target syllable; the disfluency would therefore be phonetically similar to the onset of the target syllable, because the disfluency *is* part of the target syllable.

Although, unlike Van Riper, Wingate does not believe that the disfluency would be realised as an allophone of the consonant of the target syllable which is appropriate for a [-ə] context, the suggestion is made (Wingate, 1976) that if a vowel-like sound is produced as part of the *disfluency,* it will be phonetically different from the vowel in a *fluent* production of the target syllable. Wingate (1976) emphasizes that the stutterer is not necessarily producing a schwa vowel, or what he calls a neutral vowel, as part of the disfluency, but that whatever vowel-like sound he/she is producing, it will not be the same as the vowel of the target syllable:

Actually, there is very good reason to deduce that it is incorrect to speak of the "neutral vowel" in respect to the occurrence of this "sound" in stuttering... It gives evidence that execution of the intended vowel is not proceeding as it should. In essence, this "sound" reveals that the phonatory aspect of the intended vowel has only been initiated but that it is not being developed or coordinated with proper oral shaping. (Wingate, 1976: 257).

An acoustic correlate of a lack of oral shaping might then be formants which point in the 'wrong' direction in the disfluent production compared with the transition from prevocalic consonant(s) to the vowel in a *fluent* production of the target syllable. Although Wingate (1976, 1977) presents no acoustic evidence in support of his comments, the acoustic analysis of preschool children labelled as stutterers in Stromsta (1965) shows that the formant transitions within the disfluency are 'abnormal' compared with the corresponding transitions in the fluent production of the target syllable and this result has also been found for certain types of disfluencies produced by adults (Stromsta & Fibiger, 1980).

In the experimental section of this chapter, the task will be to use acoustic and electropalatographic techniques to test some of the hypotheses discussed above. The first section will consider whether stuttering can be characterised as a breakdown in coarticulation, as described in Van Riper's framework. If Van Riper is wrong, this may support Wingate's view that stuttering is a breakdown in transition between the prevocalic consonants and the following vowel, in which the disfluency is part of the target syllable. In the second part of the experimental section, the object will be to test whether formant transitions in the production of the disfluency are different compared with those of the target syllable, a characteristic which is described by Stromsta (1983) as the 'core' of stuttering behaviour. A correlate of 'abnormal formant transitions' may be the production of a vowel which is not phonetically equivalent to the vowel in a fluent production of the target syllable, as Wingate seems to imply.

METHOD

36 adult, male and female stutterers all attending speech therapy clinics around Edinburgh and Cambridge were recorded in a sound treated recording studio. Each subject read a list of 200 English monosyllables one at a time following the offset of a 1 kHz tone from a frequency generator. The tone, which was activated by the experimenter following the production of each word by the subject, was designed to prevent coarticulation across word boundaries. The monosyllables included all phonotactically legal prevocalic consonant sequences followed by Received Pronunciation (R.P.) /i/ (Scots /i/) as in *heat*, R.P. /uː/ (Scots /u/) as in *pool*, R.P. /ɒ/ (Scots /ɔ/) as in *not*. The vowels were chosen for two reasons. First, because there is no phonemic overlapping between the vowel phonemes; second, they are sufficiently far apart on the vowel quadrilateral to exert different coarticulatory effects on the preceding consonant(s).

For the electropalatographic recording, two subjects, one male, one female, were selected from the population of 36 stutterers. In choosing the subjects, it was necessary to ensure that the majority of their disfluencies were realised as some form of lingual-palatal contact. An upper plaster cast impression was made for each subject and from this an acrylic palate containing 62 silver electrodes extending as far back as the junction of the hard and soft palate. These two subjects read the same list of 200 monosyllables described above; in addition, a Reading University electropalatograph connected to a Commodore 3032 computer was used at a sampling rate of 100 Hz to store the palatograms as a function of time. The technique of electropalatography is reported in detail in Hardcastle (1972) and so will not be repeated here.

RESULTS

Van Riper's Theory

In the corpus of stuttered speech examined, it was difficult to find any support for Van Riper's claim that stuttering is a breakdown in coarticulation. Figure 1 shows the production of a disfluency and target syllable *out* (phonologically /aut/) and a disfluency and target syllable *eel* (phonologically /il/) produced by the same subject. Van Riper's theory would predict that either the disfluency in the context of these target syllables would be realised as a schwa; or else, the supralaryngeal tract would adopt a configuration appropriate for a schwa vowel without phonation. In the spectrogram of the target syllable *out* in Figure 1, there is a concentration of energy at the onset of periodicity (B) in the 0 - 1.8 kHz range, then a trough, then another energy peak at 2.8 kHz, followed by a dip and another peak at 4 kHz. The burst-like concentration of energy (presumably a glottal stop) of the disfluency (A) shows an almost identical pattern; in particular, the trough is in the same frequency range of 1.8 kHz to 2.8 kHz. The spec-

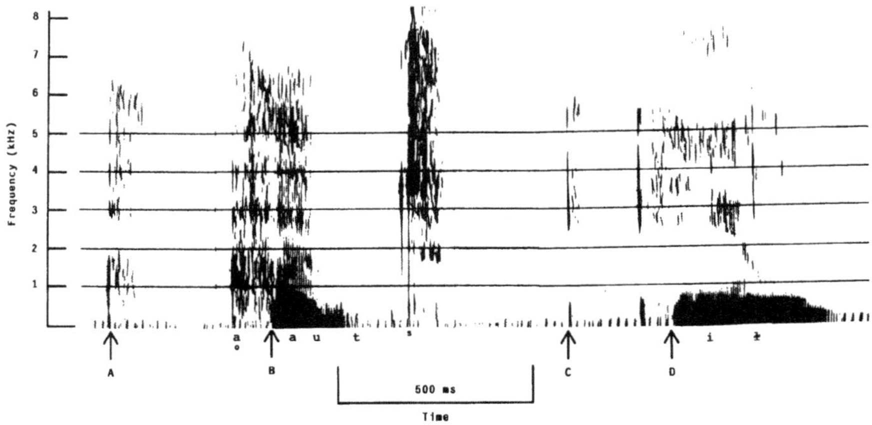

Figure 1. Spectrograms 0 - 8 kHz range, 300 Hz analysing filter, of disfluency and *out* (left) and disfluency and *eel* (right) produced by the same subject. The energy distribution at the onset of the disfluency before *out* (A) is similar to the energy distribution of the onset of periodicity in the target syllable *out* (B). Similarly, the energy distribution at the onset of the disfluency before *eel* (C) is similar to that at the onset of periodicity in the target syllable *eel* (D).

trogram suggests therefore that the shape of the supralaryngeal tract at the release of the disfluency (A) is not dissimilar to the supralaryngeal tract shape at the onset of periodicity in the target syllable (B). The same figure shows a spectrogram of a disfluency and target syllable *eel.* At the onset of periodicity in the target syllable *eel* (D), the first two formants are around 300 Hz and 2.5 kHz. At the onset of the disfluency (C), the burst-like concentration of energy is distributed in a similar frequency region, suggesting again that the supralaryngeal tract shape at this point is not dissimilar to that at the onset of periodicity in the target syllable; above all, there is a similar trough between 600 Hz and 2.5 kHz.

It seems unlikely based on this evidence that anything resembling a schwa vowel, or schwa 'burst' (i.e. the release of a glottal stop with the supralaryngeal tract in an appropriate configuration for a schwa vowel) was produced in the contexts of target syllables *out* and *eel.* Furthermore, if the same schwa burst had been produced in both these contexts, it would be difficult to explain why the spectra at the glottal bursts are so different: in the glottal release of the *out* disfluency, there is an energy peak between 1 kHz and 2 kHz; in the glottal release of the *eel* disfluency, there is a trough in this frequency region.

The analysis above is corroborated by a spectrographic study of disfluencies produced by a Cantonese stutterer discussed in Harrington (1984). This study presented spectrograms of two disfluencies produced in the context of target syllables /sœŋ/ and /se/ in a fluent production of the former, /s/ would be realised as [s̹] because of the rounded [œ] vowel, but not in the latter. In Figure 2, the spectra labelled (A) and (B) were taken 50 msec

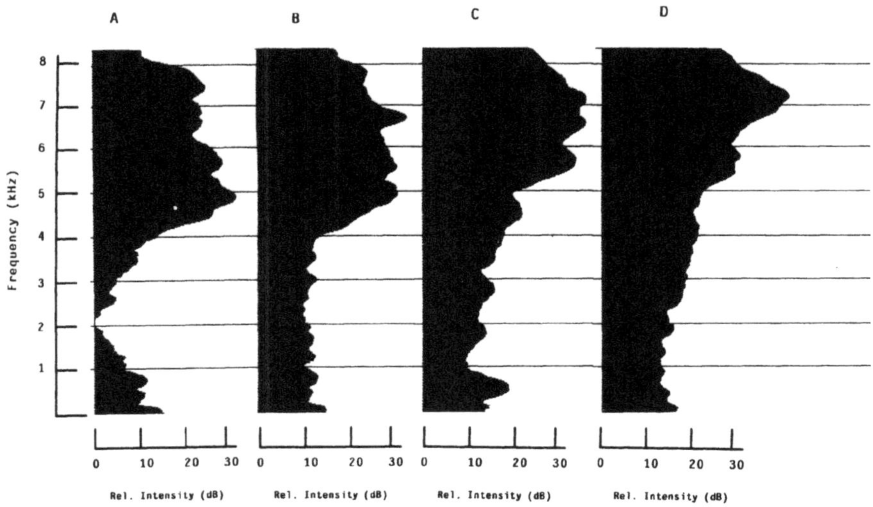

Figure 2. Amplitude sections, 0 - 8 kHz range, 300 Hz analysing filter, taken 50 ms following the onset of a prolonged /s/ before /sœŋ/ (A) and /se/ (C); and 50 ms before the onset of periodicity in the target syllables /sœŋ/ (B) and /se/ (D). The higher intensity of spectral energy in the 4 kHz - 5 kHz range of A and B compared with C and D suggests the production of a more rounded [s̫] in the prolonged /s/ before /sœŋ/ compared with the prolonged /s/ before /se/.

following the onset of the prolongation before /sœŋ/ and 50 msec before the onset of periodicity in a fluent production of /sœŋ/ respectively; similarly, the spectra labelled (C) and (D) were taken 50 msec following the onset of the prolongation before /se/ and 50 msec before the onset of periodicity in a fluent production of /se/ respectively. It is well-known that the superimposition of lip-rounding will tend to lower the frequency distribution of the energy (Fant 1960: 64, Lindblom and Sundberg 1971: 116): since the intensity of the spectrum (A) is greater in the 4kHz-5kHz range compared with (C) this suggests that the disfluency produced in the context of target syllable /sœŋ/ was produced with a greater degree of lip rounding than the disfluent [s] production in the context of target syllable /se/. Furthermore, the similarity of the shape of the spectra (A) and (B) suggests that the degree of lip rounding did not change from the beginning of the prolonged /s/ to the fluent transition from /s/ to /œ/ contrary to the predictions made by Van Riper.

The results of the electropalatographic analysis support the conclusions from the acoustic study discussed above. Figure 3 shows palatograms of a disfluency produced in the context of target syllable *speed*. The disfluency was realised as a prolonged version of the closure phase of [p] in the absence of audible sound. The offset of the closure and the onset of the (perceptually fluent) target syllable is correlated with frame 260, the production of the [i] vowel, which shows extensive contact laterally from the front to

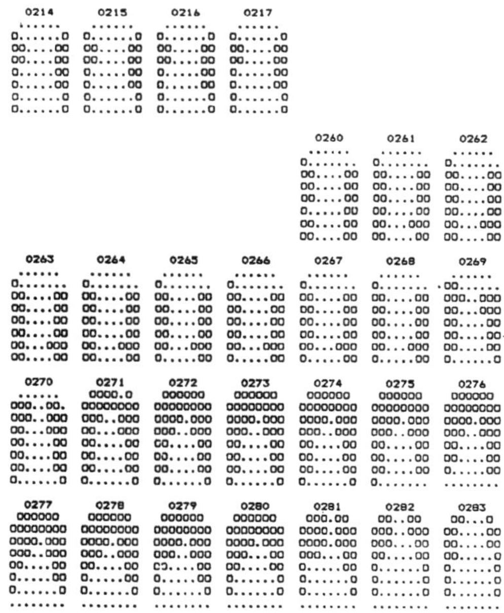

Figure 3. Palatograms, sampling rate 100 Hz, of a prolonged bilabial stop closure and the subsequent production of [id] of *speed*. Frames 214-217 show the onset of a prolonged bilabial stop closure. The release of the bilabial closure and onset of the [i] vowel is at frame 260; the onset of the [d] closure is at frame 269. The extensive lateral contact at the onset of the prolonged closure (frames 214-217) suggests that the tongue was raised in anticipation of the following [i] vowel.

the back of the palate. Prior to this (in the production of the prolonged bilabial closure), the palatograms show a similar location of lateral contact, although the total area of contact is slightly less compared with the fluent production of the [i] vowel. What this suggests is that during the production of the bilabial closure, the sides of the tongue were raised towards the palate: the bilabial closure was actually slightly palatalised. By contrast, Van Riper's theory would predict that the tongue should adopt a configuration appropriate for a schwa vowel. On the basis of the above evidence, there seems to be no justification for such a theory.

Formant Frequency Transitions

Of 200 monosyllables produced by 36 stutterers (i.e. 7200 utterances), a total of 313 (i.e. just over 4% of the utterances) were disfluently produced by 15 subjects. The acoustic analysis of these disfluencies in this section show that the acoustic vowel onglide[2] could be realised as part of the disfluency, but not the acoustic vowel target[3]. In Figure 4, for example, at the offset of the prolonged [ɹ] (A), F2 falls from 1.4 kHz to .9 kHz and an

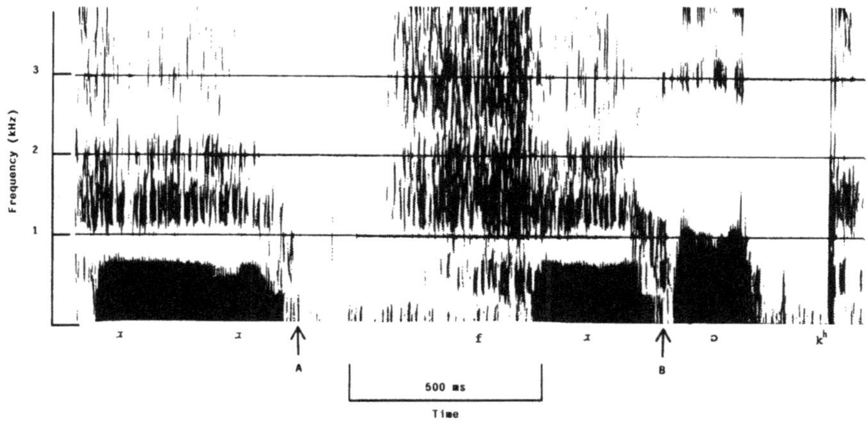

Figure 4. Spectrogram, 0 - 4 kHz range, 300 Hz analysing filter of a disfluency and *frock*. At the offset of the first prolonged [ɹ], F2 falls from 1.4 kHz rises to around 0.9 kHz (A) as in the transition from [ɹ] to [ɔ] (B).

almost identical F2 transition is shown from [ɹ] to [ɔ] in the subsequent production of *frock* (B). There is, therefore, nothing 'abnormal' about the acoustic vowel onglide at the offset of the prolonged [ɹ] (A); the only abnormality is that the acoustic vowel target is not produced as part of the disfluency.

An analysis of other disfluencies did show differences comparing the acoustic vowel onglide of the disfluency with that of a subsequent fluent production of the target syllable and there were three ways in which these differences were manifested. First, the acoustic vowel onglide of the disfluency would bend in the direction of the acoustic vowel target, but not reach the frequency values of the acoustic vowel target. Such an example is shown in Figure 5 which is a spectrogram of a disfluency and target syllable *weed*. At the offset of the first prolonged [w], F2 rises to around 1.5 kHz, whereas in the transition from [w] to [i], a target value of 2.8 kHz is reached. Second, following the release of the consonant in the disfluency, the formants might remain level in contrast to the clear transition shown in the production of the target syllable. Figure 6 shows a spectrogram of part of the disfluency and target syllable *see*. In the transition from [s] to [i], F2 rises, whereas in the disfluency, F2 remains more or less level at a frequency of around 1.5 kHz. Finally, there were some examples in which the formants at the release of the consonant of the disfluency would point in the 'wrong' direction compared with the formant transitions from the prevocalic consonant(s) to the vowel in the target syllable: in the fluent transition from [l] to [u] of *look* in Figure 7, F2 falls; at the offset of the disfluent [l] however, F2 falls but then rises.

The reason why the acoustic vowel onglide in the disfluency can be different compared with the onglide in the fluent transition from /C/ to /V/ in figures 5 and 6 can probably be explained with

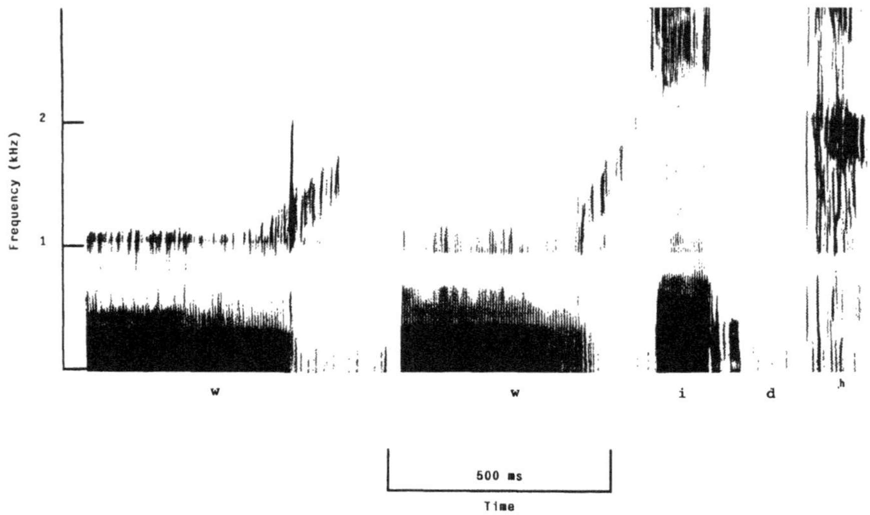

Figure 5. Spectrogram, 0 - 3 kHz range, 300 Hz analysing filter of a disfluency and *weed*. At the offset of the first prolonged [w], F2 rises to around 1.5 kHz whereas in the transition from [w] to [i], F2 rises to 2.8 kHz.

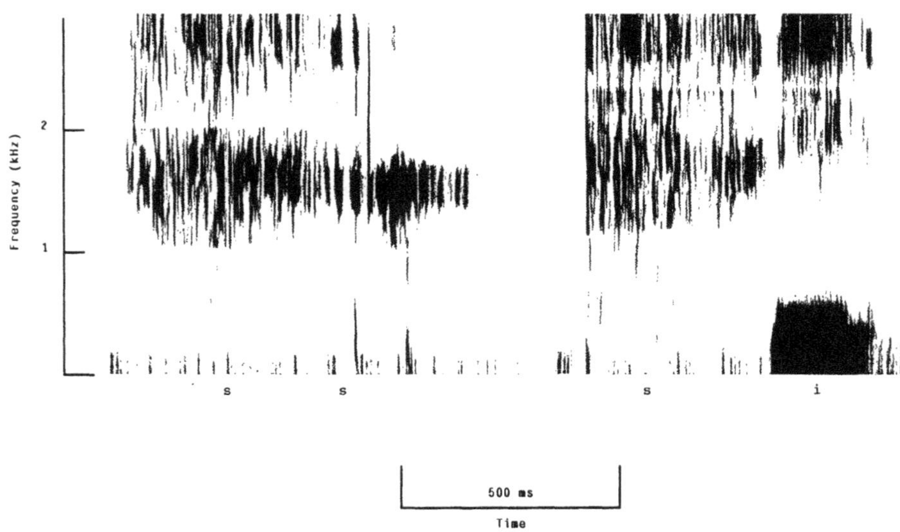

Figure 6. Spectrogram, 0 - 3 kHz range, 300 Hz analysing filter of a disfluency and *see*. In the transition from [s] to [i], F2 rises from 1.5 kHz to 1.8 kHz. At the offset of the prolonged [s], F2 is level at around 1.5 kHz.

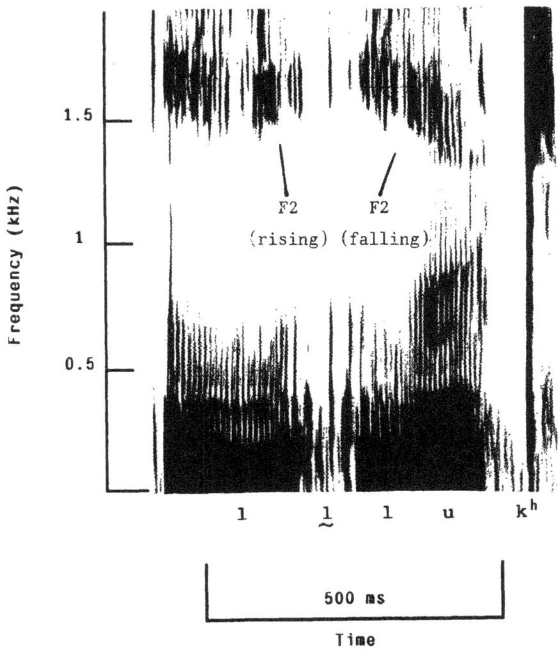

Figure 7. Spectrogram, 0 - 2 kHz range, 300 Hz analysing filter of a disfluency and *look*. At the offset of the first [l], F2 falls then rises, probably because an alveolar closure is being made once more for [l], whereas in the transition from [l] to [u] F2 falls.

reference to the point at which the disfluency 'breaks off' in an attempted production of the target syllable. The data in the former section and the acoustic analysis in this section suggest that a disfluency can be realised as any part of the target syllable from its acoustic onset up to its acoustic vowel target (see in particular Figure 4). However, many disfluencies end in silence well before the acoustic vowel target is reached. If the disfluency breaks off close to the beginning of the acoustic vowel onglide, the formants may show no transition as in Figure 6. If slightly more of the syllable is produced as part of the disfluency, but the disfluency still breaks off well before the acoustic vowel target, as in Figure 5, only the first part of the acoustic vowel onglide will be realised in the disfluency. The maximum 'domain' of a disfluency is shown in Figure 4 which includes all of the acoustic vowel onglide.

This still does not provide an adequate explanation for the formants of the acoustic vowel onglide of the disfluency which point in a different direction compared with those of a fluent transition from /C/ to /V/, as in Figure 7. As Nolan has suggested[4], this can probably be explained by a repetition of the prevocalic consonant(s) following the vowel-like sound of the disfluency. In the spectrogram in Figure 7, F2 of [l] in the disfluency begins to fall as in the target syllable for an initial transition towards the [u] vowel. But unlike the transition of the target syllable, F2 rises, probably because the tongue is returning towards a configuration for [l]. This is why the offset of the F2 transition of the disfluency is at about the same frequency value as the onset of [l] of the target syllable. Furthermore, the frequency of F2 at the offset of the disfluent [l] is around 1.8 kHz, which has been reported to be the locus frequency of alveolars (Delattre, Liberman & Cooper, 1955).

DISCUSSION

There seems to be no basis for Van Riper's (1982) claim that stuttering can be explained as a breakdown in coarticulatory timing. This is because in the production of a /C_0V/ target syllable, in which /C_0/ stands for 1, 2 or 3 consonants, the disfluency can consist of a realisation of /C_0/ which *is* phonetically appropriate for the context /-V/.

The data also suggest that the acoustic vowel target is not realised in the production of a disfluency. Thus, in the production of a /C_0V/ target syllable, the disfluency can consist not only of a realisation of /C_0/ which is phonetically appropriate for the context /-V/ but also (and maximally) of all of the acoustic vowel onglide. Sometimes only part of the acoustic vowel onglide will be produced in the disfluency, in which case the formants may point towards, but not reach, the acoustic vowel target as in Figure 5; or if production of the disfluency breaks off at the beginning of the acoustic vowel onglide, the formants at the offset of the disfluency may remain level as in Figure 6. The pattern of the formants in the acoustic vowel onglide of the disfluency will only be different if the consonant is repeated, as in Figure 7: in this case, the formants following the release of the first consonant will be deflected back towards its locus frequency. Whether the spectrogram in Figure 7 shows the same kind of abnormal transitions to which Stromsta (1965, 1983) refers cannot be determined since no acoustic data are presented in Stromsta (1965).

Finally, Howell, Williams and Vause (see Chapter 29, this volume) argue that the frequent production of vowel-like sounds of disfluencies with low amplitude and short duration can cause them to be perceived as neutral (i.e. schwa-like) even if their spectra suggest otherwise. Figures 5 and 6, however, suggest that the second formant of the acoustic vowel onglide of the disfluency may also be responsible for the perception of a neutral vowel: in these spectrograms, the offset of F2 of both the prolonged [s] and prolonged [w] is at 1.5 kHz, the theoretically predicted second resonance of [ə] for an adult, male vocal tract (Fant, 1960). That the second formant of the acoustic vowel onglide in the disfluency does not *necessarily* terminate at values appropriate for [ə] is clearly shown in Figure 4; whether the majority of disfluencies which break off in the middle of the acoustic vowel onglide (e.g. Figure 5) terminate with formant frequencies appropriate for [ə] is the subject of further investigation.

ACKNOWLEDGEMENTS

I am grateful to Francis Nolan for the loan of the electropalatographic equipment from the Phonetics Laboratory at Cambridge University and to Alan Kemp for reading an earlier draft of this chapter.

NOTES

[1] Throughout this chapter, a distinction is made between production of the *stuttering disfluency,* or simply the *disfluency* and the *target syllable* to which such a disfluency relates. If a stutterer is given a list of monosyllables to read one at a time following the offset of a tone, production of disfluent speech following the offset of the tone is the stuttering disfluency; the target syllable is the word which is to be read, but which is not produced.

[2] Following Lehiste and Peterson (1961), the vowel/diphthong in CVC syllables (where C can be any number of consonants and V is a vowel or diphthong) can be segmented acoustically into an *onglide, target* and *offglide.* The onglide designates the initial formant transitions following the release of the consonant; the target is the point at which the formant frequencies correspond most closely to those of the same vowel when produced in isolation. The offglide is the final transition from the target to the following consonant(s).

[3] See note 1 above.

[4] Personal communication, Francis Nolan, Department of Linguistics, University of Cambridge.

REFERENCES

Delattre, P.C., Liberman, A.M. & Cooper, F.S. (1955). Acoustic loci and transitional cues for consonants. *Journal of the Acoustical Society of America, 27,* 769-773.

Fant, G. (1960). *Acoustic Theory of Speech Production.* The Hague: Mouton.

Harrington, J.M. (1984). The implications of stuttering for speech production: evidence from English and Cantonese. *Edinburgh University, Department of Linguistics Work in Progress, 17,* 39-58.

Hardcastle, W.J. (1972). The use of electropalatography in phonetic research. *Phonetica, 25,* 197-215.

Lehiste, I. & Peterson, G. (1961). Transitions, glides and diphthongs. *Journal of the Acoustical Society of America, 33* (3), 268-277.

Lindblom, B. & Sundberg, J. (1971). Acoustical consequences of lip, tongue, jaw, and larynx movement. *Journal of the Acoustical Society of America, 50,* 1166-1179.
Stromsta, C. (1965). A spectrographic study of dysfluencies labeled as stuttering by parents. *De Therapia Vocis et Loquellae, 1,* 317-320.
Stromsta, C. & Fibiger, S. (1980). *Physiological correlates of the core behavior of stuttering.* Paper presented to the 18th Congress of the International Association of Logopaedics and Phoniatrics.
Stromsta, C. (1983). *Phonatory reaction time of stutterers as a function of masking and therapeutic intervention.* Paper presented to the 19th Congress of the International Association of Logopaedics and Phoniatrics.
Van Riper, C. (1973). *The Treatment of Stuttering.* New Jersey: Prentice-Hall.
Van Riper, C. (1982). *The Nature of Stuttering.* (2nd edition) New Jersey: Prentice-Hall.
Wingate, M.E. (1976). *Stuttering: Theory and Therapy.* New York: Irvington.
Wingate, M.E. (1977). Immediate source of stuttering. In R.W. Rieber & J. Wollock (Eds.), *The Problem of Stuttering: Theory and Therapy.* New York: Elsevier, North Holland Inc.

Chapter 31

Stuttering as a Prosodic Disturbance: A Link between Speech Execution and Emotional Processes

Günther Bergmann

INTRODUCTION

Investigating stuttering as a prosodic disturbance points to an earlier hypothesis on speech behavior of stutterers. On the basis of clinical observations, the hypothesis has been put forth that the speech of stutterers is "monotonous" in the sense that it exhibits reduced pitch variability even in episodes free of stuttering (Scripture, 1925; Travis, 1927).

Contrary to this hypothesis, Schilling (1962) found no difference between stutterers and nonstutterers with respect to mean fundamental frequency of speech and range of Fo. A number of recent studies using a more sophisticated instrumentation showed that stutterers as a group did not differ from nonstutterers in their production of mean fundamental frequency and variability of fundamental frequency (Lechner, 1979; Schäferskupper, 1982; Schmitt & Cooper, 1978). In our own study mentioned below, we investigated among other questions stutterers' fundamental frequency production and found no differences to other speakers (cf. Bergmann, 1986). Only Healey (1982) found stutterers to have a smaller range of fundamental frequency; there was no difference in mean fundamental frequency.

These attempts in the study of prosodic patterns of stutterers apparently suffer a lack of generalizability since aberrant patterns have only been observed in singular studies. One possible explanation is that it seems misleading to look for general deficits in stuttering, irrespective of differences in the reading or speaking material, of task difficulties, and of situational differences in the experimental setting of data acquisition. This lack of generalizability has often been stated in empirically oriented stuttering research (e.g. Van Riper, 1982). Sometimes this has been attributed to more or less unexplainable interindividual differences in stutterers, sometimes to differences in the predominant symptoms and/or to stuttering severity in general.

The same problem with limited validity possibly arises in the research on irregularities of speech motor execution related to the segmental level of execution processes. In the following it is argued that stuttering occurrence is related to a suprasegmental level of speech motor execution, i.e. to certain prosodic features and to suprasegmental timing processes of speech. Empirical evidence for this view from our own research will be given. Furthermore, the attempt will be made to link the hypothesis of stuttering as a prosodic disturbance to emotional, situation-dependent factors of communication. Although we are widely speculating in this respect, there is considerable empirical support for this point of view, not only from research in stuttering but also from research in the social psychology of language (cf. Bergmann & Forgas, 1985).

STUTTERING AND SEGMENTAL EFFECTS IN SPEECH

Recently, great interest has developed in the study of the neuromuscular coordination in the speech of stutterers on a segmental level. Two main paradigms of research are considered: reaction time studies of the initiation and termination of voicing and the study of segmental coordinative timing processes, especially the voice-onset-time (VOT) production. By a number of authors (cf. Starkweather, 1982) aberrant timing patterns have been observed in CVC clusters of perceptually fluent productions of stutterers as well as differences in the VOT productions of stutterers and nonstutterers. Negative results with respect to VOT-differences were received by Watson and Alfonso (1982) and by Borden, Baer and Kenny (1984). The latter concluded that stutterers yielded VOTs well within normal limits when speaking fluently.

With respect to negative results in the study of VOT irregularities in stutterers, Healey and Gutkin (1984) speculated that the position of words in between carrier phrases could be the reason for missing positive results. Thus, they pointed to possibly involved suprasegmental effects. In their study they analyzed VOT data for words in utterance-initial positions, which were expected to more likely show timing irregularities. Their results demonstrated significantly longer VOTs in voiced stops but not in voiceless stops for stutterers. As a carrier phrase they used sentences like "Pea is a word", "Do is a word", etc., with the critical monosyllablic word always in the initial position. These critical words are clearly the accented words of always the same carrier phrase. Thus, suprasegmental effects are mingled with the segmental effects studied and many possibly contribute to the observed timing irregularities.

While in VOT studies a more or less natural speaking task is used, the dependent variables obtained by reaction time paradigms are even less comparable to normal speech, thus causing doubts about the generalizability of the general deficits often mentioned. Despite the prevailing equivocal results of voice-initiation-time, (VIT) and voice-termination-time (VTT) studies (reviewed elsewhere; Andrews et al., 1983; Bergmann, 1985, 1986; Starkweather, 1982) three major objections may be raised. First, the phonatory reaction to auditory pure-tone cueing is a different behavior modality compared to self-generated phonation, i.e. the neurophysiological processes may involve completely different pathways. Secondly, suprasegmental effects may again be involved. In the reaction time task, the critical word or syllable in the response mode is strongly "accented", although there is no suprasegmental embedding. Thirdly, the speech or speech-like quick reaction is an especially demanding, stressful task for stutterers. Thus, we can hardly expect stutterers to behave similar to fluent speakers. On the other hand, an extremely high activation level cannot be considered typical for any stuttered nor perceptually fluent production of stutterers. Perkins (1981), Ciambrone, Adams and Berkowitz (1983), and Andrews et al. (1983) warned to draw extensive conclusions from VIT investigations.

STUTTERING AND PROSODY

In the cited research on segmental effects in stuttering, some suspicion has been raised that suprasegmental effects may have been involved in the irregularities observed. Turning to research that addresses the question of prosodic disturbances in stuttering, a theoretical framework for this perspective has been proposed by Wingate in several publications (1976, 1979, 1982). Wingate (1976, p. 260) described stuttering as a "prosodic defect" manifested "as an intermittent disorder of actualizing stress increase". Thus, stuttering is viewed as a defect in the transition to stressed syllables. The significance of stressed syllables as the most likely location for stuttering to occur is difficult to prove because in both English and German stressed syllables are also word initial syllables in about 80% of cases. Addressing the question of the loci of stuttering to be related to grammar or to prosody, i.e. the important role of stressed syllables, Wingate points to a lack of research in languages other than English and states that "comparable material from other languages would be of considerable value to our understanding of linguistic determinants in stuttering" (Wingate, 1979, p. 283).

Wingate (1979) discussed earlier investigations addressing the question of loci of stuttering being related to grammar or to prosody. There has been considerable agreement between various studies indicating that stuttering is associated more frequently with "content" words than with "function" words and with word positioning at the beginning of sentences. Wingate raised doubts about the relevance of grammatical class per se and points to accent structures as being involved in these effects (compare Hejna, 1972).

Additionally, Wingate (1982) discussed a study by Shapiro (1970) concerning this question. He pointed out that the early position effect on stuttering occurrence may be related to the accent structure of sentences used in this experiment. Still, empirical evidence that is directly related to stuttering as a prosodic disturbance is rare.

Two experiments have been conducted by the author (Bergmann, 1986) to provide more empirical evidence for the prosodic disturbance hypothesis of stuttering. In the first study, the stuttering frequency at the loci of central accentuation was examined. The appropriate accent patterns were varied by the use of different context questions so that the sentence accent fell on two different words of the same sentence.

At first, most of the nine subjects (with the exception of two) produced sentence accent almost entirely correctly. Even six accent placement errors (in the case of two subjects) were a very small number compared to the 58 correct accent productions. Thus, we cannot speak of a general inability of stutterers to realize appropriate accent patterns, which is what we had expected. On the other hand, stutterers showed significant difficulties in the fluent execution of these accent patterns. Disfluencies have been counted at three points of the sentences: the beginning, the sentence accent location, and the word that bears the sentence accent in the other version (depending on the context question). Stuttering disfluencies have been categorized according to a modification of the Johnson, Darley, and Spriestersbach (1963) schema proposed by Bergmann (1984). A highly significant difference in stuttering frequency between accented and not accented words has been demonstrated. The extent of difference is almost stable irrespective of the overall stuttering frequency. All stutterers showed significantly more disfluencies on the accented words than on the same words not being accented.

In the second experiment, the predominance of stressed syllables for stuttering incidence was examined. A poem with a regular metre (iambic) was used for material. This offered the advantage that the stressed syllables could be unambiguously identified from the metrical structure and that stressed and unstressed syllables occurred with an approximately equal number. Subjects were 13 adult male (moderate and moderate-to-severe) stutterers and six nonstutterers. Results of stuttering frequencies at stressed and unstressed syllables are given in Table 1 in absolute values; because of the approximately equal number of cases direct comparisons are possible.

Results showed that a significant difference could be confirmed: all subjects (with the exception of one) stuttered drastically less at unstressed syllables than at stressed syllables. These results strongly confirmed Wingate's hypothesis that stuttering incidence is predominantly located on stressed syllables. Furthermore, the stress timing structure realized in the poem was investigated in those lines showing no audible disfluencies. The stress timing structure was analyzed by calculating the time intervals between Fo peaks of stressed syllables (as a measurement for the tendency for isochrony; all further details see Bergmann, 1986). While there was no difference in the mean peak-to-peak intervals

Table 1. Number of disfluent syllables in poem reading in experiment II. The analyzed part of the poem contained 60 stressed and 70 unstressed syllables; Thus, absolute comparisons between the last two columns are possible.

Subject No.	Poem	in %	Stressed syllables in poem	Unstressed syllables in poem
1	22	17	12	10
2	8	6	6	2
3	5	4	1	4
4	10	8	8	2
5	2	2	2	0
6	10	8	8	2
7	2	2	1	1
8	41	32	32	9
9	1	1	1	0
10	30	23	16	14
11	18	14	18	0
12	7	5	6	1
13	38	19	28	10
Mean	14.9		10.7	4.2
S.D.	13.8		10.2	4.8

between stutterers and nonstutterers, stutterers showed a significantly greater variability of their stress timing structure (the standard deviation of peak-to-peak intervals was nearly twice as large as for nonstutterers; complete results in Bergmann, 1986).

The result last mentioned in our study indicates the functional relevance of stressed syllables for obtaining fluency. Stressed syllables determine the timing patterns of sentences and therefore affect overall fluency. This is at least true for languages like German or English (cf. Allen, 1972, 1975; Jassem, Hill & Witten, 1984). Stressed syllables generate a speech rythm that "functions mainly to organize the information bearing elements of the utterance into a coherent package, thus permitting speech communication to proceed efficiently" (Allen, 1975, p. 84). This aspect of speech rhythm and fluency seems to be essential for stuttering. Cooper and Allen (1977) studied the sentence timing structure of stutterers. They asked their subjects to repeat the same sentence a number of times with the same timing structure (stressed syllable intervals) and found a significantly greater variability in stutterers' productions compared to nonstutterers. The results of this study are in agreement with our findings cited above.

So far we may conclude that relevant prosodic features for stuttering occurrence are sentence accent structures and stressed syllables in particular. The appropriate timing of stressed syllables in utterances is directly related to the whole timing structure in connected speech. Disruptions at these central points of stress therefore disturb overall fluency patterns of speech. A linkage to segmental effects in stuttering may lie in the fact that stressed syllables and stressed vowels in particular require more precise phonatory and articulatory movements than unstressed syllables (formant structure), thus causing a greater effort in phonatory and articulatory coordination (for example, compare the discoordination hypothesis by Perkins et al., 1976; Perkins, 1981). A further argument for the relevance of stressed syllables is related to emotional factors - a point we will later turn to. We will now leave the level of speech production processes in stuttering and deal with inferences of speaking situations considered as communication.

STUTTERING AND COMMUNICATION

This chapter is introduced by a personal observation from the beginning of our experiments on stutterers' prosody mentioned above. Since high quality recordings were essential for the subsequent digital speech analysis, the stutterers were recorded in a sound-isolated booth. There was no direct contact with the experimenter, neither visual nor auditory. Subjects even received their instructions from a tape recording, and spoke into a microphone.

Surprisingly, some subjects did not stutter at all during the various reading tasks. When the subjects were asked to describe their experiences during the experiment, after leaving the booth, they again stuttered in their customary way. Eventually, the experimental arrangement was changed, and a co-experimenter sat with the subjects face-to-face in the booth. His only function was to follow the text as the subjects read. Once this procedure was adopted, stuttering again occurred at a level which was usual for the subjects' normal interactions, and the experiment could be conducted as planned.

From this observation a small experimental demonstration has been derived (see also Bergmann & Forgas, 1985). In order to explore this effect of a more or less "communicative" setting more systematically, we introduced several further variations into the experimental setting. Six male stutterers performed a reading task, first reading a fable in the isolated reading situation without a co-experimenter. Afterwards they were interviewed about their reactions to the experiment. About four weeks later the same subjects returned to the laboratory, and they again performed the same reading task, this time in a non-isolated speaking situation with a co-experimenter also sitting in the booth. A second interview was conducted afterwards.

The number of disfluent syllables was counted from audio recordings for each condition using the same categorization scheme proposed by Bergmann (1984). Since the fable first read by subjects contained 130 syllables, a section of the interview of the same length was selected for evaluation. This section was taken from the middle of the interview. In Table 2, the absolute values of stuttering frequency in these different situations can be compared. Absolute values without further conversions are used since they express most clearly the differences between these situations.

As Table 2 clearly shows, there was a very noticable difference in stuttering between the isolated speaking situation and the

Table 2. Number of disfluent syllables in each of four speaking situations.

Subject No.	(1) Isolated Speaking (Fable)	(3) First Interview	(2) Non-Isolated Speaking (Fable)	(4) Second Interview
1.	27	42	33	49
2.	3	21	21	19
3.	0	11	6	11
4.	2	32	18	29
5.	0	27	28	32
6.	2	24	19	22
Mean values	5.7	26.2	20.8	27.0
Mean values without subject 1.	1.4	23.0	18.4	22.6

Three speaking conditions have been varied:
(1) Isolated speaking: Reading a fable when sitting in a sound-isolated booth without co-experimenter (i.e. sitting alone in the booth and being recorded).
(2) Non-isolated speaking: Reading a fable when sitting in the booth face-to-face to a co-experimenter.
(3) and (4) Interpersonal communication: Being interviewed by the experimenter about one's experiences with stuttering in a natural setting (no tape recording equipment; normal room).

following interview (interpersonal communication situation). Five of the six subjects stuttered hardly at all during the isolated reading task. Only subject 1 showed substantial stuttering. The increase in stuttering in the post-experimental interview cannot be fully explained by the differences in the material (fable vs. speaking one's own experiences). As the right side of the table shows, the same stutterers reading the same material also produced a significantly higher rate of stuttering when a co-experimenter sat with them in the booth. While there is a difference in stuttering rate as a function of the material (reading vs. speaking), the major effect illustrated by Table 2 is between isolated vs. interpersonal speaking situations. We must also remember that the non-isolated speaking situation created here is much more restrictive than normal everyday interactions.

It seems most likely that the situations summarized in Table 2 differed in terms of the subjectively experienced communication responsibility of the speakers. In a completely isolated, non-social situation, communication responsibility is minimal: there is no immediate reaction to what is said, and the material itself is not personally relevant. When another person shares the same space, communication responsibility is likely to be dramatically increased. Even though the message is not personally relevant, the onus is now on the speaker to communicate it clearly and effectively to another individual who is monitoring this performance. Finally, face-to-face interviews represent the highest level of communication responsibility. Here, the speaker is both personally involved in the message, and his performance is directly evaluated by an attentive audience. The data in Table 2 generally support such an interpretation.

This interpretation would be highly speculative in the light of only weak empirical bases. On the other hand, there has been extensive empirical research on situational factors and stuttering frequency. In the first place stuttering frequency seems to depend on the speaking modality. Most stutterers produce less stuttering in an oral reading task than in spontaneous speech (Van Riper, 1982; Kroll & Hood, 1976). Stuttering is also reduced when reading meaningless materials such as syllables or numbers (Bloodstein, 1975). Other studies, for example Bardrick and Sheehan (1956), showed that emotionally loaded words produced more stuttering than either ordinary communication or nonsense material. These findings are consistent with the view that stuttering incidence is related to the degree of subjectively experienced communication responsibility on the part of the speakers. Communication responsibility (and stuttering) is clearly reduced when the spoken material is either meaningless, or is not the speaker's own communication. Thus, the extent of stuttering depends not only on the meaningfulness or propositionality, but also on the affective loading of the communicational content.

Secondly, social aspects of situations play an important part for the frequencies of stuttering occurrence. There are several studies showing that stuttering varies depending on the characteristics of the surrounding social situation. For example, Van Riper (1982) reports that the identity of the communication partner has a noticeable effect on stuttering frequency. Stuttering incidence was found to increase across situations in the following order: speaking to an audience, speaking to a stranger (one of the opposite sex is particularly demanding), speaking to a therapist, speaking to a close friend, and speaking alone (cf. Young, 1985). Other situational features, such as status differences, sexual composition of the dyad and behavior setting may also influence the occurrence of stuttering. Unfortunately, research is not always unequivocal on these various points, probably because the stutterers' subjective perception and interpretation of a confronting situation are more important in eliciting stuttering behavior than the objective features of the situations commonly studied.

A point of special interest is the speaking behavior of stutterers when speaking alone, which would of course be in strong accord with a social-situational account of this disturbance. In general, one cannot speak of a total absence of stuttering when speaking alone. On the other hand, stuttering is often drastically reduced in this condition (e.g. Van Riper, 1982; Wingate, 1976). It should be mentioned that empirical evidence is difficult to obtain because it is hardly possible to realize a totally isolated speaking situation in an experimental setting.

In the important study by Rasdol'skij (1965), a self-monitoring instruction (speaking alone) was given to children and adults, ranging in age from 2 to 6 years (pre-school children), from 7 to 12 years (school children), from 13 to 17 years (teenagers), as well as 18 years and older (adults). He compared stuttering frequency in children and adults when alone and speaking in a social interaction situation. Only 22 out of the total of 125 subjects did not stutter when speaking alone. However, most subjects did stutter much less when speaking alone, and the size of this effect was also found to be age dependent. Most preschool children showed no or only little improvement when speaking alone. Most of the school children in turn stuttered noticeably less when alone, and most of the teenagers and adults in fact stuttered significantly less in the isolated speaking situation. A drastic reduction (but not complete elimination) of stuttering in isolated speech by adults has been confirmed in several studies (Porter, 1939; Hahn, 1940; Svab, Gross & Langova, 1972). These results are consistent with the view that a person's increasing sophistication in differentiating between social situations with increasing age may be intimately related to the situation-dependent incidence of stuttering.

However, the apparent persistence of stuttering in isolated speaking situations requires additional explanation. For one thing, demand characteristics in these studies might have caused the stutterers to expect observation by an anticipated audience. Even without such demand characteristics, an isolated stutterer can still modify the relevant situational components by subjectively representing an audience, or by intensified monitoring of his own speech. The importance of self-monitoring and attempts at control has been frequently noted in stuttering research (Krause, 1982). We may then conclude that stuttering frequency seems to be specifically associated with the social nature of the situations, although the removal of an audience does not reliably result in its complete elimination.

There is additional evidence supporting this assumption from social psychology research on social situations. In these studies, the "difficulty" of several interaction situations has been explored and systematically described (e.g. Argyle, Furnham & Graham, 1981; Brown & Frazer, 1979; Bryant and Trower, 1974; Zimbardo, 1982). Considerable agreement between these empirical attempts has been reached that a hierarchy of "difficult" situations exists, similar to the hierarchy summarized by Van Riper (1982, cited above) for frequencies of stuttering occurrence in social situations. Furthermore, the occurrence of disfluencies of normally fluent speakers is related to this hierarchy of "difficult" situations. On the other hand, a large number of social psychology researchers have pointed out that subjective determinants are of special relevance for experiencing a social situation as difficult. These determinants can be described as internal representations of social episodes on the background of personal needs and prior interaction experiences (e.g. Richardson & Tasto, 1976; Forgas, 1982, 1983; for a detailed review see Bergmann & Forgas, 1985).

On the basis of this social psychology research, a hypothetical model of stuttering incidence in social interactions has been proposed (Figure 1). We must take into account at least three aspects of a communicative encounter if we wish to link situations to speech disfluencies. The first aspect is *situation perception*, or the way a person perceives and cognitively represents a particular social episode. The other two subjective aspects are *message content*, and the perceived *consequences of the communication*. These three aspects must always be considered in conjunction. For example,

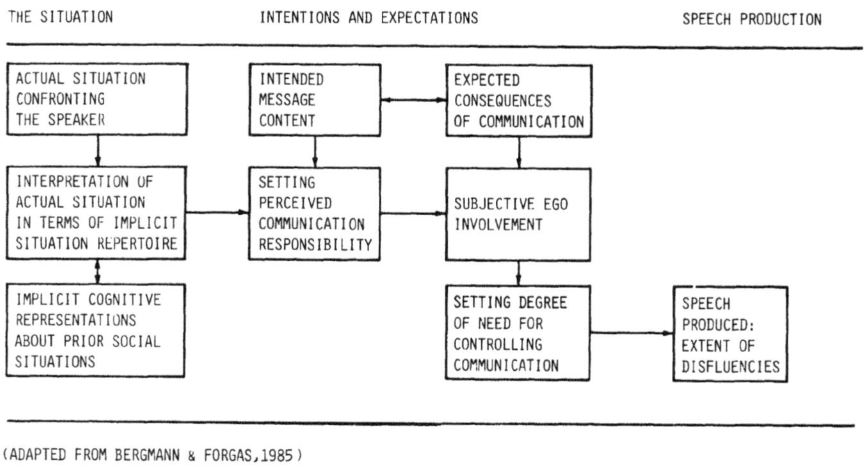

Figure 1. A hypothetical linking situational variables to the occurrance of stuttering.

stuttering frequency could be very high even in an episode generally considered easy, such as a conversation with a friend, if the content of the message is emotionally important. Communication with a stranger, normally a "difficult" episode, may in turn cause no problems if the message content is neutral and no further interaction is expected.

The combination of subjective aspects and characteristics of the situations determine the degree of subjective *communication responsibility* and *ego-involvement* in a specific interaction. For example, in a highly restricted experimental setting (as shown in our experimental demonstration) without any direct interaction, the communication responsibility may be low, since all communicative characteristics of the situation may be regarded as mediated by the machinery. Ego-involvement at the same time is at its lowest, since material read from cards is emotionally irrelevant and has no real communicative function. One can efficiently discuss situational characteristics, known as "difficult" for stutterers, within these terms.

Distraction from the interpersonal characteristics of an encounter seems a common feature of many therapeutic aids. Instrumental speech aids, such as metrical pacing, auditory masking and delayed auditory feedback were often found to improve the fluency of stutterers directly and very drastically. One likely explanation is that these aids reduce the interactional characteristics of the communication (Krause, 1976; Fiedler & Standop, 1978). Similar processes may also account for the improvements achieved with such techniques as shadowing, speaking in chorus and even singing, where stuttering normally does not occur. In all of these techniques clients are brought to subjectively define the speaking situation as non-interpersonal (on the other hand, these techniques cause changes in motor execution processes of speech).

The crucial variable which is also regarded as being linked to stuttering symptomatology is the *need for controlling communication* (e.g. Stäcker, Kriebel & Bergmann, 1982). The great importance of control, particularly the control of affective expression in stuttering, has been well-documented in the research by Krause (1980, 1982). Among other things, Krause found that stutterers use reduced expression of affect even in the nonverbal modalities. Stutterers also tend to occupy more speaking floortime than their partners, even when they are not stuttering. Krause interpreted these manifestations as symptoms of a chronically defensive coping strategy, particularly oriented towards avoiding expression of affect. As a result, even situations not commonly seen as demanding may require considerable effort of affect control for stutterers. In the concluding chapter we wish to center the affect control hypothesis of Krause on the speaking behavior of stutterers.

SPECULATIONS ON STUTTERING, PROSODY, AND AFFECT CONTROL

At first, we wish to return to the relevance of stressed syllables for the occurrence of stuttering. Stressed syllables are not only important for the rhythmic organization of speech fluency. Stressed syllables bear a lot of information about a speaker's emotional state. Some empirical results are to be included, originally belonging to the domain of research on vocal communication.

We have shown that emotional and attitude-related pragmatic functions of speech may be identified from certain aspects of intonation contours and from the range of fundamental frequency (Ladd, Silverman, Tolkmitt, Bergmann & Scherer, 1985). The acoustic parameters in this research have been digitally manipulated on sentence accent and stress structures. Even if we consider the emotional expression in speech to be much more pervasive and long-lasting in comparison to the rather molecular element of stress structures, this addresses the relative importance of these elements of speech in communication. Furthermore, it has been revealed that certain aspects of the stress structure of utterances are essential for the linguistic functions of intonation (e.g. Ladd, 1983; Liberman & Pierrehumbert, 1984) as well as for the pragmatic and emotional functions of intonation (Ladd et al., 1985; cf. the recent review by Frick, 1985, on the role of prosodic features in communicating emotion). Because of the relative importance of stress structures for communication, these elements of speech may be controlled fairly well on part of the speaker.

As has been pointed out, stressed syllables are of special relevance for organizing overall fluency of speech. If we follow the affect control hypothesis and relate this hypothesis to the speaking behavior of stutterers, these central points may be overcontrolled because of their communicative functions. Overcontrol processes may disturb the quick and precise timing processes that are normally highly automatized and function without voluntary control. Thus, stuttering symptoms can be seen as a result of an overcontrol strategy of speech in social situations. Therefore, the parts of ongoing speech that are mainly effected by disfluencies are those that are important for affective and pragmatic components of communication. In this sense, we proposed to link stuttering as a prosodic disturbance to aspects of speech motor organization on the one side and to emotional aspects of communication on the other side. Of course, some elements of the proposed model are hypothetical at present. This mainly concerns the affect control hypothesis related to the speaking behavior of stutterers. On the other hand, it seems to be fruitful to connect various aspects of research, those of speech motor control in stuttering, prosodic disturbances in stuttering, social psychology research in communication, and person-oriented approaches to stuttering behavior. We feel that an integration of different levels of analysis and of different areas of research may help to come closer to a unified view of stuttering.

REFERENCES

Allen, G.D. (1972). The location of rhythmic stress beats in English speech. Parts I & II. *Language and Speech, 15,* 72-100, 179-195.

Allen, G.D. (1975). Speech rhythm: its relation to performance universals and articulatory timing. *Journal of Phonetics, 3,* 75-86.

Andrews, G., Craig, A., Feyer, A.M., Hoddinott, S., Howie, P. & Neilson, M. (1983). Stuttering: A review of research findings and theories circa 1982. *Journal of Speech and Hearing Disorders, 48,* 226-246.

Argyle, M., Furnham, A. & Graham, J.A. (1981). *Social situations.* Cambridge: Cambridge University Press.

Bardrick, R.A. & Sheehan, J.G. (1956). Emotional loadings as a source of conflict in stuttering (abstr.). *American Psychologist, 11,* 391.

Bergmann, G. (1984). Vorschläge für eine kontrollierte und standardisierte Diagnostik des Stotterns. *Die Sprachheilarbeit, 29,* 167-176.

Bergmann, G. (1985). Apparative Sprechhilfen und Theorien des Stotterns: Ein Literaturüberblick. *Beiträge zur Phonetik und Linguistik, 43,* 7-94.

Bergmann, G. (1986). Studies in stuttering as a prosodic disturbance. *Journal of Speech and Hearing Research, 29,* 290-300.

Bergmann, G. & Forgas, J.P. (1985). Situational variation in speech dysfluencies in interpersonal communication. In J.P. Forgas (Ed.), *Language and social situations.* New York: Springer. 229-252.

Bloodstein, O. (1975). *A Handbook on stuttering.* Chicago, Ill.: National Easter Seal Society for Crippled Children and Adults.

Borden, G.J., Baer, T. & Kenney, U.K. (1984). Onset of voicing in stuttered and fluent utterances. *Haskins Laboratories: Status Report on Speech Research SR-79/80,* 65-80.

Bryant, B. & Trower, P. (1974). Social difficulty in a student sample. *British Journal of Educational Psychology, 44,* 13-21.

Ciambrone, S.W., Adams, M.R. & Berkowitz, M. (1983). A correlational study of stutterers' adaptation and voice initiation times. *Journal of Fluency Disorders, 8,* 29-37.

Cooper, M.H. & Allen, G.D. (1977). Timing control accuracy in normal speakers and stutterers. *Journal of Speech and Hearing Research, 20,* 55-71.

Fiedler, P.A. & Standop, R. (1978). *Stottern.* München: Urban & Schwarzenberg.

Forgas, J.P. (1982). Episode cognition: Internal representations of interaction routines. In L. Berkowitz (Ed.), *Advances in experimental social psychology.* New York: Academic Press. 59-101.

Forgas, J.P. (1983). Social skills and the perception of interaction episodes. *British Journal of Clinical Psychology, 22,* 195-207.

Frick, R.W. (1985). Communicating emotion: The role of prosodic features. *Psychological Bulletin, 97,* 412-429.

Hahn, E.F. (1940). A study of the relationship between the social complexity of the oral reading situation and the severity of stuttering. *Journal of Speech Disorders, 5,* 5-14.

Healey, E.C. (1982). Speaking fundamental frequency characteristics of stutterers and nonstutterers. *Journal of Communication Disorders, 15,* 21-29.

Healey, E.C. & Gutkin, B. (1984). Analysis of stutterers' voice onset times and fundamental frequency contours during fluency. *Journal of Speech and Hearing Research, 27,* 219-225.

Hejna, R.F. (1972). The relationship between accent or stress and stuttering during spontaneous speech. (Abstr.) *ASHA, 14,* 479.

Jassem, W., Hill, D.R. & Witten, I.H. (1984). Isochrony in english speech: its statistical validity and linguistic relevance. In D. Gibbon & H. Richter (Eds.), *Intonation, accent and rhythm.* Berlin: De Gruyter. 203-225.

Johnson, W., Darley, F. & Spriestersbach, D. (1963). *Diagnostic methods in speech pathology.* New York: Harper and Row.

Krause, R. (1976). Probleme der psychologischen Stottererforschung und Behandlung. *Zeitschrift für Klinische Psychologie und Psychotherapie, 24,* 128-143.

Krause, R. (1980). Stuttering and nonverbal communication: Investigations about affect inhibition and stuttering. In H. Giles, W.P. Robinson & P.M. Smith (Eds.), *Language. Social psychological perspectives.* Oxford: Pergamon. 261-266.

Krause, R. (1982). A social psychological approach to the study of stuttering. In C. Fraser & K.R. Scherer (Eds.), *Advances in the Social Psychology of Language.* Cambridge: Cambridge University Press. 77-122.

Kroll, R.M. & Hood, S.B. (1976). The influence of task presentation and information on the adaptation effect in stutterers and normal speakers. *Journal of Communication Disorders, 9,* 95-110.

Ladd, D.R. (1983). Phonological features of intonational peaks. *Language, 59,* 721-759.

Ladd, D.R., Silverman, K.E.A., Tolkmitt, F., Bergmann, G. & Scherer, K.R. (1985). Evidence for the independent function of intonation contour type, voice quality, and Fo range in signalling speaker affect. *Journal of the Acoustical Society of America, 78,* 435-444.

Lechner, B.K. (1979). The effects of delayed auditory feedback and masking on the fundamental frequency of stutterers and nonstutterers. *Journal of Speech and Hearing Research, 22,* 343-353.

Liberman, M. & Pierrehumbert, J. (1984). Intonational invariance under changes in pitch range and length. In M. Aronoff & R. Oehrle (Eds.), *Language Sound Structure.* Cambridge, MA: MIT Press.

Perkins, W.H. (1981). Implications of scientific research for treatment of stuttering - A lecture. *Journal of Fluency Disorders, 6,* 155-162.

Perkins, W.H., Rudas, J., Johnson, L. & Bell, J. (1976). Stuttering: Discoordination of phonation with articulation and respiration. *Journal of Speech and Hearing Research, 19,* 509-522.

Porter, H.V.K. (1939). Studies in the psychology of stuttering: XIV. Stuttering phenomena in relation to size and personnel of audience. *Journal of Speech Disorders, 4,* 323-333.

Rasdol'skij, W.A. (1965). Wie sprechen Stotternde, wenn sie alleine sind (in Russian). *Zhurnal Nevropatologii i Psikhiatrii, 65,* Heft 11, 1717-1720. (German translation by S. Mika; also cited in Wingate, 1976, p. 25.)

Richardson, F.C. & Tasto, D.L. (1976). Development and factor analysis of a social anxiety inventory. *Behavior Therapy, 7,* 453-462.

Schäfersküpper, P. (1982). *Pathophysiologie und Therapie des Stotterns.* Berlin: Marhold.

Schilling, A. (1962). Untersuchungen über die Monotonie bei Stotterern. *Proceedings of the 4th International Congress of Phonetic Sciences in Helsinki, 1961.* Paris: Mouton. 374-386.

Schmitt, L.S. & Cooper, E.B. (1978). Fundamental frequencies in the oral reading behavior of stuttering and nonstuttering male children. *Journal of Communication Disorders, 11,* 17-23.

Scripture, E.W. (1925). Das Stottern. *Archiv für psychiatrische Nervenkrankheiten, 72,* 108-113.

Shapiro, C.W. (1970). *Phrasal stress patterns of the fluent speech of stutterers and nonstutterers.* M.A. thesis, State University of New York of Buffalo.

Stäcker, K.H., Bergmann, G. & Kriebel, R. (1982). Sprechflussstörungen. In G.O. Kanter & F. Masendorf (Eds.), *Brennpunkte der Sprachheilpädagogik und Leseforschung.* Berlin: Marhold. 1-50.

Starkweather, C.W. (1982). Stuttering and laryngeal behavior: A review. *ASHA Monograph, No. 21.*

Svab, L., Gross, J. & Langova, J. (1972). Stuttering and the social isolation: Effect of social isolation with different levels of monitoring on stuttering frequency. *Journal of Nervous and Mental Disease, 155,* 1-5.

Travis, L.E. (1927). A phono-photographic study of stutterer's voice and speech. *Psychological Monographs, 36,* 109-141.

Van Riper, C. (1982). *The nature of stuttering.* Englewood Cliffs, New Jersey: Prentice-Hall, Inc.

Watson, B.C. & Alfonso, P.J. (1982). A comparison of LRT and VOT values between stutterers and nonstutterers. *Journal of Fluency Disorders, 7,* 219-241.

Wingate, M.E. (1976). *Stuttering. Theory and treatment.* New York: Irvington.

Wingate, M.E. (1979). The loci of stuttering: Grammar or prosody? *Journal of Communication Disorders, 12,* 283-290.

Wingate, M.E. (1982). Early position and stuttering occurrence. *Journal of Fluency Disorders, 7,* 243-258.

Young, M.A. (1985). Increasing the frequency of stuttering. *Journal of Speech and Hearing Research, 28,* 282-293.

Zimbardo, P.G. (1982). Shyness and the stresses of the human connection. In L. Goldberger & S. Breznitz (Eds.), *Handbook of stress: Theoretical and clinical aspects.* New York: Free Press. 466-481.

Author Index

Subject Index

T

V

Druck: Novographic, Ing. Wolfgang Schmid, A-1230 Wien.

GPSR Compliance
The European Union's (EU) General Product Safety Regulation (GPSR) is a set of rules that requires consumer products to be safe and our obligations to ensure this.

If you have any concerns about our products, you can contact us on

ProductSafety@springernature.com

In case Publisher is established outside the EU, the EU authorized representative is:

Springer Nature Customer Service Center GmbH
Europaplatz 3
69115 Heidelberg, Germany

www.ingramcontent.com/pod-product-compliance
Lightning Source LLC
Chambersburg PA
CBHW071306180926
51613CB00001B/140
* 9 7 8 3 2 1 1 8 1 9 7 1 5 *